1989
YEAR BOOK OF
SPORTS
MEDICINE®

The 1990 Year Book® Series

Year Book of Anesthesia®: Drs. Miller, Kirby, Ostheimer, Roizen, and Stoelting

Year Book of Cardiology®: Drs. Schlant, Collins, Engle, Frye, Kaplan, and O'Rourke

Year Book of Critical Care Medicine®: Drs. Rogers and Parrillo

Year Book of Dentistry®: Drs. Meskin, Ackerman, Kennedy, Leinfelder, Matukas, and Rovin

Year Book of Dermatology®: Drs. Sober and Fitzpatrick

Year Book of Diagnostic Radiology®: Drs. Bragg, Hendee, Keats, Kirkpatrick, Miller, Osborn, and Thompson

Year Book of Digestive Diseases®: Drs. Greenberger and Moody

Year Book of Drug Therapy®: Drs. Hollister and Lasagna

Year Book of Emergency Medicine®: Dr. Wagner

Year Book of Endocrinology®: Drs. Bagdade, Braverman, Halter, Horton, Kannan, Korenman, Molitch, Morley, Rogol, Ryan, and Sherwin

Year Book of Family Practice®: Drs. Rakel, Avant, Driscoll, Prichard, and Smith

Year Book of Geriatrics and Gerontology: Drs. Beck, Abrass, Burton, Cummings, Makinodan, and Small

Year Book of Hand Surgery®: Drs. Dobyns, Chase, and Amadio

Year Book of Hematology®: Drs. Spivak, Bell, Ness, Quesenberry, and Wiernik

Year Book of Infectious Diseases®: Drs. Wolff, Barza, Keusch, Klempner, and Snydman

Year Book of Infertility: Drs. Mishell, Lobo, and Paulsen

Year Book of Medicine®: Drs. Rogers, Des Prez, Cline, Braunwald, Greenberger, Wilson, Epstein, and Malawista

Year Book of Neonatal and Perinatal Medicine: Drs. Klaus and Fanaroff

Year Book of Neurology and Neurosurgery®: Drs. Crowell and Currier

Year Book of Nuclear Medicine®: Drs. Hoffer, Gore, Gottschalk, Sostman, Zaret, and Zubal

Year Book of Obstetrics and Gynecology®: Drs. Mishell, Kirschbaum, and Morrow

Year Book of Occupational Medicine: Drs. Emmett, Brooks, Harris, and Schenker

Year Book of Oncology: Drs. Young, Longo, Ozols, Simone, Steele, and Weichselbaum

Year Book of Ophthalmology®: Dr. Laibson

Year Book of Orthopedics®: Drs. Sledge, Poss, Cofield, Frymoyer, Griffin, Hansen, Johnson, Springfield, and Weiland

Year Book of Otolaryngology–Head and Neck Surgery®: Drs. Bailey and Paparella

Year Book of Pathology and Clinical Pathology®: Drs. Brinkhous, Dalldorf, Grisham, Langdell, and McLendon

Year Book of Pediatrics®: Drs. Oski and Stockman

Year Book of Plastic, Reconstructive, and Aesthetic Surgery®: Drs. Miller, Bennett, Haynes, Hoehn, McKinney, and Whitaker

Year Book of Podiatric Medicine and Surgery®: Dr. Jay

Year Book of Psychiatry and Applied Mental Health®: Drs. Talbott, Frances, Freedman, Meltzer, Schowalter, and Yudofsky

Year Book of Pulmonary Disease®: Drs. Green, Ball, Loughlin, Michael, Mulshine, Peters, Terry, Tockman, and Wise

Year Book of Rehabilitation®: Drs. Kaplan, Frank, Gordon, Lieberman, Magnuson, Molnar, Payton, and Sarno

Year Book of Speech, Language, and Hearing: Drs. Bernthal, Hall, and Tomblin

Year Book of Sports Medicine®: Drs. Shephard, Eichner, Sutton, and Torg, Col. Anderson, and Mr. George

Year Book of Surgery®: Drs. Schwartz, Jonasson, Peacock, Shires, Spencer, and Thompson

Year Book of Urology®: Drs. Gillenwater and Howards

Year Book of Vascular Surgery®: Drs. Bergan and Yao

1989

The Year Book of
SPORTS MEDICINE®

Editor-in-Chief

Roy J. Shephard, M.D., Ph.D., D.P.E.
Director, School of Physical and Health Education, and Professor of Applied Physiology, Department of Preventive Medicine and Biostatistics, University of Toronto

Editors

Col. James L. Anderson, PE.D.
Director of Physical Education, United States Military Academy

Edward R. Eichner, M.D.
Professor of Medicine and Chief, Section of Hematology, University of Oklahoma Health Sciences Center, Oklahoma City, Oklahoma

Francis J. George, ATC, PT
Head Athletic Trainer, Brown University

John R. Sutton, M.D.
Professor of Medicine; Consultant in Intensive Care and Coronary Care; McMaster University Medical Center, Hamilton, Ontario

Joseph S. Torg, M.D.
Professor of Orthopedic Surgery, and Director, Sports Medicine Center, University of Pennsylvania School of Medicine

Year Book Medical Publishers, Inc.
Chicago • London • Boca Raton • Littleton, Mass.

Printed in U.S.A.

International Standard Book Number: 0-8151-7739-9

International Standard Serial Number: 0896-4475

Editor-in-Chief, Year Book Publishing: Nancy Gorham
Sponsoring Editor: Judy L. Plazyk
Senior Medical Information Specialist: Terri Strorigl
Assistant Director, Manuscript Services: Frances M. Perveiler
Assistant Managing Editor, Year Book Editing Services: Elizabeth Griffith
Production Coordinator: Max F. Perez
Proofroom Supervisor: Barbara M. Kelly

Table of Contents

The material in this volume represents literature reviewed through January 1989.

Journals Represented

Year Book Medical Publishers subscribes to and surveys nearly 850 U.S. and foreign medical and allied health journals. From these journals, the Editors select the articles to be abstracted. Journals represented in this YEAR BOOK are listed below.

Acta Cytologica
Acta Physiologica Scandinavica
American Heart Journal
American Journal of Cardiology
American Journal of Epidemiology
American Journal of Medicine
American Journal of Obstetrics and Gynecology
American Journal of Perinatology
American Journal of Roentgenology
American Journal of Sports Medicine
American Review of Respiratory Disease
Annales de Chirurgie de la Main
Annals of Internal Medicine
Annals of Sports Medicine
Archives of Internal Medicine
Archives of Orthopedic and Traumatic Surgery
Arthroscopy
Athletic Training
Australian Family Physician
Australian Journal of Science and Medicine in Sport
British Journal of Radiology
British Journal of Sports Medicine
British Medical Journal
Calcified Tissue International
Canadian Family Physician
Canadian Journal of Sports Sciences
Canadian Journal of Surgery
Chest
Chirurg
Circulation
Clinica Chimica Acta
Clinical Orthopaedics and Related Research
Clinical Radiology
Clinical Science
Ergonomics
European Journal of Applied Physiology and Occupational Physiology
European Journal of Clinical Investigation
European Respiratory Journal
Fertility and Sterility
Foot and Ankle
French Journal of Orthopedic Surgery
Injury
International Journal of Cardiology
International Journal of Eating Disorders
International Journal of Sports Medicine
Journal of Adolescent Health Care
Journal of Applied Sport Sciences Research
Journal of the American College of Cardiology

Journal of the American Medical Association
Journal of the American Podiatric Association
Journal of the Applied Physiology
Journal of Biomedical Engineering
Journal of Bone and Joint Surgery (American volume)
Journal of Bone and Joint Surgery (British volume)
Journal of Cardiopulmonary Rehabilitation
Journal de Chirurgie
Journal of Clinical Endocrinology and Metabolism
Journal of Clinical Immunology
Journal of Gerontology
Journal of Hypertension
Journal of Internal Medicine
Journal of Laboratory and Clinical Medicine
Journal of Occupational Medicine
Journal of Orthopaedic Research
Journal of Orthopaedic and Sports Physical Therapy
Journal of Pharmacology and Experimental Therapeutics
Journal of Sports Medicine and Physical Fitness
Journal of Sports Sciences
Journal of Trauma
Lancet
Mayo Clinic Proceedings
Medical Journal of Australia
Medicine and Science in Sports and Exercise
Muscle and Nerve
National Strength and Conditioning Association Journal
New England Journal of Medicine
Obstetrics and Gynecology
Pediatric Emergency Care
Physician and Sportsmedicine
Physiotherapy
Physiotherapy Canada
Postgraduate Medicine
Proceedings of the Finnish Dental Society
Prosthetics and Orthotics International
Radiology
Research Quarterly for Exercise and Sport
South African Medical Journal
Topics in Emergency Medicine
Western Journal of Medicine

Publisher's Preface

We are delighted to welcome Roy J. Shephard, M.D., Ph.D., D.P.E., as Editor-in-Chief of the YEAR BOOK OF SPORTS MEDICINE. An Editor of the YEAR BOOK since its second edition in 1980, Dr. Shephard now assumes the larger role of defining the overall scope of the volume, refining its organization as changes develop in the field, and recruiting new members of the Board of Editors, all as necessary. We welcome him in this capacity and extend our sincere appreciation for his excellent efforts with the 1989 edition.

We are also pleased to welcome John Sutton, M.D., and Edward R. Eichner, M.D. as new board members. Drs. Sutton and Eichner selected and commented on material related to general medicine, replacing in this capacity Lewis J. Krakauer, M.D., who retired with the 1987 edition.

Finally, we owe another thanks to Dr. Shephard for his good humor and understanding about our unfortunate misspelling of his name on the cover of the 1988 YEAR BOOK. What a way to welcome an Editor-in-Chief! Our sincere apologies.

Introduction

It is exciting to be serving my first full year as Editor-in-Chief of the YEAR BOOK OF SPORTS MEDICINE. I have been particularly pleased during my first year of office to have the continuing strong and experienced support of Col. James Anderson in the area of sports biomechanics, Dr. Joseph Torg in the area of sports injuries, and Frank George in the field of athletic training. It has also been a pleasure to welcome two new members to the editorial team, both well-recognized and accepted among sports physicians throughout the world: Dr. John Sutton in the area of general medicine, and Dr. Edward Eichner in the areas of hematology and internal sports injuries. The editorial team now spans a broad spectrum of interests, opinions, and geographic representation.

The continuing strong demand for the series endorses both the vision of Dr. Krakauer in founding it and the wise guidance he gave to its early development. For the busy practitioner, to have such a ready and convenient access to 300–350 of the top current articles in sports medicine is an invaluable resource; the brief digests allow for speedy reading, and the critical comments from acknowledged experts bring to light potential criticisms of research that could easily have been overlooked by the generalist. It is also a pleasure to acknowledge here the major contributions made by Judy Plazyk and other members of the YEAR BOOK staff who have dealt so efficiently with the logistics of abstracting and assembling a truly international volume.

It would perhaps be invidious to attempt to single out the most interesting new developments in what continues to be an exponentially growing field of knowledge. However, I can mention some personal highlights. It has been exciting to see the rapid progress in our understanding of interactions between immune function and exercise, with potential applications in the treatment of both cancer and the acquired immunodeficiency syndrome. Illicit drug use has made depressing headlines over the year, and there continue to be important articles on steroids, human growth hormone, and blood doping, with an emphasis on methods of detection that can be applied on a large scale. Cardiac rehabilitation now concerns more than simply the myocardial infarction patient; the cardiac transplant patient must also be considered. Debate continues over the possible linkage between anorexia nervosa and compulsive running, and in the environmental field there has been exciting new work on simulated Everest climbs, hypothermia, and usage of glycogen stores. Other interesting areas include new concepts on warming up and rehabilitation of shoulder and back injuries; also, there is a variety of fascinating contributions from the orthopedic surgeons.

I hope you will find this year's research in sports medicine as interesting and as challenging as I have done. If you have any suggestions as to how future editions of the book can be shaped to meet your particular needs, I will be delighted to consider your suggestions; I look forward to hearing from you.

Roy J. Shephard, M.D., Ph.D., D.P.E.

xiii

Prescribing Exercise for the Senior Citizen: Some Simple Guidelines

Roy J. Shephard, M.D., Ph.D., D.P.E.

School of Physical and Health Education, and Department of Preventive Medicine and Biostatistics, Faculty of Medicine, University of Toronto.

Introduction

As a person becomes older, the various body systems begin to lose their functional capacity (1) and guidelines for active recreation must become progressively more conservative. Nevertheless, too many senior citizens and their family physicians are influenced by the popular notions that it is time to "slow down" and "take a well-earned rest." Appropriately selected and prescribed active recreation not only remains possible for the older adult, but it can make an important contribution to sustenance of the waning physiologic capacity.

In this editorial, we will look at the older person's need of anaerobic power, muscular strength, and aerobic power; discuss the optimum training plan and the likely response of an older person; note the specific concerns aroused by an adverse environment; and comment on the need for detailed laboratory testing and medical supervision. The comments will relate mainly to the "young-old" who continue to function with little physical restriction of their activity; however, brief comments will also be made on activities suitable to the "middle-old" and the "old-old" who have some limitation of their daily activities.

Anaerobic Power and Strength

Younger individuals often enjoy exploiting their muscular strength, engaging in bouts of exercise in which their maximum anerobic power is deployed (for example, a vigorous sprint up several flights of stairs). The ability to undertake such activity diminishes with age, owing in part to a progressive wasting of the body muscles, with an associated decrease of lean body mass (2, 3). The coordination of muscle contraction also becomes less effective in the elderly, leading to slower and less efficient movements (4–6); enzyme changes may slow the speed of muscle contraction (7); and stiffness of the muscles and joints may sometimes lead to increasing dissipation of the available physical energy against internal resistance (8).

From a practical point of view, the prescription of anaerobic types of activity becomes progressively less desirable as a person gets older. Over-vigorous twisting and turning or excessive straining can lead to various musculoskeletal injuries, including hernias and back problems. Moreover, during anaerobic effort the systemic blood pressure of an older adult increases to a greater extent than would be anticipated in a younger person (9); this represents an attempt to sustain blood flow through working muscles that are contracting at a large fraction of their maximum force, and the resulting increase of double-percent throws a heavy load on the aging heart (10). In the few patients in whom atherosclerosis has not developed, both peak heart rate and ventricular contractility are surprisingly well maintained (11). However, if the coronary vessels are narrowed by atherosclerosis, as is more likely in an older person, the added cardiac burden may be sufficient to induce a reduction of peak heart rate and stroke volume, electrocardiographic signs of ischemia (12, 13), anginal pain, or even some form of "heart attack" (myocardial infarction or electrical failure) (14–16).

Nevertheless, if the exercise prescription places an undue emphasis on an aerobic form of exercise such as distance jogging rather than on muscle-building activities, an undesirable weakening of the muscles can develop, particularly in the arms. It is thus important for an older person to undertake sufficient muscular activity to counter the age-related tendency toward a progressive loss of contractile protein from the lean tissue compartment, thereby conserving sufficient strength in the major muscles to deal with occasional emergencies.

The rise of blood pressure during bouts of both isometric and heavy rhythmic activity is a progressive, time-related change that is dependent also on the fraction of the maximum voluntary force that the individual exerts (17). The safe approach to exercise prescription is thus to ensure that any isometric contractions are held for only a few seconds, that the carrying of excessive weights is avoided, and that rest pauses are introduced into any more sustained bout of isotonic muscular activity (14).

All-out sprinting carries additional risks of physical injury in an older person because of poor vision, deteriorating balance, and failure to allow a "warm-up" of muscles and tendons that are becoming progressively stiffer through organic changes in collagen molecules (18, 19). There is finally some evidence that all-out activity without a warm-up exacerbates the risk that exercise will precipitate a cardiac emergency (20).

Aerobic Power

The type of physical activity best suited to the overall health needs of an older person is aerobic exercise involving the large muscles of the body: brisk walking, vigorous swimming, and cross-country skiing, for example. The main determinant of the ability to undertake such types of activity is the maximum oxygen intake, i.e., the ability of the heart and lungs to transport oxygen from the atmosphere to the working tissues (21). The oxygen cost of walking is similar in young adults and in healthy older people (22), but problems of gait may increase the energy consumption in the more frail elderly at any given speed of movement (23).

The rate of loss of oxygen transport with aging is typically about 5% per decade of adult life (24); thus, a speed of walking that would be considered a very moderate exercise for a young person can become an effective training stimulus in an older person. On the other hand, an effective training program can boost the older person's maximum oxygen intake by as much as 20% (25), giving the senior citizen who has optimized personal fitness an exercise tolerance and functional capacity matching that of a sedentary person who is 10–20 years younger in terms of calendar age. Plainly, exercise prescription for the elderly must take more account of functional than of calendar age.

Even if oxygen transport has developed to match that of a younger person, the elderly exerciser should approach most types of exercise more cautiously than would a young adult. For example, vigorous swimming remains an excellent source of large muscle activity; however, in recommending such a program, care must be taken to ensure that an older individual does not have a history of dizziness, loss of consciousness, or syncopal attacks caused by aortic stenosis or disorders of heart rhythm (26). Postural hypotension (27) can be a source of difficulty on leaving the pool, particularly if hypotensive drugs are being administered; also, an elderly person has an increased risk of slipping on a wet pool deck.

Similarly, cross-country skiing remains an excellent source of winter recreation for the elderly, providing large muscle exercise during the coldest months of the year; nevertheless, a greater vulnerability of the aged to cold (28) and a more ready fracture of bones that have already lost much of their calcium and organic matter through the processes of osteoporosis and osteopenia (29, 30) calls for care, particularly on icy slopes.

Moderate rates of cycling continue to provide a good stimulus to the heart and lungs, but deterioration of vision, hearing, and balance increase the risk of accidents and falls in many older people (31–33), whereas weakening of the thigh muscles can lead to an excessive rise of blood pressure (17) if an older person attempts to hurry the climb up a steep hill or forces the pace against a strong headwind. At the same time, the progressive loss of aerobic power makes fast walking a progressively more effective method of cardiorespiratory training for the elderly. Brisk walking has several advantages over jogging as far as the senior citizen is concerned. The mechanical impact that is sustained by the aging knees and vertebral column is only about a third as great when walking as when jogging, and there is much less danger that a walker will slip or fall. Stress ruptures of aging tendons and bones are also less likely.

Walking is an activity that can be combined with a variety of pleasurable outdoor relaxations, such as a study of the local fauna, flora, or architecture, and this increases the likelihood that motivation, always a problem in exercise prescription, will be sustained. Walking can also be incorporated into the normal weekly round of visits to the shops, library, and local church or synagogue, a technique that lessens the likelihood that the activity will be neglected. Further, the duration of individual walking bouts can be sufficient to help in creating a negative energy balance, thus making appreciable inroads on the middle-aged accumulation of body fat over exercise programs as short as 3 months (34).

In the frail elderly with problems of knee instability, potential alternatives to walking are exercises in a heated pool (35) and chair exercises (36).

Training Plan

Although a clear experimental proof of the optimal regimen has yet to be provided, most exercise physiologists seem agreed that an effective training plan stresses an individual to at least 60% of maximum oxygen intake for 30 minutes or more per session (21); this implies increasing the heart rate of the exerciser about 60% of the way from the resting to the maximum value. If the intent of the program is to develop cardiorespiratory fitness, sessions are recommended 4–5 times per week, whereas at least 3 sessions per week are desirable for the maintenance of physical condition (37).

If these general principles of exercise prescription are applied specifically to elderly patients, some modifications may be necessary. If the person concerned has been inactive for many years, an exercise intensity equivalent to 60% of maximum oxygen intake may initially prove too vigorous; however, in such individuals, a slow training response may result from a surprisingly low intensity of exercise, perhaps as little as 50% of maximum oxygen intake (25). The patient may also find it difficult at first to sustain vigorous activity over a 30-minute session. An initial target prescription might thus be to cover a distance of 0.8 km (half a mile) in 15 minutes. The time allowed to walk this distance could be progressively shortened to 10 minutes over a couple of weeks; if this amount and intensity of effort are tolerated without difficulty, the measured distance could then be extended to 1.6 km (1 mile), to be covered in 20 minutes. The time allowed would next be reduced progressively to 15 minutes for the same distance, and the distance would then be extended to 2.4 km (1.5 miles). By prescribing alternately an increasing speed and an increasing distance, the patient could gradually be brought to the desired target of covering 3.2–4.0 km (2–2.5 miles) in 30 minutes on a regular basis (38). Occasional duplication of the exercise sessions on good walking days would soon enable the exerciser to enjoy a worthwhile country walk of 6.4–8 km (4–5 miles), provided that a generous lunchtime rest period was allowed.

Formal stretching and warm-up exercises are less essential for walking than for a jogging program. Nevertheless, the first few minutes of exercise should be kept to a moderate walking pace, with the patient picking up speed once the limbs have become comfortably warm. Likewise, if the body becomes hot over the exercise period (as it should do if an effective dose of training has been undertaken), the final few minutes of activity should be devoted to a "warm-down" at a progressively slower speed. The warm-down allows opportunity for a return of fluid from the legs to the central part of the circulation, reducing the likelihood that fainting or abnormalities of cardiac rhythm will develop during the recovery period (39). A warm-down also helps to remove lactate from muscles that have been working beyond their anaerobic threshold (40), and it lessens the chances that the active parts will develop stiffness and muscle pain. The ideal dose of exercise should leave the patient no more than comfortably tired the following day.

Training Response

There has been considerable discussion of the likely response of an elderly person to a training program. Some of the reactions associated with effective training, such as a thickening of the ventricular wall and a development of limb muscle mass, plainly require the synthesis of new protein, and it might be imagined that such changes would proceed more easily in a young person than in an older person.

There is probably some truth to this view, and if gains of fitness are expressed in absolute terms, the response to a given dose of training is certainly reduced with aging (25, 41, 42). Nevertheless, senior citizens can make substantial gains of both oxygen transport and muscle strength in response to a vigorous and progressive training regimen. Indeed, in percentage terms, the gains are as large as would be anticipated in a young adult. Moreover, the flexibility of the joints is improved, much of the adult accumulation of subcutaneous fat is metabolized (34), and the loss of minerals from the limb bones is checked if not corrected (43, 44).

Although a master's class athlete ages at about the same rate as a sedentary person (24), the training effect is such that on any given birthday he or she has a functional capacity corresponding to that of a sedentary person who is 10 or even 20 years younger (1). Regular exercise does not increase the age at death by more than 1–2 years (45), but the period of independent living is likely to be substantially extended (46). This has enormous practical implications for both the happiness of the senior citizen and the budget of those who must ultimately provide any necessary institutional care (47).

Environmental Concerns

Age reduces the individual's ability to adapt to an adverse environment. The older person must thus be more cautious when exercising in extremes of either heat or cold.

It is well established that heat waves in the United States are associated with an increased death rate among the elderly (48–50). Under hot environmental conditions, it is necessary to direct blood flow to the skin (to dissipate heat) as well as to the working muscles; this requirement imposes an added workload on the heart at all ages, and a proportion of the more vulnerable individuals succumb to the added stress. The risks of the North American summer are still not sufficiently appreciated. However, a combination of a hot, humid afternoon, bright sunlight, and inadequate fluid replacement can severely tax the cardiac reserve of a senior citizen who has incurred some coronary atherosclerosis (14). A poor sweating response because of lack of recent training, obesity, and an unwillingness to wear minimal light clothing compound the problem.

Cold weather can be equally hazardous for the elderly. Poor peripheral circulation increases the chances of frostbite and other local cold injuries. Inhalation of cold air may provoke bronchial spasm, overloading respiratory muscles that are already hard-pressed by chronic chest disease. Stimulation of the nerve endings in the airway and vasoconstriction of the skin blood vessels may also induce anginal pain in a cold environment. Icy sidewalks add further danger to many types of outdoor activity during the winter months. Also, the elderly are particularly vulnerable to hypothermia (28), the cold-induced syndrome of confusion, irrational behavior, and death. If the weather is very cold, an older person often lacks the fitness that would allow him or her to exercise at a sufficient rate to sustain body temperature. Excessive body cooling arises not only from exposure to high winds and ultralow temperatures but also from a loss of insulation in clothing (as a result of soaking by sweat, rain, spray, and falls into icy lakes). The thickness of the clothing that is worn should be carefully matched to the intended rate of exercise to provide adequate insulation while avoiding an accumulation of sweat and thus a degradation of insulation during the more vigorous phases of an exercise prescription.

Testing and Detailed Supervision of Activity Programs

Excessive preliminary testing and detailed medical supervision of the elderly exerciser tend to be counterproductive. Most elderly patients are affected by 1 or more chronic disorders, and in younger persons these conditions might be regarded as relative or even absolute contraindications to participation in an unsupervised training program. However, with a very few exceptions, both elderly patients and their advisers are overcautious, and the need is to increase rather than to restrict their activity.

Provided that the patient is encouraged to do just a little more than has been habitual, and that this is accomplished without inducing symptoms, it is unlikely that the overall life expectancy is shortened by the prescribed exercise. Moreover, in terms of quality-adjusted life expectancy, prospects are greatly improved by regular exercise. A much broader range of interests is available to the active individual, and it is likely that the age of institutionalization will be set back by quite a number of years. Detailed laboratory testing, medical supervision, and possible restriction of activity are thus required only by (1) an occasional patient who wishes to train hard for master's competition, and (2) persons with major symptomatic disease.

Overall Recommendation

Despite traditional concerns about the safety of exercise programs for the elderly, moderate recreational activities such as regular brisk and sustained bouts of walking can do much to develop and to sustain the fitness of an older person. Aging tissue will not be replaced, nor is there any guarantee that the overall life span will be extended. Nevertheless, functional capacity will be increased by the equivalent of up to 10–20 years, with a corresponding increase of immediate life satisfaction and enhancement of the quality of the remaining years of survival. There is also likely to be some decrease in the period for which costly institutional care is required.

Design of an appropriate exercise prescription for the senior citizen must take due account of the individual's experience and training potential. It must also recognize any physical limitations, noting the risks of overrapid progression of training and vulnerability to extremes of heat and cold. However, physicians should accept that moderate physical activity is a normal part of daily living for an older person, and they should encourage participation rather than constrain it by unnecessary restrictions, prohibitions, and the use of medical technology.

References

1. Shephard RJ: *Physical Activity and Aging,* ed 2. London, Croom Helm; Rockport, Md, Aspen Publications, 1987.
2. Korenchevsky V, in Bourne GH (ed): *Physiological Changes and Pathological Ageing.* Basel, S Karger AG, 1961, pp 40–44, 311–315.
3. Borkan GA, Hults DE, Gerzof SG, et al: Age changes in body composition revealed by computed tomography. *J Gerontol* 38:673–677, 1983.
4. Jalavisto E: The role of simple tests measuring speed of performance in the assessment of biological vigor: A factorial study in elderly women, in Welford AT, Birren JE (eds): *Behavior, Aging and the Nervous System.* Springfield, Ill, Charles C Thomas, Publ, 1973, pp 353–365.
5. Stelmach GE, Diewert GL: Aging, information processing, and fitness, in Borg G (ed): *Physical Work and Effort.* Oxford, Pergamon Press, 1977.
6. Wright GR, Shephard RJ: Brake reaction time: Effects of age, sex, and carbon monoxide. *Arch Environ Health* 33:141–150, 1978.
7. Davies CTM, White MJ: Contractile properties of elderly human triceps surae. *Gerontology* 29:19–25, 1983.
8. Allman FL: Conditioning for sports, in Ryan AJ, Allman FL (eds): *Sports Medicine.* New York, Academic Press, 1974.
9. Sheffield LT, Roitman D: Systolic blood pressure, heart rate, and treadmill work at anginal threshold. *Chest* 63:327–335, 1973.
10. Toscani A: Physiology of muscular work in the aged, in Huet JA (ed): *Work and Aging: Second International Course in Social Gerontology.* Paris, International Centre of Social Gerontology, 1971, pp 185–220.
11. Weisfeldt ML, Gerstenblith ML, Lakatta EG: Alterations in the circulatory function, in Andres R, Bierman EL, Hazzard WR (eds): *Principles of Geriatric Medicine.* New York, McGraw-Hill Book Co, 1985, pp 248–279.
12. Montoye HJ: Physical activity and health: An epidemiological study of an entire community. Englewood Cliffs, NJ, Prentice Hall, 1975.
13. Sidney KH, Shephard RJ: Training and e.c.g. abnormalities in the elderly. *Br Heart J* 39:1114–1120, 1977.
14. Shephard RJ: *Ischemic Heart Disease and Exercise.* Chicago, Year Book Medical Publishers, 1982.
15. Thompson PD, Funk EJ, Carleton RA, et al: Sudden death during jogging: A study of the Rhode Island population from 1975 through 1980. *Med Sci Sports Exerc* 14:115, 1982.
16. Siscovick DS, Weiss NS, Fletcher RH, et al: The incidence of primary cardiac arrest during vigorous exercise. *N Engl J Med* 311:874–877, 1984.
17. Lind AR, McNicol GW: Muscular factors which determine the cardiovascular responses to sustained and rhythmic exercise. *Can Med Assoc J* 96:706–712, 1967.
18. Viidik A: Experimental evaluation fo the tensile strength of isolated rabbit tendons. *Biomed Eng* 2:64–67, 1967.
19. Hall DA: Metabolic and structural aspects of aging, in Brocklehurst JC

(ed): *Textbook of Geriatric Medicine and Gerontology,* ed 2. Edinburgh, Churchill Livingstone Inc, 1978, pp 452–461.
20. Barnard RJ, MacAlpin RN, Kattus AA, et al: Ischemic response to sudden strenuous exercise in healthy men. *Circulation* 48:936–942, 1973.
21. Shephard RJ: *Endurance Fitness,* ed 2. Toronto, University of Toronto Press, 1977.
22. Waters RL, Lunsford BR, Perry J, et al: Energy-speed relationship of walking: Standard tables. *J Orthop Res* 6:215–222, 1988.
23. Paez PN, Phillipson M, Maasengkay M, et al: The physiological basis of training patients with emphysema. *Am Rev Respir Dis* 95:944–953, 1967.
24. Shephard RJ: The aging of cardiovascular function, in Eckert H, Spirduso W (eds): *Physical Activity and Aging.* Champaign, Ill, Human Kinetics Publishers, 1989.
25. Sidney KH, Shephard RJ: Frequency and intensity of training for elderly subjects. *Med Sci Sports* 10:125–131, 1978.
26. Atwood JE, Kawanashi S, Myers J, et al: Exercise testing in patients with aortic stenosis. *Chest* 93:1083–1087, 1988.
27. Lipsitz LA, Nyquist RP, Wei JY, et al: Post-prandial reduction in blood pressure in the elderly. *N Engl J Med* 309:81–83, 1983.
28. Collins KJ, Dore C, Exton-Smith AN, et al: Accidental hypothermia and impaired temperature in the elderly. *Br Med J* 1:353–356, 1977.
29. Raab DM, Smith EL: Exercise and aging effects on bone. *Top Geriatr Rehabil* 1:31–39, 1985.
30. Chestnut CH: Osteoporosis, in Andres R, Bierman EL, Hazzard WR (eds): *Principles of Geriatric Medicine.* New York, McGraw-Hill Book Co, 1985, pp 801–812.
31. Overstall PW, Exton-Smith AN, Imms FJ, et al: Falls in the elderly related to postural imbalance. *Br Med J* 1:261–264, 1977.
32. Exton-Smith AN: Musculoskeletal system: Bone aging and bone metabolic disease, in Brocklehurst JC (ed): *Textbook of Geriatrics and Gerontology,* ed 2. Edinburgh, Churchill Livingston Inc, 1978, pp 510–524.
33. Gryfe CI, Amies A, Ashley MJ: A longitudinal study of falls in an elderly population. 1. Incidence and morbidity. *Age Ageing* 6:201–210, 1977.
34. Sidney KH, Shephard RJ, Harrison J: Endurance training and body composition of the elderly. *Am J Clin Nutr* 30:326–333, 1977.
35. Lawrence G: *Aquafitness for Women.* Toronto, Personal Library Publishers, 1981.
36. McNamara PS, Otto RM, Smith TK: The acute response of simulated bicycle and rowing exercise on the elderly population. *Med Sci Sports Exerc* 17:574–579, 1985.
37. American College of Sports Medicine: *Resource Manual for Guidelines for Graded Exercise Testing and Prescription.* Philadelphia, Lea & Febiger, 1988.
38. Kavanagh T: *The Health Heart Programme.* Toronto, Van Nostrand, 1980.
39. Shephard RJ, Kavanagh T: Predicting the exercise catastrophe in the post-coronary patient. *Can Fam Physician* 24:614–618, 1978.
40. Hermansen L, Stensvold I: Production and removal of lactate during exercise in man. *Acta Physiol Scand* 86:191–201, 1972.

41. Saltin B, Hartley LH, Kilbom A, et al: Physical training in sedentary middle-aged and older men. II. Oxygen uptake, heart rate, and blood lactate concentration at submaximal and maximal exercise. *Scand J Clin Lab Invest* 24:323–334, 1969.
42. Kilbom A: Physical training in women. *Scand J Clin Lab Invest* 28(Suppl 119):1–34, 1971.
43. Smith E, Smith PE, Ensign CJ, et al: Bone involution decrease in exercising middle-aged women. *Calcif Tissue Int* 36(Suppl 1):S129–S138, 1984.
44. Chow RK, Harrison J, Sturtridge W, et al: The effect of exercise on bone mass of osteoporotic patients on fluoride treatment. *Clin Invest Med* 10:59–63, 1987.
45. Paffenbarger R, Hyde RT, Wing AL, et al: Physical activity, all-cause mortality, and longevity of college alumni. *N Engl J Med* 314:605–613, 1986.
46. Shephard RJ, Montelpare W: Geriatric benefits of exercise as an adult. *J Gerontol* 43:M86–M90, 1988.
47. Shephard RJ: *Economic Benefits of Enhanced Fitness.* Champaign, Ill, Human Kinetics Publishers, 1986.
48. Oeschli FW, Buechley RW: Excess mortality associated with three Los Angeles hot spells. *Environ Res* 3:277–284, 1970.
49. Schuman SH: Patterns of urban heat-wave deaths and precautions for prevention: Data from New York and St. Louis during July 1966. *Environ Res* 5:59–75, 1972.
50. Besdine RW, Harris TB: Alteration in body temperature (hypothermia and hyperthermia), in Andres R, Bierman EL, Hazzard WR (eds): *Principles of Geriatric Medicine.* New York, McGraw-Hill Book Co, 1985, pp 209–217.

1 Biomechanics

Introduction

The term biomechanics has been used for many years in medicine, rehabilitation, anatomy, and aerospace science, but it has been in the last half of this century that it has emerged in the field of physical education in the United States as a means to study sports-related movement of organic bodies or tissues. The nature of the body response and the determination of the mechanical properties and limits of tolerance of organic bodies and their parts are the major concerns of biomechanical research.

The studies selected for review in the YEAR BOOK OF SPORTS MEDICINE are those relating primarily to the analysis of sports performance and injuries. It must be understood that analysis of mechanical principles is but one aspect of the examination of sports performance. For a complete picture we must seek the help of the physiologist and the psychologist, as well as the physicist.

Col. James L. Anderson, PE.D.

Measurement of Discrete Vertical In-Shoe Stress With Piezoelectric Transducers
Gross TS, Bunch RP (Converse, Inc, North Reading, Mass)
J Biomed Eng 10:261–265, May 1988   1–1

Because force plate analyses fail to demonstrate discrete foot function, discrete stress transducers were used for the noninvasive measurement of in-shoe vertical plantar stress during dynamic activities. Eight transducers were developed with small piezoelectric ceramic squares used to generate a charge output proportional to vertical plantar stress. The transducers had 2.3% linearity and 3.7% hysteresis for stresses up to 2,000 kPa and loading times up to 200 msec.

The largest average peak stress was beneath the hallux. Metatarsal loading was greatest beneath the second and third metatarsal heads (Fig 1–1). Impulse data followed the trends of peak stress data. The first and third metatarsal heads contributed less to propulsion, and the fifth metatarsal acted chiefly as a support mechanism. A lateral to medial onset of loading beneath the forefoot was evident. Within-day proportional error, reflecting trial-to-trial variability, averaged 3.1%. Between-day proportional error ranged from 4.9% to 15.8% and averaged 9.9%.

The use of piezoelectric transducers appears to be a valid means of recording discrete foot function. Contributions of discrete foot structures to the braking and propulsive phases of running were readily identified.

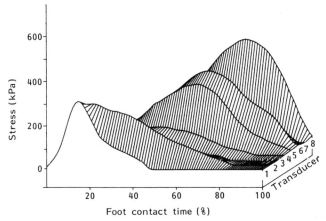

Fig 1–1.—Sample stress vs. time plot of the 8 transducers. *1*, calcaneus; *2*, fifth metatarsal base; *3*, medial midfoot; *4*, fifth metatarsal head; *5*, third metatarsal head; *6*, second metatarsal head; *7*, first metatarsal head; *8*, hallux. (Courtesy of Gross TS, Bunch RP: *J Biomed Eng* 10:261–265, May 1988.)

A Kinetic Evaluation of the Effects of In Vivo Loading on Running Shoes
Hamill J, Bates BT (Univ of Massachusetts, Amherst; Univ of Oregon, Eugene)
J Orthop Sports Phys Ther 10:47–53, August 1988   1–2

The design and construction of running shoes have greatly improved. Cushioning and control, the 2 most important functions of the shoe, depend largely on the midsole. Better-quality running shoes now contain a midsole made of ethylvinyl acetate, compression-molded ethylvinyl acetate, and polyurethane. However, these materials deteriorate with time and use. The effects of running on the shock-absorbing and stabilizing qualities of shoes were assessed.

Six healthy men who regularly ran more than 48 km per week entered the study. They were given 1 of 2 dual-density shoe models made with ethylvinyl acetate midsoles. Testing was done on a platform system connected to a digital computer. There were four 3-hour experimental sessions for each participant in addition to 2 weeks of training with the shoes. During the training period, the volunteers ran 140 km.

A breakdown in midsole material occurred, although the different cushioning systems deteriorated at the same rate. The 7.3% increase in average impact force was considerably less than that of previous reports. The runners, however, accommodated to the changes in the midsole by improvement in foot control. Because control is as important as cushioning in the prevention of injuries, loss of some degree of shock absorption may be acceptable. Changes in the midsole occurred after only 300–400 km of wear; therefore, newer materials would appear to be required for improved longevity in running shoes.

Shock Absorption During Running and Walking

Voloshin AS (Lehigh Univ, Bethlehem, Pa)
J Am Podiatr Med Assoc 78:295–299, June 1988   1–3

Walking and running, especially on hard surfaces, causes shock waves that affect the entire human musculoskeletal system. The destruction of tissue and cartilage that follows dynamic loading can be lessened by external shock absorbers—footwear that shields the system from excessive force. The shock-absorbing capacities of shoes and shoe inserts were evaluated in a group of young men in good health who walked or ran on a hard surface. Results were recorded by an accelerometer attached to each participant. A barefoot test was used as a baseline, and comparisons were made between the effects of running and walking.

Because maximum acceleration during running was 3.6 times higher on the average than during walking, running shoes should have greater shock-absorbing capacity. Knee problems result from increases in mileage or speed and changes in shoes or running surface. A change in shoes or the use of insoles can correct problems for as many as 77% of runners.

Both shoes and insoles can be evaluated according to the method described. On the basis of such tests, shoes and shoe inserts can be designed that substantially reduce shock to the musculoskeletal system. Better-quality insoles can reduce shock by as much as 30%.

The Effectiveness of Shock-Absorbing Insoles During Normal Walking

Johnson Gr (Univ of Newcastle upon Tyne, England)
Prosthet Orthot Int 12:91–95, 1988   1–4

The increased popularity of running and jogging has generated an interest in assessing skeletal shock and in developing footwear to prevent it. The value of commercial shock-absorbing insoles was studied by using them in 4 different pairs of shoes during normal walking. Axial acceleration of the leg was measured by an accelerometer mounted at the ankle. Shock was estimated by a factor identified as the rms acceleration between 50 and 150 Hz and expressed as a proportion of that between 10 and 150 Hz.

The most impressive reduction in shock was accomplished by Lightweight Sorbothane and Soft Blue Sorbothane insoles, each of which were more than 30% effective. Sorbolite, Nonshock, and the Sorbothane walking insole reduced shock by more than 20%.

A portable shock meter is now available to evaluate further studies on shock-absorbing insoles and footwear during both walking and running.

▶ Abstracts 1–1 to 1–4 concern the noninvasive measurement of in vivo compressive loading and the shock attenuation incurred on the foot in walking and running. It is interesting to note that, in one instance, piezoelectric transducers were used to determine vertical in-shoe stress and in another the experimental set-up consisted of a forced platform system interfaced with a microcomputer via an analogue to a digital converter. Yet a third method used an externally mounted lightweight accelerometer. It appears that the next steps in the quest to determine the perfect shoe, insole, or playing/running surface will be the establishment of injury thresholds as well as clinical studies designed to correlate various shock-absorbing devices with the occurrence of injury.—J.S. Torg, M.D.

Muscle Strength in the Triceps Surae and Objectively Measured Customary Walking Activity in Men and Women Over 65 Years of Age
Bassey EJ, Bendall MJ, Pearson M (Univ of Nottingham Med School; Queen's Med Centre, Nottingham, England)
Clin Sci 74:85–89, January 1988   1–5

Muscle strength declines with age. The 2 probable components of this loss are loss of motor neurons and the progressive decrease in the use of muscles with advancing age. The repetitive production of force in the triceps surae during walking may constitute a stimulus that would help to preserve the strength of the muscle in old age. If this is so, a relationship with both chosen speed of walking and amount of walking would be expected. A study was done to test this hypothesis.

Objective measurements of the maximal voluntary strength of triceps surae and the amount and speed of customary walking were made in 56 men and 66 women older than 65 years who were living independently. The men were significantly stronger, even after adjustment for body weight. Their amount of walking was similar to that of women, but their speed was significantly faster. Men were more active in leisure pursuits. Significant associations were found between strength and chosen normal walking speed for both sexes. The amount of walking was significantly but less strongly correlated with strength in men. Multiple regression analysis demonstrated that in men neither age nor amount of walking had any further effect in addition to speed; in women, age had an additional effect. The observed correlations suggest that loss of muscle strength might be reversed through increased daily activity.

▶ Maintaining the health of our aging population is something we all need to be concerned about. This excellent study helps to show that exercise such as walking at a brisk pace may help to maintain calf muscle strength and an independent life-style. Other exercise, concentrating on other muscle groups, can help the aging to maintain muscular strength and joint flexibility.—Col. J.L. Anderson, PE.D.

Age-Related Changes in Anticipatory Postural Adjustments Associated With Arm Movements
Inglin B, Woollacott M (Univ of Oregon, Eugene)
J Gerontol 43:M105–M113, July 1988   1–6

Studies suggest that poor reaction time in older adults could in many cases be the result of poor posture control. The postural control system declines with advancing age. Efficient feed-forward activation of postural muscles may be needed to execute voluntary movement skillfully. The effects of age on the feed-forward activation of postural muscles in advance of reaction time arm movements were studied.

Fifteen young persons (mean age, 26 years) and 15 older persons (mean age, 71 years) participated in the study. They were instructed to rapidly push or pull on a hand-held manipulandum. Postural muscle response-onset latencies of the lower leg were significantly elevated in older adults in 3 of the 4 conditions when compared with the young adults. Prime mover muscle response-onset latencies of the upper arm showed a large, significant increase in older adults beyond that caused by slowing of the postural response.

These findings suggest 2 conclusions: The voluntary control system may be affected to a slightly greater degree with age, resulting in slower voluntary movement in older adults, or deterioration of the postural control system with aging may slow the speed of voluntary movement by delaying the onset of the voluntary muscle response.

▶ The fact that aging has a negative effect on the voluntary control system, resulting in slower voluntary movement in older adults, is certainly not surprising. Even the effect of the deterioration of the postural control system with aging, which may slow the speed of voluntary movement by delaying the onset of the voluntary muscle response, although a new and interesting concept, cannot surprise us too much. Perhaps of more interest would be investigating effects of a muscular conditioning program to see if that will slow down the aging process or maybe reverse it and consequently decrease reaction time again.— Col. J.L. Anderson, PE.D.

Growth of Segment Principal Moments of Inertia Between Four and Twenty Years
Jensen RK, Nassas G (Laurentian Univ, Sudbury, Ont)
Med Sci Sports Exerc 20:594–604, December 1988   1–7

Many studies have been done on the moments of inertia of the body segments, but few have reported the principal moments, and none has considered the changes in the principal moments during childhood. A mathematical model was used to determine the intraindividual changes and interindividual differences in the segment principal moments during growth.

The body was modeled as 15 segments composed of transverse elliptical zones of known density (Fig 1–2). Moments and products of inertia about the segment mass centroid were determined, and the principal moments and axes were calculated from the ellipsoid of inertia. A longitudinal study of 12 boys done over a 9-year period yielded 88 annual recordings from age 4 to 20 years. Polynomial regressions fitted to the

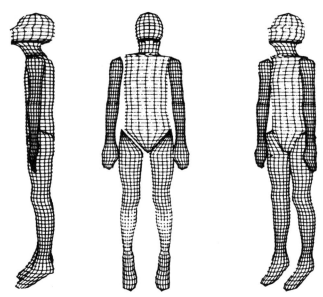

Fig 1–2.—Elliptical zone representation of segments with the body in the reference configuration. (Courtesy of Jensen RK, Nassas G: *Med Sci Sports Exerc* 20:594–604, December 1988.)

intraindividual changes demonstrated a similarity in the curves to 10 years, followed by a wide divergence of growth patterns. The changes in the principal moments across age followed principles of cephalocaudad and distal to proximal development for all 3 axes. These changes were more accentuated than those for segment length, volume, or mass.

These findings were consistent with principal moments reported for cadavers and young male adult gamma radiation scans and with estimates based on simplified models of the segments. The magnitude of the changes observed in principal moments with age makes it essential that appropriate parameters be used in analyzing or simulating the movements of children and adolescents.

▶ Authors Jensen and Nassas are to be commended for their diligence on this excellent longitudinal work. As they stated, it is clear from the results of this study that there are substantial changes in the principal moments of inertia of most segments across age. They found these changes to be much larger than for segmental length and mass, and made it clear that the patterns of interindividual difference for the different segments are consistent with principles of segment growth. These changes must be considered when joint moments are calculated. They found that there are considerable interindividual differences in the intraindividual growth patterns of principal moments, particularly after the age of 10 when, under the influence of puberty, the differences in magnitude are amplified.

This is a good example of the kind of longitudinal work that we need to help us understand the intricacies of body growth and development and the effects on body movement.—Col. J.L. Anderson, PE.D.

Spinal Effects of Head-Down Tilting: Part 1. Low Back Contour Changes
Nosse LJ, Sobush DC, McCrimmon C (Marquette Univ, Milwaukee)
Phys Ther 68:60–66, January 1988   1–8

One type of inversion appliance used to administer spinal traction inverts the user with the lower limbs extended (ILLE), whereas the other type inverts the user with the lower limbs flexed (ILLF) (Fig 1–3). Changes in spinal shape, contour, and length were studied in 25 healthy persons aged 19–39 years who had less than 20% body fat and no known cardiovascular problems. Positions were maintained for about 90 seconds before measurements were made. Low back contour was measured from S2 upward for 19 cm at 1-cm intervals.

The standing and sitting positions produced the largest and smallest mean contour values, respectively. The mean contour value with the ILLF was smaller than both supine mean contour values, but it did not differ appreciably from the ILLE value. Both the ILLE and ILLF positions significantly reduced mean contour values compared with the standing position, but neither as much as the sitting position.

These findings support using inversion therapy to reduce the depth of the low back contour when sitting is not appropriate.

▶ The inversion technique discussed in this study is used by some therapists with clients who have low back pain normally associated with nerve root compression or disk herniations. Most agree that the clients must also have healthy cardiovascular systems before inversion therapy is advised. This study was done with healthy individuals and involved only anatomical measurements of

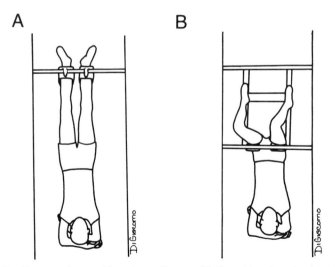

Fig 1–3.—Two general types of inversion appliances and body positions for using them. **A,** subject using ankle boots with lower limbs extended; **B,** subject using trapeze with lower limbs flexed. *PSIS,* posterior superior iliac spine. (Courtesy of Nosse LJ, Sobush DC, McCrimmon C: *Phys Ther* 68:60–66, January 1988.)

low back contour. However, we are not certain that by simply lessening the concavity the low back pain will subside. Simple deduction shows this, because sitting with hips flexed 90 degrees was the most effective position for reducing the lower back contour. However, sitting is dismissed because it is known to increase intradiskal pressure. Knowing this while planning the study, measurements of intradiskal pressures for all anatomical positions could have greatly increased the value of this investigation.

Most physicians and therapists would like to have a simple, effective way to give their patients relief from low back pain. There appears to be some help on the way. Rushatz and Peterson of West Point, NY, have developed a simple procedure that is now being tested under the name *BackMate*. Early tests have shown this procedure to bring effective relief for most patients.—Col. J.L. Anderson, PE.D.

Effect of Viscoelastic Shoe Insoles on Vertical Impact Forces in Heel–Toe Running
Nigg BM, Herzog W, Read LJ (Univ of Calgary, Alberta)
Am J Sports Med 16:70–76, January–February 1988   1–9

Insertion of viscoelastic arch supports or heel pads in running shoes is said to reduce the magnitude or loading rate of impact forces during running. Kinetic and kinematic data were collected for 14 injury-free males running heel–toe at an average speed of 4 m/s using running shoes equipped with conventional insoles or with 1 of 4 different viscoelastic insoles. Impact forces in running were compared using regular or viscoelastic soles and the possible effects on lower leg kinematics were assessed using a mechanical model (Fig 1–4).

No significant difference in maximum vertical impact forces and their time of occurrence was found on comparison of the viscoelastic insoles with regular insoles. As for kinetic results, a lower maximal vertical loading rate was found for the regular insole when inserted in a shoe with a heel stabilizer, but no systematic pattern in results was seen. Furthermore, the kinematic variables of the lower extremity were not affected by the viscoelastic insoles systematically.

It appears that viscoelastic insoles do not reduce impact force peaks for runners, nor do they seem to affect kinetic and kinematic variables during impact in a relevant way.

▶ This study calls into question the use of viscoelastic insoles in running shoes to replace the conventional insoles designed for the shoes. Although the authors make an attempt to analyze fairly the reasons for the difference between their findings and those of other researchers, it still comes down to validity and reliability of measurements. These differences between the findings of various researchers are not insignificant. Considerable amounts of money are being spent for these viscoelastic insoles that may be neither necessary nor useful.—Col. J.L. Anderson, PE.D.

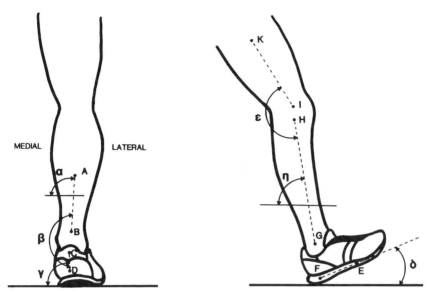

MEDIAL   LATERAL

Fig 1–4.—Illustration of the markers and angles used in the film analysis for the posterior and lateral views. (Courtesy of Nigg BM, Herzog W, Read LJ: *Am J Sports Med* 16:70–76, January–February 1988.)

Changes in the Surface Electromyogram During Increasing Isometric Shoulder Forward Flexions

Gerdle B, Eriksson N-E, Hagberg C, (Natl Inst of Occupational Health Umeå; Univ of Umeå, Sweden)
Eur J Appl Physiol 57:404–408, March 1988   1–10

When using electromyographic techniques to assess muscular load, it is necessary to determine the mathematical relationship between the torque and the amplitude of the electromyographic signal. Gradually rising isometric contractions up to 100% maximal voluntary contraction can then be used. Often, more than linear increases for the amplitude root mean square (RMS)-force regression have been described. Whether changes in power spectral density function occur during a gradually increasing isometric contraction of 10 seconds' duration was examined in 22 healthy women. They performed increasing isometric shoulder forward flexion for 10 seconds using an isokinetic dynamometer. Electromyographic (EMG) activity was measured in the trapezius, deltoid, infraspinatus, and biceps brachii. Mean torque values were calculated together with mean power frequency and RMS values from the EMG signals for each 256-ms period.

The RMS torque regressions demonstrated higher regression coefficients during the sixth to the ninth second than during the first 5 seconds. There was no significant correlation between mean power frequency for the 4 muscles and the torque. A gradual decline in mean power frequency was found from the sixth second.

The reduction in power spectral density function may have contributed to the significantly higher regression coefficient for the RMS torque regression at the high output part of the gradually increasing isometric contraction.

▶ This study is included here for the benefit of those researchers who wish to collect data concerning maximal voluntary contractions of various muscle groups using surface EMG. The validity and reliability measurement problems cannot be taken lightly. For certain, more studies are necessary to determine the causes of the downward shift in power spectral density function during isometric increasing contractions. The following study (Abstract 1–11) by the same authors, is another attempt to clarify the causes.— Col. J.L. Anderson, PE.D.

Surface EMG Recordings During Maximum Static Shoulder Forward Flexion in Different Positions
Gerdle B, Eriksson N-E, Brundin L, Edström M (Natl Inst of Occupational Health, Umeå, Sweden)
Eur J Appl Physiol 57:415–419, March 1988   1–11

Recent research has demonstrated that significant changes occur throughout the range of motion during maximum isokinetic plantar flexions. How position in the range of motion influences the power spectral density function during static shoulder forward flexion was investigated in 23 healthy women who performed maximum static shoulder forward flexions in 3 positions—45, 65, and 90 degrees of shoulder flexion.

An isokinetic dynamometer was used, and the women were seated in a chair specially constructed to enable adequate fixation. The elbow was extended, and the hand was pronated. Electromyographic (EMG) signals were obtained from the descending portion of the right trapezius, the anterior portion of the right deltoid, the right infraspinatus, and the common belly of the right biceps brachii. The 4 EMG signals and the torque and shoulder angle were computer analyzed.

For each 256 ms, mean power frequency, root mean square value, and mean torque were determined. In the trapezius and biceps brachii, the mean power frequency did not change between the positions. The deltoid and infraspinatus had significantly greater mean power frequencies at 90 degrees than at 45 degrees of flexion. The hypothesis that significant differences in mean power frequency exist between the 3 different positions was confirmed for 2 of the 4 muscles studied.

▶ This study presents more information concerning the difficulty and possible measurement complications that one may experience when using surface electrodes for electromyographic studies. Considerations such as standardization of range of motion, effects of changed muscle length, position of the electrodes

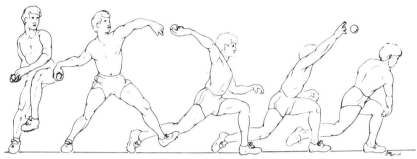

Fig 1–5.—Five phases of pitching baseball (from *left* to *right*): wind-up, early cocking, late cocking, acceleration, and follow-through. *Wind-up or preparation:* preliminary activity dominated by flexion of upper extremity, with both hands holding ball. *Early cocking:* period of abduction and external rotation of shoulder that begins as ball is released from nondominant hand. *Late cocking:* contact of forward foot with ground divides this stage from early cocking. Late cocking continues until maximum external rotation at shoulder is attained. *Acceleration:* starts with posture of maximum abduction and external rotation at shoulder and continues until release of ball, as ball leaves fingers. *Follow-through:* final interval of motion as arm flexes and internally rotates across chest and is decelerated. (Courtesy of Glousman R, Jobe F, Tibone J, et al: *J Bone Joint Surg* 70:220–226, February 1988.)

in relation to the innervation zone, and distance between the electrodes are also possible causes for the observed differences in mean power frequency.—Col. J.L. Anderson, PE.D.

Dynamic Electromyographic Analysis of the Throwing Shoulder With Glenohumeral Instability
Glousman R, Jobe F, Tibone J, Moynes D, Antonelli D, Perry J (Centinela Hosp, Inglewood, Calif)
J Bone Joint Surg 70:220–226, February 1988   1–12

Throwing and pitching are complex mechanisms that need a high level of neuromuscular coordination of the shoulder muscles. Flexibility and stability of the shoulder are required in most competitive sports. The sequence of activation of the muscles of the shoulder that occurs during pitching in throwers with instability of the shoulder was analyzed.

Fifteen athletes skilled in throwing who had chronic anterior instability of the shoulder were assessed by dynamic intramuscular electromyography while pitching a baseball. The pitch was divided into 5 parts (Fig 1–5). Results were compared with previously studied uninjured athletes.

Activity mildly increased in the biceps and supraspinatus in the first group as compared with the second group. Similar patterns of activity were seen in the deltoid. In the first group the infraspinatus had increased activity during early cocking and follow-through but decreased activity during late cocking. The pectoralis major, subscapularis, latissimus dorsi, and serratus anterior in injured athletes all had markedly decreased activity. A difference between the 2 groups was noted in all shoulder muscles except for the deltoid.

The increased activity levels of the biceps and supraspinatus in the first group may compensate for anterior laxity. The reduction in activity in the pectoralis major, subscapularis, and latissimus dorsi added to the anterior instability by decreasing the normal internal-rotation force needed in the late cocking and acceleration phases. Reduced activity of the serratus anterior might decrease protraction of the scapula, causing the glenoid fossa to remain behind the forward-flexing humerus during late cocking. Decreased protraction of the scapula increases anterior laxity because of increased stress of the humeral head on the anterior part of the glenoid labrum and capsule.

There was a difference between injured and uninjured pitchers in all of the shoulder muscles tested except for the deltoid. The neuromuscular imbalance seen in throwing athletes who have instability of the shoulder is either part of the primary pathology or a secondary phenomenon. These data provide a basis for the development of a rehabilitation program for patients with chronic anterior instability of the shoulder.

▶ At West Point, shoulder injuries from all causes have replaced knee injuries as the most serious and most prevalent joint injury. There has been some debate as to whether this is because of the emphasis that was put on running over development of upper body muscular strength and endurance during the 1970s and early 1980s. The concern for knee injuries during the 1960s led to some great improvements in surgical repair and rehabilitation techniques. We can only hope that the same thing will happen for the benefit of those who injure their shoulders.— Col. J.L. Anderson, PE.D.

Fine Structural Changes in Electrostimulated Human Skeletal Muscle: Evidence for Predominant Effects on Fast Muscle Fibres
Cabric M, Appell H-J, Resic A (Univ of Split, Yugoslavia; German Sports Univ, Cologne, West Germany; Gen Hosp Split)
Eur J Appl Physiol 57:1–5, January 1988   1–13

Knowledge of the effects of electrical stimulation of locomotor muscles is based mostly on animal experiments involving long-term stimulation with low frequencies. The effects of electrical stimulation on human muscles were studied morphologically with particular attention to differential effects on muscle fiber types.

Six male physical education students aged 19–22 years were subjected to electrical stimulation of relatively high frequency and current amplitude for 19 days. A quantitative study of several morphological parameters was done on biopsy samples from the gastrocnemius, using stereologic methods at light and electron microscopic levels. Muscle fiber size was increased, as was nuclear volume, suggesting that a proliferation of nuclei had occurred. An increased content of nuclear DNA was also noted. The size of single myonuclei was increased, and their heterochromatin fraction was reduced; these changes were most pronounced in type

II fibers. The increase in the mitochondrial fraction was also greatest in this type of fiber.

▶ The Russians have used electrical stimulation of locomotion muscles to train their athletes for a number of years. When Butler, the gymnastics coach at West Point, visited the USSR to study their athletic training techniques in the early 1980s, electrical stimulation was demonstrated on him. He reported that there was nothing comfortable about it. He was not certain what frequency he was subjected to, but he was pleased when the treatment ceased.— Col. J.L. Anderson, PE.D.

Mechanical Muscular Power Output and Work During Ergometer Cycling at Different Work Loads and Speeds
Ericson MO (Karolinska Inst, Stockholm)
Eur J Appl Physiol 57:382–387, March 1988   1–14

The cycle ergometer has been widely used in applied human physiology. The magnitude of the instantaneous muscular power output at the hip, knee, and ankle during ergometer cycling at different workloads and speeds was investigated.

Six healthy individuals pedaled a weight-braked cycle ergometer at 0, 120, and 240 W at 60 rpm. They also pedalled at 40, 60, 80, and 100 rpm against the same resistance, giving power outlets of 80, 120, 160, and 200 W, respectively. The cyclists were filmed and pedal reaction forces recorded from a force transducer mounted in the pedal. The muscular work for the hip, knee, and ankle muscles was determined using a model based on dynamic mechanics.

The increase in total work during 1 pedal revolution was directly proportional to significantly increased workload but did not increase with increased pedaling rate at the same braking force. Hip and ankle extension work proportionally declined with increased workload.

Instantaneous muscular power output increased as expected in all major muscle groups because of increase in work on the ergometer. However, the power increase from increased workload was not so significant for the hip and knee flexor muscles as for the other muscle groups. The major output response to increased workload was noted in the hip, knee, and ankle extensor muscles. Pedaling rate did not change the relative proportion of total work at the different joints studied.

▶ The purpose of this study was to calculate the magnitude of net mechanical muscular power output and work generated at the hip, knee, and ankle during cycling at different workloads and speeds. Another sub-purpose was to investigate how the power production relationship between the different lower limb muscle groups was affected by changes in workload and pedaling rate. Although the design of this study was adequate, it is flawed because of too few subjects and the need for improved data collection, e.g., automatic pedal force and kinematic recording devices. The author also recognizes the need for a method to determine the gross work caused by co-contraction from antagonistic muscles.— Col. J.L. Anderson, PE.D.

Moments of Force, Power, and Muscle Coordination in Speed-Skating
de Boer RW, Cabri J, Vaes W, Clarijs JP, Hollander AP, de Groot G, van Ingen Schenau GJ (Univ of Calgary; Free Univ, Brussels; Free Univ, Amsterdam)
Int J Sports Med 8:371–378, December 1987   1–15

Most knowledge of the stroke mechanisms in speed-skating has been derived from film analysis. Such experiments yield no information on the source of generation of energy. Another interesting phenomenon in speed-skating—the hampered knee extension connected to the absence of plantar flexion of the foot—has also been analyzed in film studies only. The patterns of moments of force and power output at the ankle, knee, and hip during speed-skating were studied by biochemical analysis.

Two well-trained speed-skaters underwent biomechanical analysis incorporating push-off forces, cinematographic data, and link segment modeling. Muscle coordination was studied by electromyography and muscle contraction velocities.

During push-off, the body center of gravity (cg) was accelerated with respect to the point of application of the push-off force, with a forward gliding skate. The velocity of cg was a result of rotation of segments. Because of the absence of plantar flexion of the foot, the knee extension range was limited. The short, explosive push-off resembles a catapult-like action. The knee extensor muscles—the vastus medialis and rectus femoris—were prestretched in the gliding phase by the antagonistic action of the gastrocnemius and biceps femoris. In this phase, the skater rotated cg from the lateral to the medial side of the skate to reach the optimal push-off angle.

Muscle coordination in speed skating was strongly coupled to the constraints inherent to the transformation of rotational energy into velocity of cg with this type of movement. The power output in the push-off was generated mainly by the monarticular extensor muscles gluteus maximus and vastus medialis.

▶ This study included only 2 subjects, and they were well-trained speed-skaters, so the results cannot be generalized to other populations of skaters. However, coaches and trainers of speed-skaters can find some useful information here to help them in correcting the form of their athletes and to help them to skate more efficiently.— Col. J.L. Anderson, PE.D.

Clinical Biomechanics of Skiing
Macintyre JG, Matheson GO (BC Sports Medicine Clinic, Vancouver)
Can Fam Physician 34:107–114, January 1988   1–16

Lower leg alignment is an important factor in skier comfort, safety, and performance. Recent advances in ski boot technology have provided adjustment for individual variations in lower leg alignment. It is important to understand the mechanics of how a ski turns to appreciate the significance of the leg-boot-ski interface and the ways in which abnormal biomechanics can affect this relationship.

Physicians must approach a skier's problems with an understanding of the basics of lower limb biomechanics and the clinical and technical presentations of malalignment. Basic problems, such as difficulty in initiating a turn, catching edges, washing-out of the tails of the skis, painful cramping or pressure points in the feet, and knee pain can all be symptoms of an underlying biomechanical problem. Compensation for tibial alignment is accomplished through adjusting the angle of the boot cuff, whereas in-boot orthotic footbeds are used to correct excessive pronation resulting from varus deformities of the tibia and foot. A proper corrective orthotic is particularly important for skiers with persistent boot-fitting difficulties and competitive skiers whose technique suffers from uncorrected alignment problems.

Abnormalities of lower leg alignment can lead to a number of skiing problems. Tibia vara may cause difficulties in turning and riding a flat ski unless the boot cuff is adjusted properly to the lower leg. Varus deformities in the foot can result in boot-fitting difficulties, foot and knee pain, and the inability to edge a ski turn properly. Compensation with an appropriately posted, corrective, orthotic device may allow skiing participation with greater comfort and better performance.

▶ This paper is an excellent example of how the sports medicine physician and coach or trainer must work together to help correct certain biomechanical structural problems to allow the athlete to improve his or her performance. Today, more and more physicians are working in sports medicine not only to treat sports injuries but also help to prevent them and improve performance.—Col. J.L. Anderson, PE.D.

Vertical and Radial Motions of the Body During the Take-Off Phase of High Jumping
Dapena J, Chung CS (Indiana Univ, Bloomington)
Med Sci Sports Exerc 20:290–302, June 1988   1–17

The most important part of the high jump is the takeoff, because the height cleared is decided primarily by the vertical velocity generated during this phase. A study was done to achieve a better understanding of the functions of eccentric and concentric muscular conditions during takeoff.

A film analysis of 7 high jumpers was done. The radial velocity of the center of mass with respect to the supporting foot was observed to be more negative or less positive than the vertical velocity throughout the takeoff phase, which favored faster eccentric or slower concentric conditions of the leg muscles. The radial distance from the hip of the takeoff leg to the center of mass ($R_{G/H}$) first decreased by 0.03 m because of negative radial motions of the arms and swinging leg. This contributed to a smaller negative radial velocity of the hip (V_{RH}) and therefore to slower eccentric conditions of the muscles of the takeoff leg. Thus it may have helped to cushion the initial impact with the ground. Subsequently, $R_{G/H}$ increased by 0.12 m because of positive radial velocities of the arms, the swinging leg, and the head and trunk. This contributed to larger negative and later to smaller positive V_{RH} values, and therefore to faster eccentric and slower concentric conditions of the muscles of the takeoff leg.

By placing the muscles of the takeoff leg in faster eccentric or slower concentric conditions, high jumpers can increase the ground reaction force and the height of the jump.

▶ There is much more to this research paper than can be adequately presented in this short abstract. Coaches and trainers should study the entire paper to better understand the vertical and radial motions of the body during the take-off phase in high jumping. It is significant that this research was supported by a grant from the United States Olympic Committee and The Athletics Congress.— Col. J.L. Anderson, PE.D.

Load- and Skill-Related Changes in Segmental Contributions to a Weightlifting Movement
Enoka RM (Univ of Arizona, Tucson)
Med Sci Sports Exerc 20:178–187, April 1988   1–18

As a measure of the rate of work performance or energy flow, the power output of muscle is thought to limit human performance, particularly if the event is of short duration. Because muscle-produced power is limited by the metabolic rate of adenosine triphosphate (ATP) production and the rate at which the myofilaments can convert chemical energy into mechanical work, the extent to which power output may limit performance depends on how closely the muscle activity approaches either of these rate-limiting capabilities. An exemplary short-duration, high-power, weightlifting event was studied to determine whether the ability to lift heavier loads and whether variations in the level of skill are accompanied by quantitative changes in selected aspects of lower extremity joint power-time histories.

Six experienced weightlifters, 3 skilled and 3 less skilled, did the double-knee-bend execution of the pull in Olympic weightlifting, a movement that lasts almost 1 second. Skilled athletes lifted heavier loads by increasing the average power, but not the peak power, around the knees and ankles. The changes with load were more subtle than a mere quantitative scaling and also appeared to be associated with a skill element in the form of variation in the duration of the phases of power production and absorption. Similarly, statistical differences resulting from skill did not involve changes in the magnitude of power but, rather, the temporal organization of the movement. The ability to execute the double-knee-bend movement successfully depends on an athlete's ability to both generate a sufficient magnitude of joint power and to organize the phases of power production and absorption into an appropriate temporal sequence.

▶ This research shows that weightlifting is not merely a sport requiring brute strength alone. High levels of skill are also important. The author reported, for example, that as the load increased from 69% to 77%, the skilled athletes increased the average knee power for the first 2 phases. When the load went from 77% to 86%, rather than increasing the power the skilled lifters varied the timing. The significance of this observation lies in the nature of the movement, the double-knee-bend technique of the pull, a technique that requires considerable practice before mastery and one demanding substantial control of knee motion.—Col. J.L. Anderson, PE.D.

Limited Joint Mobility in Power Lifters

Chang DE, Buschbacher LP, Edlich RF (Univ of Virginia)
Am J Sports Med 16:280–284, May–June 1988   1–19

Power lifting has been associated with muscle hypertrophy and marked increases in lean body cell mass. Although the flexibility of power lifters has not been scientifically documented, the flexibility of weight lifters reportedly is the same as or better than that of nonlifters. The flexibility of 10 power lifters was compared with that of 10 age-matched nonlifters not involved in competitive sports. Goniometric measurements, the behind-the-back-reach test, and the sit-and-reach test were used.

No significant differences were found between functional extensibility and goniometric measurements of the power lifters' and nonlifters' right and left sides. Nonlifters had significantly more extensibility in the behind-the-back-reach test than did the lifters, but the extensibility of the lifters in the sit-and-reach test was significantly greater than that of the nonlifters. All goniometric measurements of shoulder range of motion were significantly greater for the nonlifters than the lifters (Fig 1–6). Nonlifters were also significantly more supple than the lifters in elbow and wrist flexion. Goniometric measurements for hip flexion, internal and external rotation of the hip, and knee flexion were significantly greater for nonlifters. The sit-and-reach test was the only measurement that showed the flexibility of power lifters to be greater than that of nonlifters.

▶ The significance of this study is that it points out the lack of balance present in power lifters' training programs. This is because of the failure of power lifters to include stretching in their workouts. It has been shown that the incidence of strains and sprains in athletes can be reduced when a stretching exercise program is made a part of the overall workout. Power lifters commonly

SHOULDER JOINTS

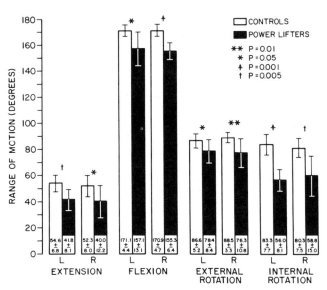

Fig 1–6.—All goniometric measurements of the shoulder range of motion were significantly greater for the nonlifters than those for the power lifters. (Courtesy of Chang DE, Buschbacher LP, Edlich RF: *Am J Sports Med* 16:280–284, May–June 1988.)

experience low back pain, shoulder pain, and knee injuries. Stretching should be used by power lifters to reduce the threat of these injuries.—Col. J.L. Anderson, PE.D.

Kinematic Analysis of Human Upper Extremity Movements in Boxing
Whiting WC, Gregor RJ, Finerman GA (Univ of California, Los Angeles)
Am J Sports Med 16:130–136, March–April 1988   1–20

Three-dimensional (3-D) analyses in sports have proved useful in assessing movement patterns and relating movements to potential injury mechanisms. Such techniques were applied to boxing to develop an analysis model and protocol for assessment of the 3-D kinematics of the human upper extremity during boxing.

Using 2 synchronized cameras, 4 experienced boxers were filmed throwing a series of punches at a practice bag. Three-dimensional coordinates of each boxer's shoulder, elbow, wrist, and glove were used to calculate the linear and angular kinematics of the upper extremity. Average velocities at contact were 5.9–8.2 m/s, with peak velocities of 6.6–12.5 m/s reached 8–21 ms before hand/glove contact with the bag (Fig 1–7). Significant differences in shoulder and wrist velocities, elbow angle excursions, and elbow angular velocities were noted when hooks and

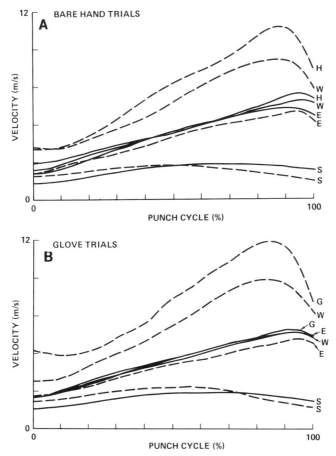

Fig 1–7.—Average joint center velocity curves for bare-handed trials (**A**) and gloved trials (**B**). Body marker designations are shown as: hand *(H)*, wrist *(W)*, elbow *(E)*, shoulder *(S)*, and glove *(G)* for both jobs *(solid lines)* and hooks *(dashed lines)*. (Courtesy of Whiting WC, Gregor RJ, Finerman GA: *Am J Sports Med* 16:130–136, March–April 1988.)

jabs were compared. There were few differences when the kinematics of gloved punches were compared with bare-handed punches.

The findings can be used in a kinetic model of punch impact and its relationship to potential injury mechanisms.

▶ Some will no doubt be surprised to see this study of boxing included in this YEAR BOOK. Discussion of the sport of boxing seldom is carried out in a rational, thoughtful way. Most people have made up their minds about boxing, either pro or con, and do not want to be confused with the facts. Few researchers have looked at boxing the way we have looked at other sports in an attempt to make the sport safer. There are few scientific data available that can be applied in the design of gloves and headgear to lessen the impact of punches. The

American Medical Association has sent mixed signals. In a 1983 issue of *JAMA* the AMA Council on Scientific Affairs, Advisory Panel on Brain Injury in Boxing, stated: "Some would favor banning boxing completely, but this is not a realistic solution to the problem of brain injury in boxing. Moreover, the sport does not seem any more dangerous than other sports presently accepted by society." A few years later, with little additional research, the AMA called for the banning of boxing. The authors of this study are to be commended for trying to bring out some facts to allow reasoned decisions to be made in place of the purely emotional ones that are prevalent today.—Col. J.L. Anderson, PE.D.

2 Women in Sports

Introduction

Until relatively recent times the exhibition of physical prowess was considered the sole domain of the male. Since about 1900 women began to be viewed as capable of holding their own in physical competition, but they have still been limited by prejudicial societal patterns of culture, ethics, and morals. The last half of this century has seen a major change in the United States in the quantity and quality of opportunities for women to participate in sports.

Researchers are now working to catch up in the level of understanding of women's sports performance. More and more, we are beginning to identify the differences as well as the similarities between men and women and how they relate to performance in sports. There are real physiologic and psychological differences between men and women. It is difficult to identify what the *real* differences are because they tend to be masked by differences caused by the sociocultural prejudices that have limited women's full participation in sports.

Studies selected for review in the YEAR BOOK OF SPORTS MEDICINE represent some of the kinds of work being done all over the world to help us better understand and develop the physiologic and psychological capabilities of women who wish to participate in sports.

Col. James L. Anderson, PE.D.

Women in Sport
Fardy HJ (Taree, New South Wales)
Aust Fam Physician 17:183–186, March 1988   2–1

Women with sports injuries usually seen by general practitioners tend to be recreational athletes who are serious about their sport and need accurate, appropriate care and advice. A review of data on women in sports was conducted from the point of view of general practitioners who rarely treat elite athletes but often see patients with health concerns about their sport.

Several studies have demonstrated a higher injury rate for women than for men in various sports. Many are overuse injuries resulting from differences in female anatomy. Whereas there is a rapid increase in cardiovascular fitness in women, there is not a parallel increase in the strength of the musculoskeletal system and tendons.

Certain injuries are unique to women, such as forceful vaginal douches in waterskiing, breast contusions, and vulvovaginal injuries. Among women participating in athletic training for endurance events, 25% to 40% of those considered highly trained have fewer than 3 menses a year. There is no adequate explanation for amenorrhea or oligomenorrhea associated with exercise. The choice of contraception for exercising women is complicated by the tendency for menstrual irregularities and amenorrhea, and by the effects, if any, of contraception method on athletic performance. It is inadvisable for women to begin a sports training program during pregnancy. A high level of maternal fitness, however, does not affect pregnancy outcome. The most important consideration for exercise during pregnancy is that the exercise program be individualized in consultation with an obstetrician. Breast problems in exercising women are usually not serious but can cause marked discomfort.

Women consulting their general practitioner about exercise should be encouraged and given advice that considers their medical history and state of health. They should be advised that a regular pattern of exercise with a slowly increasing intensity of effort is the best way to maintain an exercise habit. Most women benefit greatly in physical and mental well-being from regular exercise.

▶ What this author calls the recreational athlete is the same as I call the Weekend Athlete, and they are the athletes who suffer the most injuries and are most often seen by the general practitioner. Weekend Athletes do not have coaches or trainers, and they sustain most of their injuries because they look at their sports participation as their conditioning program and do not condition themselves to play their sports. General practitioners should encourage Weekend Athletes to get into shape to play their sport, rather than to play their sport to get into shape.— Col. J.L. Anderson, PE.D.

Benefits and Risks of Running Among Women: An Epidemiologic Study
Marti B (Univ of Berne, Switzerland)
Int J Sports Med 9:92–98, April 1988   2–2

The suggested benefits of a high level of exercise or fitness are less well documented for women than for men. A group of Swiss women runners entering a popular 16-km road race was studied to determine some of the suggested health benefits and potential risks of recreational running in women. Questionnaires were given to 428 runners; the response rate was 86%.

The estimated endurance capacity of women runners (VO_{2max} equivalents) was superior to the endurance capacity of females and males in the general population (Fig 2–1). The best predictor of a runner's VO_{2max} was the habitual weekly training distance. Training and life-style characteristics of the runners explained part of the difference in VO_{2max} seen between runners and women in the general population. Running was positively associated with weight loss and with quitting smoking. However, in the year preceding the race, 40% of the female contestants had running-related injuries or complaints, 17% sought medical help, and

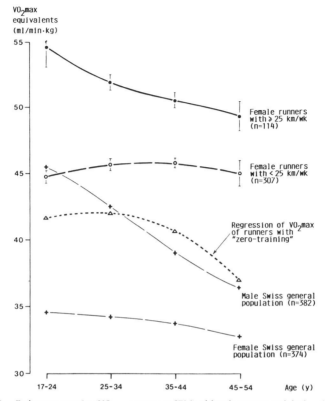

Fig 2–1.—Endurance capacity (VO$_{2max}$; means ± SEM) of female runners with high mileage, moderate mileage, and hypothetical "zero training" compared with male and female general population (Courtesy of Marti B: *Int J Sports Med* 9:92–98, 1988.)

14% had to interrupt running for an average of 6 weeks. The sites and types of injury showed specific female properties. Female runners had significantly less outpatient physician visits than the general population, but highly active runners had more visits than moderately active runners because of running-related complaints.

Apparently, female runners have a high endurance capacity and low body weight, and almost none smoke. However, they have relatively frequent running-related injuries and therefore have more medical consultations.

▶ It is well known that women sustain more overuse injuries than do men. At West Point when men and women cadets participate in the same running conditioning program during their first 7 weeks after enrollment, women experience a stress fracture injury rate that is approximately 10 times higher than that for men. We believe that the primary reason is because, in our culture, women do not exercise as rigorously during the first 17 years of their lives as men do. If this is what causes the higher injury rate among women, we should see a decrease in the stress fracture rate after another 10 or so years. It should be pointed out that we have observed little change during the past 12 years.— Col. J.L. Anderson, PE.D.

Adolescent Females' Readiness to Participate in Sports: Sex and Race Differences in the Preparticipation Athletic Examination
Durant RH, Linder CW, Sanders JM Jr, Jay S, Brantley G, Bedgood R (Med College of Georgia, Augusta; Univ of Arkansas)
J Adolesc Health Care 9:310–314, July 1988   2–3

The increasing number of adolescent girls participating in athletics has caused concern about their susceptibility to injury. Whether girls differ from boys in the severity and frequency of abnormalities on the preparticipation athletic examination (PAE) was determined.

Standardized PAEs were performed on 1,259 high school athletes. Girls had significantly fewer orthopedic problems than boys on the health history and physical examination. Girls also had a lower percentage of abnormalities of the hips, knees, and ankles. Black boys had significantly higher rates of hip abnormalities than white boys, and black girls had a higher rate of knee abnormalities than white girls. Significantly more boys than girls were referred for further assessment before participation in athletic activities.

Adolescent girls appear to have fewer physical problems on the PAE than boys. Therefore, they might be at lower risk of athletic injury. The types of problems noted in girls on the PAE, however, suggests that they may benefit from participation in more aerobic and strength training before the sports season.

▶ The authors of this study quote findings of one of my studies that I did in 1979 using data collected in 1976–1978. I stated then that when women are involved in a vigorous, physically demanding conditioning program equal in duration and intensity to that of men, there will be a significantly higher injury rate, and that the rate will increase over time. This is partly because of physiologic differences and partly the result of sociocultural differences. Ten years later we have seen no change in the differences in injury rates. If our society encourages our female children to be physically active from a very early age, we can greatly reduce those injuries that are the result of sociocultural differences. However, only evolution can change the physiologic differences.— Col. J.L. Anderson, PE.D.

Physiological Responses to Treadmill Exercise in Females: Adult-Child Differences
Rowland TW, Green GM (Baystate Med Ctr, Springfield, Mass)
Med Sci Sports Exerc 20:474–478, July 1988   2–4

Most studies of differences between children and adults in physiologic response to treadmill exercise have involved men and boys. Prepubertal boys had greater oxygen consumption ($\dot{V}O_2$) per body weight at all work levels, including $\dot{V}O_{2max}$; higher levels of ventilation ($\dot{V}_E$) per kg at submaximal and maximal speeds; inferior breathing efficiency; and higher heart rates at all exercise levels. The variations between women and girls were investigated.

Eighteen premenarchal girls and 18 young women underwent treadmill testing to exhaustion. The girls had significantly higher oxygen consumption and ventilation per body weight at maximal and submaximal speeds, except at the lowest workload. When $\dot{V}O_2$ was related to body surface area, differences in submaximal running economy disappeared. The girls had a higher respiratory rate and lower tidal volume per kg at a given ventilation and an inferior breathing efficiency. The absolute ventilatory breakpoint was higher in the girls, but when this parameter was expressed as percent $\dot{V}O_{2max}$, the difference was not significant. Girls, however, had a higher heart rate at the ventilatory breakpoint.

The physiologic differences between premenarchal girls and women during treadmill exercise are similar to those reported previously between boys and men. The energy cost of treadmill running was higher in girls. This difference became more pronounced as speed increased.

▶ The findings of this study comparing premenarchal girls with young women running on a treadmill are about the same as those of other authors who compared prepubertal boys with young men. The differences in both groups are probably the result of the more efficient running styles of men and women as compared with boys and girls.—Col. J.L. Anderson, PE.D.

Biomechanical Studies of Elite Female Distance Runners
Williams KR, Cavanagh PR, Ziff JL (Univ of California, Davis; Pennsylvania State Univ, University Park)
Int J Sports Med 8:107–118, November 1987   2–5

Little is known about how biomechanical aspects of running style influence the ability to achieve maximum potential. Fourteen elite female distance runners were filmed while running on a treadmill (Fig 2–2).

The runners were mainly midfoot strikers. Ground reaction force measurements showed peaks of 3.3 times body weight in the vertical component, 0.8 in the braking phase, and 0.3 mediolaterally. Asymmetry was most evident in the mediolateral component. More abduction during foot placement was related to greater rearfoot motion and greater change in the mediolateral component of velocity. There were few correlations between biomechanical variables and running economy. The elite runners tended to be shorter and lighter than typical female nonathletes. They had shorter legs and considerably less iliac-crest fat. Compared with elite male runners performing at the same velocity, the women had more hip flexion, greater angular velocities in hip flexion and extension, and longer stride lengths relative to leg length. Vertical oscillation was less in women than in men.

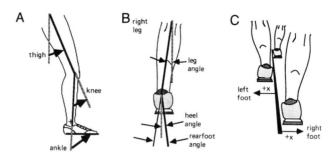

Fig 2–2.—Conventions used for angular kinematic measurements for **A**, sagittal plane angles; **B**, leg, heel, and rearfoot angles; and **C**, crossover of the feet relative to a midline. Note the opposite reference axes for crossover for the left and right sides of the body. (Courtesy of Williams KR, Cavanagh PR, Ziff JL: *Int J Sports Med* 8:107–118, November 1987.)

It has been proposed that females are at increased risk of musculoskeletal injury during weight-bearing activities such as running, but the present data suggest that elite female runners are not typical of the female population. They may in fact be more similar to elite males with regard to relative pelvic width, a factor implicated in injury in female athletes.

▶ Because of the paucity of studies on women's distance running, this work will be helpful for those persons who work with elite women runners. However, the sample size used for this study was small and care should be taken in generalizing the results to a larger population. More studies such as this need to be done for us to better understand how biomechanical aspects of running style affect a runner's ability to achieve maximum potential. As useful as this study may be in understanding elite women runners, that is a very small percentage of the population of female runners. The larger percentage of the population may demonstrate entirely different biomechanical running styles that are less mechanically efficient and may cause the runners to be more prone to injury. It is important that we study and come to understand the running mechanics of both populations. The study reviewed in Abstract 2–6 used recreational runners as subjects.—Col. J.L. Anderson, PE.D.

Knee Muscle Torques in Patellofemoral Pain Syndrome
MacIntyre D, Wessel J (Univ of British Columbia, Vancouver)
Physiother Canada 40:20–24, January–February 1988   2–6

Patellofemoral pain syndrome is characterized by diffuse pain around the patella secondary to abnormal patellar tracking. Malalignment, arthralgia, or runner's knee are all names applied to the syndrome. Pain is made worse by activities that load the patellofemoral joint in flexion and those worsening any biomechanical abnormalities that are present. Peak concentric and eccentric torques of the quadriceps and hamstrings were compared in 20 female recreational runners aged 15–36 years, 8 of whom had right patellofemoral pain syndrome.

The runners were tested on an isokinetic dynamometer at an angular velocity of 200 degrees per second. There were no significant group differences in peak torques or hamstring/quadriceps ratios. However, the concentric H/Q ratio was beyond the normal range in affected athletes. Peak torques differed significantly in the 2 muscles and between concentric and eccentric contractions. Eccentric contractions produced greater peak torques in both groups, especially for the quadriceps muscle.

Further study is needed of force-velocity relationships of concentric/eccentric contractions in different muscle groups in both normal persons and those with pathology.

▶ Here is a study of recreational runners, the type that most general practitioners normally treat. The authors studied the muscle groups acting on the patella in order to better understand the often reported patellofemoral pain syndrome, a common complaint of recreational runners. This study would have benefited had a protocol been used similar to that described in Abstract 2–5. The combination of the 2 protocols might have allowed us to understand the effect that mechanical running styles have on the cause of patellofemoral pain syndrome.—Col. J.L. Anderson, PE.D.

Cardiac Frequency and Caloric Cost of Aerobic Dancing in Young Women
Nelson DJ, Pels AE III, Geenen DL, White TP (Univ of Michigan)
Res Q Exerc Sport 59:229–233, September 1988   2–7

Aerobic dancing reportedly is intense enough to yield beneficial physiologic adaptations, but variable results are reported. The heart rate and oxidative energy cost of this activity were determined in 13 women enrolled in aerobic dance classes at a university. The classes met for 50 minutes twice weekly, and each included 35 minutes of actual dancing.

Heart rates were significantly elevated (Fig 2–3). Exercisers reached 40% of heart rate reserve after the 10-minute warm-up phase, and the reserve varied from 50% to 70% during the dance phase. Heart rates declined markedly during the 5-minute cool-down phase. The estimated total caloric cost of the entire session was 317 kcal. During actual dancing the caloric cost was about 8 kcal/minute.

These exercisers previously had engaged regularly in low-level aerobic activities and, as a result, had oxygen uptake values at the high end of the range for college-age women. Aerobic dancing reportedly promotes cardiovascular endurance.

▶ This study is included because of the popularity of aerobic dance as an exercise activity for so many young and not-so-young adults. It is important for everyone to know that there are great differences in the intensity levels of various aerobic dance classes. I would consider the one reported on here to be of moderate intensity because the heart rate usually stayed somewhere between 60% and 70% of the heart rate reserve. In some classes the heart rates of well-conditioned athletes stay above 80% of heart rate reserve. There is no

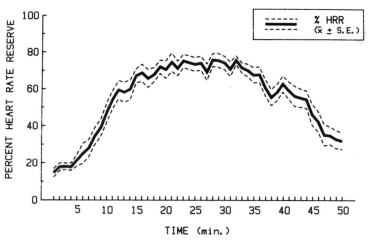

Fig 2–3.—Cardiac frequency, expressed as a percentage of heart rate reserve, recorded during aerobic dance class. The first 10 minutes consisted of warm-up exercises, followed by a 35-minute main dancing phase and a 5-minute cool-down. (Courtesy of Nelson DJ, Pels AE III, Geenen DL, et al: *Res Q Exerc Sport* 59:229–233, September 1988.)

doubt that aerobic conditioning can be improved this way. It is important, however, that the participants become involved in classes that will stress, but not overstress, their cardiovascular systems. It is also important that the aerobic dance instructor be well trained to recognize the abilities of the participants.—Col. J.L. Anderson, PE.D.

Endogenous Hormones Subtly Alter Women's Response to Heat Stress
Carpenter AJ, Nunneley SA (US Air Force School of Aerospace Medicine, Brooks AFB, Tex)
J Appl Physiol 65:2313–2317, November 1988   2–8

Women's resting core temperature rises by 0.5 F during the menstrual cycle. The impact of this temperature increase on thermoregulation during exercise and heat stress is still debated. The effects of the normal hormone changes associated with the menstrual cycle on the thermoregulatory responses of women to work in heat were investigated.

The thermoregulatory reactions of menstruating women to exercise in dry heat were assessed 3 times during the cycle: at menstrual flow, 3–5 days during midcycle ovulation, and in the middle of the luteal phase. After acclimation, the 8 individuals underwent heat stress tests consisting of a 2-hour cycle ergometer exercise at 30% maximal O_2 consumption in the heat.

At rest, rectal temperature was lowest at ovulation and significantly increased in the luteal phase. During steady-state exercise, both rectal and mean skin temperatures were lowest at ovulation and significantly higher in the luteal phase. No differences were found between phases with regard to total sweat loss, degree of sweating on the chest and thigh, or metabolic rate. All women were able to complete the 2 hours of exercise despite higher rectal and mean skin temperatures.

The menstrual cycle alters temperature regulation with obvious changes in sweat output or steady-state metabolic rate. These changes are so subtle that they could be missed if hormonal status is not carefully monitored concomitant with heat stress tests. The magnitude of the changes noted in this series was small and did not impair the women's ability to work in dry heat.

▶ From a practical sense rather than a theoretical sense, the important finding of this study is that there is no evidence that a woman's menstrual phase has any significant effect on her tolerance for physical work and heat stress, which is heavily dependent on aerobic fitness, heat acclimation, and individual variation in heat stress response. Of course, physiologists will continue to study the mechanism behind the observed differences in temperatures during the 3 phases of the menstrual cycle. This mechanism is not understood, although this study did show that the differences in temperature over the 3 phases were not because of changes in sweat production.— Col. J.L. Anderson, PE.D.

Relationship of Estrogen to Strength, Percent Body Fat and Oxygen Uptake in Women
Rice PL (Murray State Univ, Murray, Ky)
J Sports Med 28:145–150, June 1988   2–9

Most previous work on estrogen and physical performance has concentrated on physical performance during different phases of the menstrual cycle and the response of various sex hormones to different levels of physical performance. Several studies have shown estradiol levels to increase acutely during exercise but to be slightly suppressed after long-term exercise programs. The relationship of estradiol to measures of strength, percent body fat, and oxygen uptake was determined in 21 active and sedentary women aged 20–40 years.

Active women exercised regularly 4 times a week for 30 minutes and had been exercising for at least 1 year. None was an intercollegiate athlete. The sedentary women were involved in no regular physical activity. There was a significant correlation between estradiol level and percent body fat in active women. Strength and estradiol level showed significance in sedentary women. Active women had higher oxygen consumption and lower percent fat than sedentary women but similar estradiol levels and strength. Physical performance measures did not significantly predict the estradiol level in either group.

Because research on female hormones and their relationship to physical performance is limited, further study is needed.

▶ One of the major physiologic variables differentiating men and women are the sex hormones. There is evidence that testosterone may have effects on strength development, but there has been little research investigating the effects of estrogen on various physical performance measures. I agree with this author that further study of female hormones and their relationship to physical performance is necessary if we are to better understand the physiologic capabilities of women.—Col. J.L. Anderson, PE.D.

Dynamic Strength and Work Variations During Three Stages of the Menstrual Cycle
Dibrezzo R, Fort IL, Brown B (Univ of Arkansas, Fayetteville)
J Orthop Sports Phys Ther 10:113–116, October 1988   2–10

The increase in the number of women participating in strenuous and physically exhausting activities has raised concerns about physiologic and biomechanical responses in women. Some studies state that there are no significant differences in work capacity or strength in any phase of the menstrual cycle, whereas others contradict these findings. The effects of 3 different phases of the menstrual cycle on dynamic strength and work performance of the knee flexors and extensors were investigated.

Twenty-one women aged 18–36 years were tested for dynamic strength and endurance on a Cybex II isokinetic dynamometer at speeds of 60, 180, and 240 degrees per second. Each woman was assessed within 24 hours of onset of menses, at the time of ovulation, and during the luteal phase. Strength was evaluated by peak torque values of knee flexion and extension at the 3 speeds. Flexion and extension endurance ratios and a work ratio were calculated at a speed of 240 degrees per second.

There were no significant differences among the strength variables during the 3 phases of the menstrual cycle. Endurance ratios showed that peak torque values were less than two thirds of original strength at the end of 20 repetitions. Flexors were observed to fatigue slightly less than extensors. No significant differences in work ratios among the 3 phases were noted.

These data show that the physical capabilities of women are far greater than previously believed. Active women with a normal menstrual cycle should experience no discernible change in strength and work performance as a result of cycle changes.

▶ I'm not certain where these authors have been, but at least 13 years ago we reported that women's physical performance capabilities are far greater than previously believed. However, the authors have reconfirmed that active women with normal menstrual cycles should experience no major change in strength and work performance as a result of cycle changes.—Col. J.L. Anderson, PE.D.

Menarche in Athletes: The Influence of Genetics and Prepubertal Training
Stager JM, Hatler LK (Indiana Univ, Bloomington)
Med Sci Sports Exerc 20:369–373, August 1988   2–11

It is unclear whether the later menarche seen in competitive athletes is caused by genetic or environmental factors related to intense prepubertal training. The importance of these factors on age of menarche was investigated by questionnaire in 263 competitive swimmers and 71 women without athletic experience. Similar questionnaires were then sent to the sisters of both groups.

Complete data were obtained from 140 athlete/sister pairs and 43 control/sister pairs. The athletes were older at menarche than their sisters, nonathletes, and nonathletes' sisters. The sisters of athletes were significantly older at menarche than the control women and their sisters, whereas the age of menarche of the nonathletes and their sisters did not differ. The sisters of the athletes were likely to be athletes, whereas those of the nonathletes tended to be nonathletic. The athletes differed from their sisters who trained before menarche and from those who did not train in the prepubertal period. Control women did not differ from any of their sister groups or from the untrained sisters of athletes. Significant correlations were noted between athletes and their sisters who trained before menarche and control women and their sisters who did not.

Interpretation of these findings is difficult because of the tendencies within families either to participate in sports or not. Swimmers were older at menarche than their sisters, and athletes' sisters were older at menarche than all nonathletic controls, but the data cannot rule out either of the 2 seemingly opposing explanations for later menarche among athletes.

▶ This is one of those cause-and-effect problems that will take more research before a definitive answer is found. It has seemed obvious from previous data, however, that rigorous prepubertal training does appear to delay the onset of menstruation. However, it is also true that the cause/effect relationship has not been proven. Maybe the important question is whether it makes any difference if reproductive maturity is delayed.—Col. J.L. Anderson, PE.D.

Prediction of $\dot{V}O_{2max}$ During Cycle Exercise in Pregnant Women
Sady SP, Carpenter MW, Sady MA, Haydon B, Hoegsberg B, Cullinane EM, Thompson PD, Coustan DR (Miriam Hosp, Providence, RI; Womens and Infants Hosp, Providence; Brown Univ)
J Appl Physiol 65:657–661, August 1988   2–12

Both the popular press and professional publications advocate physical activity during pregnancy. Individualized exercise prescriptions typically specify the intensity, duration, and frequency of physical activity. Exercise intensity, usually expressed as a percentage of maximal oxygen uptake ($\dot{V}O_2$ $_{max}$), is determined from equations relating heart rate to percent $\dot{V}O_2$ $_{max}$. Such equations, however, were derived from nonpregnant women. It was hypothesized that a $\dot{V}O_2$ $_{max}$ prediction derived from pregnant women would be more accurate in this population.

Maximal oxygen uptake was measured during stationary cycling in 40 pregnant women at a mean gestational age of 26 weeks. Data from 30 women were used to develop an equation to predict the percent $\dot{V}O_2$ $_{max}$ from submaximal heart rates. This equation and the submaximal $\dot{V}O_2$ were then used to predict $\dot{V}O_2$ $_{max}$ in the remaining 10 women. The accuracy of this procedure was compared with that of the Åstrand nomogram and the $\dot{V}O_2$ vs. heart rate ($\dot{V}O_2$-HR) curve.

The $\dot{V}O_2$ $_{max}$ values estimated by the new equation were only 3.7 $\pm$ 12.2% higher than actual values. The Åstrand method overestimated $\dot{V}O_2$ $_{max}$ by 9%, and the $\dot{V}O_2$-HR curve underestimated it by 1.6 $\pm$ 10.3%. Both methods correlated well with the actual values when all 40 women were considered, but the $\dot{V}O_2$-HR curve method had a lower standard error of prediction than the Åstrand method. In 10 nonpregnant sedentary women an equation relating percent $\dot{V}O_2$ $_{max}$ to heart rate was found almost identical to that obtained in the pregnant women, suggesting that pregnancy does not change this relationship.

Extrapolating the $\dot{V}O_2$-HR curve to an estimated maximal heart rate is the most accurate way to predict $\dot{V}O_2$ $_{max}$ in pregnant women. The derived equation yielded better results than the Åstrand method, and it should be used to predict $\dot{V}O_2$ $_{max}$ in pregnant women when exercise at only 1 power output is feasible. Alternatively, protocols in which the $\dot{V}O_2$ and heart rate response can be obtained at several submaximal outputs to construct individual $\dot{V}O_2$-HR curves should be used, as these can be extrapolated to an age-estimated maximal heart rate and give the best prediction of $\dot{V}O_2$ $_{max}$.

▶ This is a start in devising better methods of individualized exercise prescriptions for pregnant women. It is well established that women should continue to exercise throughout pregnancy after consultation with their physician. However, more study needs to be done to improve the accuracy of the exercise prescription and to explain the intensity, duration, and frequency of exercise.— Col. J.L. Anderson, PE.D.

The Effect of Participation in a Regular Exercise Program Upon Aerobic Capacity During Pregnancy
South-Paul JE, Rajagopal KR, Tenholder MF (Uniformed Services Univ of the Health Sciences, Bethesda, Md)
Obstet Gynecol 71:175–179, February 1988   2–13

The health and fitness of pregnant women at the onset of gestation affect the course and outcome of the pregnancy. Whether pregnancy reduces physical fitness as measured by maximal oxygen consumption between the second and third trimesters, and whether maintaining a regular exercise program during the second half of pregnancy influences fitness, were determined in 23 women at the beginning of the second trimester.

Patients were randomly assigned to either a nonexercising or an exercising group. They completed a maximal progressive exercise test on a cycle ergometer at 20 weeks and 30 weeks, during which time pulmonary parameters or aerobic capacity were assessed.

The exercising women had greater improvement in aerobic capacity than the nonexercising women, manifested by increases in tidal volume and oxygen consumption and a stable ventilatory equivalent for oxygen. Pregnancy did not decrease the maximal oxygen consumption between the second and third trimesters, during which detraining could have been substantial. Fitness may be improved by participation in a supervised exercise program.

▶ This study again points out the value of exercising during pregnancy. In fact, none of the women in this study was previously trained and the average baseline oxygen consumption was in the low range for both groups. Yet, when placed in a supervised exercise program, the exercise group improved their fitness, as demonstrated by increased maximal oxygen consumption per kilogram of body weight. (See Abstract 2–14.)—Col. J.L. Anderson, PE.D.

Fetal Heart Rate Response to Maternal Exertion
Carpenter MW, Sady SP, Hoegsberg B, Sady MA, Haydon B, Cullinane EM, Coustan DR, Thompson PD (Brown Univ)
JAMA 259:3006–3009, May 27, 1988   2–14

Doppler monitoring of fetal heart rates, showing fetal bradycardia during vigorous maternal exercise, has given rise to concern for fetal safety. Because Doppler measurement of fetal heart rate during maternal exertion is difficult, 2-dimensional ultrasonic imaging was used to record the fetal heart rate and determine the effect of submaximal and maximal maternal exertion and the incidence of fetal bradycardia.

Forty-five women with a mean gestation of 25 weeks performed exercise tests twice on separate days using a cycle ergometer. Resting measurements were taken with the women seated on the ergometer for 10 minutes. They underwent 85 submaximal and 79 maximal cycle ergometer tests (Fig 2–4).

Fetal cardiac activity was monitored continuously and videotaped during exercise and rest periods using a linear array 2-dimensional ultrasound system. The average fetal heart rate did not change during maternal exertion, but 15 of 16 postexercise episodes of bradycardia occurred within 3 minutes after maximal maternal exertion. There were 18 episodes of fetal bradycardia; 1 occurred during exercise.

Brief submaximal exercise up to 70% of maximal aerobic power seems to have no effect on fetal heart rate. Maximal exertion, on the other hand, is commonly followed by fetal bradycardia. The significance of this

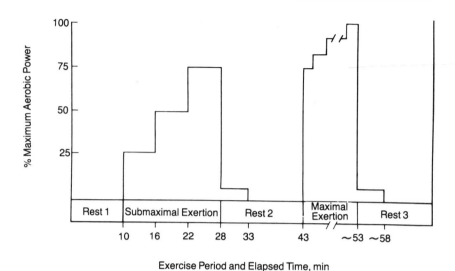

Fig 2–4.—Exercise protocol: Duration of rest and exercise periods and associated percentage of maximal aerobic power. (Courtesy of Carpenter MW, Sady SP, Hoegsberg B, et al: *JAMA* 259:3006–3009, May 27, 1988.)

bradycardia is as yet unknown, but it seems prudent to recommend that pregnant women limit vigorous exercise to activities requiring heart rates of no more than 150 beats per minute and conclude their exertion with a cool-down period.

▶ Although the significance of fetal bradycardia is not yet known, it is prudent that pregnant women be advised to keep their exercise heart rate below 150 beats per minute until more information is available. Of course, a gradual cool-down is always recommended as part of any exercise routine.—Col. J.L. Anderson, PE.D.

Effects of Supine Exercise on Fetal Heart Rate in the Second and Third Trimesters

Nesler CL, Hassett SL, Cary S, Brooke J (Oregon Health Sciences Univ, Portland; HealthLink, Portland)

Am J Perinatol 5:159–163, April 1988   2–15

Several investigators have monitored fetal heart rate (FHR) as a way to assess fetal hypoxia or distress in response to maternal exercise. An early study reported little effect on FHR, whereas later studies yielded conflicting results when using the FHR response to exercise as a screening test for uteroplacental insufficiency. Recent studies have noted minimal or no change in FHR, whereas others have reported a transient increase in baseline FHR. The effect of brief periods of mild, supine exercise on FHR in the late second trimester and mid third trimester was studied.

Twenty-five healthy, regularly exercising women, 12 in the late second trimester and 13 in mid third trimester, were studied. Although significant increases in maternal mean arterial pressure and pulse occurred, the exercise intensity was mild, with the average percent maximal pulse being $46 \pm 5\%$ in the second trimester group and $49 \pm 5\%$ in the third trimester group. Small increases in FHR were observed in both groups, which were insignificant statistically and physiologically. No patient experienced significant FHR abnormalities as a consequence of the exercise sequence.

These results indicate that pregnant women may continue submaximal supine exercise of short duration through the 36th week of gestation without harmful effects to the fetus.

▶ This study agrees with the one immediately preceding (Abstract 2–14) that moderate exercising by pregnant women does not cause increases in the FHR. However, this study differs from the preceding one in that these women were exercising while in a supine position instead of on a cycle ergometer. It appears from comparison of these 2 studies that the more vigorous exercise program used by Carpenter et al. demonstrated no more danger to the fetus than did the more conservative program described above.—Col. J.L. Anderson, PE.D.

Stress Fractures in Pregnancy
Moran JJM (St John's Hosp, Santa Monica, Calif)
Am J Obstet Gynecol 158:1274–1277, June 1988   2–16

As a result of participation in jogging and aerobic exercise, more stress fractures are occurring in women. However, such injuries in pregnant women can be unrelated to these activities. In 2 instances, stress fracture of the pubic bone was sustained during delivery.

Woman, 35, gravida 2, para 2, had an uncomplicated prenatal course and labor. Delivery was complicated by outlet forceps delivery of the vertex in the occipitoanterior position because of terminal fetal bradycardia. Anesthesia was induced with a pudendal block. The infant weighed 3,108 gm. The mother had no complaints until she began walking on the first postpartum day, when she experienced left-sided pelvic, pubic, and left thigh pain. Endometritis and infection of the episiotomy site were ruled out, and the patient was believed to have symphyseal separation. Treatment involved local heat and bed rest. About 2 weeks later an x-ray study of the pelvis showed a healing stress fracture at the junction between the left superior and inferior rami. No evidence of osteoporosis or symphyseal separation was found. After 6 weeks of rest the patient could walk with limited discomfort and had no pubic tenderness. Subsequently, the fracture healed completely.

The 2 main corrective measures recommended for stress fracture of the pubic bone sustained at delivery were rest and respite from weight-bearing activity.

▶ This author reports on 2 stress fractures of the pubic bone that occurred during delivery. Both women had complicated deliveries, and neither was athletic before pregnancy. Stress fractures occur in men and women subjected to repetitive muscle pull on bones during exercise, especially if not well conditioned. It appears here that labor and delivery can be as much a stress with muscle action on various bones, especially the pelvis, as for exercising athletes.— Col. J.L. Anderson, PE.D.

Eccentric and Concentric Torque and Power of the Knee Extensors of Females
Rizzardo M, Wessel J, Bay G (Workers' Compensation Board Rehabilitation Clinic, Richmond, BC; Univ of Alberta, Edmonton; Fraser Valley Orthopedic and Sports Medicine Clinic, Abbotsford, BC)
Can J Sport Sci 13:166–169, June 1988   2–17

The relationship between force-velocity characteristics of eccentric and concentric contractions appears to vary with different muscles. Limited data are available on the eccentric force-velocity characteristics of in vivo human muscle at velocities of more than 115 degrees per second. The peak torque-velocity and the power-velocity relationships of eccentric and concentric contractions of the knee extensors were compared in 21 women aged 19–28 years who had no history of knee pain or abnormality.

Eccentric and concentric contractions of the knee extensors of the dominant leg were tested on an isokinetic dynamometer at 60, 120, and 180 degrees per second. Eccentric peak torque was higher than concentric at each velocity tested, whereas eccentric power was significantly higher only at the 2 greater velocities. Eccentric torque increased from 60 to 120 degrees per second, but decreased again at the highest velocity. Both concentric and eccentric power increased with velocity.

▶ The results of this study compare very favorably with our results with members of our knee rehabilitation group. We normally expect the concentric contraction to be between 67% and 75% of the eccentric contraction.— Col. J.L. Anderson, PE.D.

Leg Power Characteristics of Female Firefighter Applicants
Misner JE, Boileau RA, Plowman SA, Elmore BG, Gates MA, Gilbert JA, Horswill C (Univ of Illinois; Ball State Univ, Muncie, Ind; Northern Illinois Univ, DeKalb)
J Occup Med 30:433–437, May 1988   2–18

Leg power is important in many firefighting tasks, such as climbing, lifting, and dragging objects. Leg power was characterized in 200 women taking a firefighter applicant physical performance test. The final study group included 150 women aged 20–42 years. In addition to physical work capacity and the Wingate Anaerobic Test, leg press and vertical jump tests were administered.

The women tested were the best of more than 1,000 applicants. Nine independent variables entered into a multiple regression analysis (age, height, weight, fat-free weight, percent fat, leg press strength, vertical jump, maximal physical work capacity, stair climb) explained 45% of the variance in mean power, 40% of that in peak power, and 16% of that in percent fatigue. Fat-free weight was the single variable most important for mean power and peak power. Physical work capacity accounted for the most variation in percent fatigue. The stair-climbing test did not relate closely to any of the variables.

These data support the practice of job-related testing of physical performance. It is possible to select women who can compete with the average man on tasks requiring leg strength and power. Leg power is best predicted by fat-free weight and leg strength.

▶ Some of our previous work with fire departments does not agree that leg power is the limiting factor for women who want to be firefighters. Although it is true that it is possible to select women who can compete with some men on tasks requiring leg strength and power, those tasks are not the ones that women have the most difficulty performing. Rather, our work showed that grip strength is the single most limiting factor for women who want to be firefighters or members of emergency rescue units.—Col. J.L. Anderson, PE.D.

Body Composition and Performance Characteristics of Collegiate Women Rugby Players
Sedlock DA, Fitzgerald PI, Knowlton RG (Purdue Univ; US Army Research Inst; Southern Illinois Univ, Carbondale)
Res Q Exerc Sport 59:78–82, March 1988   2–19

Rugby players are not supervised by experienced personnel, because it is not a collegiate varsity sport in the United States, but these players must meet high physical demands to compete successfully. Nineteen members of a university women's rugby club were examined. The women (mean age, 21 years) weighed 64 kg and were 165 cm tall. Body composition was measured in the last week of the competitive season.

Individuals playing forward were heavier than the backs. The backs had less relative fat, fat mass, and fat-free mass than the forwards. Body mass index was significantly lower for the backs. The forwards had greater maximal alactic anaerobic power and also higher values for peak oxygen uptake. Expressed relative to body weight, however, peak oxygen uptake was similar in the 2 groups. There were no significant differences in isometric knee extension, elbow extension, or agility.

Physical and Physiologic Characteristics of Female Athletes

Sport (study)	Age (yr)	Height (cm)	Weight (kg)	%fat	$\dot{V}O_2$ max (ml $\cdot$ kg^{-1} $\cdot$ min^{-1})	HR max (b $\cdot$ min^{-1})
Rugby (present)	20.6	165	64.4	21.0	42	189
Basketball (Sinning, 1973)	20.7	166	61.3	20.8	43	186
Master's swimming, not highly trained (Vaccaro et al., 1984)	20–29	171	64.7	19.2	31	177
Master's swimming, trained (Vaccaro et al., 1984)	20–29	165	55.8	14.8	44	179
College varsity (Katch, et al., 1973)	21.3	164	59.0	20.6	44	—
PE majors, nonvarsity (Katch, et al., 1973)	19.8	164	61.8	24.6	38	—

*Values represent means.
(Courtesy of Sedlock DA, Fitzgerald PI, Knowlton RG: *Res Q Exerc Sport* 59:78–82, March 1988.)

These body composition and performance data are similar to those reported for women in other sports (table). The similarities between backs and forwards presumably reflect training methods, whereas the differences provide part of the basis by which players are selected for particular positions.

▶ What strikes me about the data shown in the table is the relatively low levels of $VO_{2\ max}$ for all of the athletes listed. We have found that women cadets normally average about 44 ml · kg^{-1} · min^{-1} after 2 weeks of training at West Point. They show about a 5-point increase after 6 weeks.—Col. J.L. Anderson, PE.D.

The Body Type of Female Hockey Players Involved in Different Playing Positions and Levels of Competition
Wilsmore RG (Univ of Wollongong, New South Wales)
Aust J Sci Med Sport 19:26–28, December 1987   2–20

Studies of athletes in different sports suggest that the best performers in a given event come from relatively specific somatotypes, although there are exceptions. Female field hockey players, like swimmers, tend to be ectomesomorphs. Eighty-five female field hockey players of varying ability were somatotyped, using the Heath-Carter system of classifying physique.

No significant somatotype differences were found in relation to grade of competition. Athletes playing as backs had higher endomorphy ratings than those playing as halves or forwards. The latter groups had lower ectomorphy ratings than the backs. At higher levels of competition the backs and halves were more mesomorphic than the forwards were, and the forwards and halves were more ectomorphic than the backs. Mesomorphy predominated in all players.

Female field hockey players tend to be mesomorphic. Somatotype is not a limiting factor in play at higher levels of competition, but it does have a role in distinguishing between various positions.

▶ Although somatotyping may be a factor in selecting field hockey players for positions, I cannot imagine that it can be the most important factor. Certainly, there are other physiologic performance variables such as speed, stamina, and stick handling skills that will rank well above somatotype in selecting the best players.—Col. J.L. Anderson, PE.D.

The Female Bodybuilder: A Morphological, Cardiorespiratory and Strength Performance Comparison With Non-Weight Trained Female Athletes
Carlson JS, MacDonald WA, Payne WR (Footscray Inst of Technology, Mel-

40 / Sports Medicine

Aust J Sci Med Sport 29:7–11, March 1988   2–21

Although bodybuilding is a competitive sport in 122 countries, inadequate experimental research has been done on this group of athletes, and only 1 study has been reported on female bodybuilders. A study was conducted to quantify morphological, cardiorespiratory, and strength performance data on 16 female bodybuilders and 16 non-weight-trained female athletes. Body composition, physical size and structure, bone diameters and limb volumes, and isotonic strength, maximal oxygen uptake, and resting blood pressure were determined.

The bodybuilders had significantly lower body fat levels (18.4%) compared with non-weight-trained athletes (26.5%). Bodybuilders expressed significantly higher strength scores on all isotonic measures. Non-weight-trained athletes had larger limb volumes and slightly higher fat-free mass than the bodybuilders. There was no significant difference in maximal oxygen uptake between the groups.

These data indicate differences in morphological measurements and cardiorespiratory performance between female bodybuilders and non-weight-trained female athletes. These differences were accounted for largely by the differences in body fat content. Strength differences appeared to be a function of the sport-specific training.

▶ Bodybuilding for both men and women requires about as much concern for nutritional intake as it does for weight lifting. Although the percent fat for women bodybuilders in this study was 18.43%, other studies have shown percent body fat of women bodybuilders to be at about 13%. Today, there is significant concern about drug use by both men and women bodybuilders. The concern is that men are taking steroids and women are using male hormones.— Col. J.L. Anderson, PE.D.

The Influence of Resistive Exercise on Somatotype and Selected Skinfolds in College Women
Pardee S, Eisenman PA (Univ of Utah)
J Sports Med 28:93–98, March 1988   2–22

Intense resistive exercise training is accepted as a way to develop muscle mass and thus alter the physique of men, but its effect on women is less well known. Whether participation in 6 weeks of resistive exercise training would change the somatotype ratings and skinfold values of college-aged women was examined in 40 women. Thirty were assigned to a resistive exercise group and 10 served as controls.

Training resulted in significant increases in static knee flexion and extension strength. Static elbow extension strength in the exercise group did not increase significantly, and no significant changes were found in any of the 3 components of the Heath-Carter somatotypes (Fig 2–5). Of the skinfolds assessed, only the calf skinfold decreased significantly with

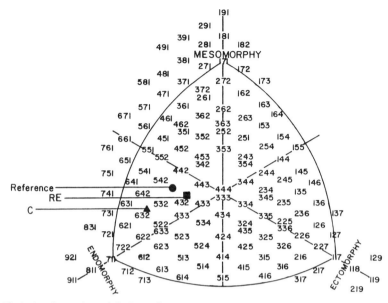

Fig 2–5.—Comparison of the RE and C group somatotypes with a female reference somatotype. (Modified from deGaray AL, Levine L, Carter JEL (eds): *Genetic and Anthropological Studies of Olympic Athletes.* New York, Academic Press, 1974.) (Courtesy of Pardee S, Eisenman PA: *J Sports Med* 28:93–98, March 1988.)

training. Only the correlations between the initial rating of endomorphy and changes in elbow extension strength, subscapular skinfold, suprailiac skinfold, and calf skinfold thickness were statistically significant.

Although college-aged women may experience significant strength increases with short-term resistive exercise, changes in somatotype are not likely to occur. Initial somatotype ratings also do not appear substantially to influence training outcomes.

▶ The failure to produce changes in the somatotypes of the women should not be too surprising to most of us. Women gain strength through weight training over a period as short as 6 weeks, their body mass is not significantly altered, and certainly not their somatotype. It takes long-term, very dedicated training and proper nutritional control to make significant changes in somatotypes, especially for women.—Col. J.L. Anderson, PE.D.

Muscle Hypertrophy in Men and Women
Cureton KJ, Collins MA, Hill DW, McElhannon FM Jr (Univ of Georgia, Athens)
Med Sci Sports Exerc 20:338–344, August 1988   2–23

It is believed that women experience less skeletal muscle hypertrophy consequent to heavy-resistance training than do men. A study was conducted to test this hypothesis using both traditional indirect indicators and direct measures of muscle size. Seven men and 8 women were studied before and after a 16-week weight-training program; 3 men and 4 women served as controls. They trained 3 days per week^{-1} at 70% to 90% of maximum voluntary contraction using exercise designed to produce hypertrophy of the upper arm and thigh.

In the study group, strength significantly increased on both elbow and knee flexion and extension tests. Absolute changes were significantly greater in the men than in the women in 2 of the 4 tests, whereas percentage changes were not significantly different. Substantial muscle hypertrophy occurred in the upper arms of both men and women, as evidenced by significant increases in upper arm circumference, bone-plus-muscle cross-sectional area (CSA) as estimated by anthropometry, and muscle CSA determined from computed tomographic scanning. Changes in men and women were not significantly different, except for the absolute increase in estimated bone-plus-muscle CSA, which was significantly greater in men. There was no muscle hypertrophy in the thighs of either men or women, evidenced by nonsignificant changes in thigh circumference, bone-plus-muscle CSA, and muscle CSA. Changes in men and women in body weight, fat-free weight, and fat weight were insignificant. It would appear that relative changes in strength and muscle hypertrophy consequent to weight training are similar in men and women.

▶ This study confirms what I said about the preceding review (Abstract 2–22), i.e., changes in body weight, fat-free weight, and fat weight are insignificant after a 16-week, rigorous, weight-training program. Although both men and women gained strength, there would be not enough change to produce a different somatotype rating.—Col. J.L. Anderson, PE.D.

Comparison of Male and Female Functional Capacity in Pull-Ups
Ricci B, Figura F, Felici F, Marchetti M (Univ of Rome)
J Sports Med 28:168–175, June 1988   2–24

Assessment of physical fitness has long disregarded biomechanical considerations that would allow greater understanding of differences between the sexes. Assessment of the shoulder has traditionally involved different evaluations based solely on gender. For males, pull-ups are included; for females, they are not.

During the positive work phase of pull-ups, integrated electromyographic signals (EMGs) were obtained from selected muscles of the upper chest, shoulder, upper back, and arm in 1 man and 1 woman of comparable age, height, and body mass. Displacement of body mass, acceleration and velocity of body mass, and force and power were calculated. Forward and reverse grasps on the horizontal bar were additional variables.

Regardless of bar grasp, the data failed to show sex differences in the EMG and biomechanical aspects of pull-up performance, assuming that applied force and power, and therefore number of completions of pull-ups of the free-hanging body, were expressed as a function of mass being displaced.

The methodology used in this study can be applied in larger, more detailed pull-up studies.

▶ From West Point we reported in 1976 that the difference between men and women in functional capacity in pull-ups is mostly the result of sociocultural bias because young girls were never asked to lift their bodies using only their arms. Only the most recent fitness test designed for the President's Council for Physical Fitness and Sports includes pull-ups for young women as an alternative for the flexed-arm hang. Young women who have been gymnasts during their childhood have no difficulty doing pull-ups. However, we found in our research conducted from 1973 to 1976 that more than 90% of female high school varsity letter winners could not do even 1 pull-up.—Col. J.L. Anderson, PE.D.

Caloric Intake, Stress, and Menstrual Function in Athletes
Schweiger U, Herrmann F, Laessle R, Riedel W, Schweiger M, Pirke K-M
(Max-Planck-Institut für Psychiatrie, Munich, West Germany)
Fertil Steril 49:447–450, March 1988   2–25

The cause of amenorrhea and other menstrual disturbances in athletes is unknown. In addition to acute and chronic effects of exertion, other associated behavioral variables (e.g., stress and nutrition) may play a key role. Eighteen endurance-trained athletes and 25 age-matched, nonathletic women were evaluated to link information about nutrition and stress with quantitative assessment of endocrine menstrual function.

Four athletes had no increases in 17β-estradiol and progesterone concentrations during the observation period, indicating that neither follicular growth nor luteinization occurred. Compared with nonathletic women, the remaining 14 athletes with cyclic gonadal function had normal estradiol values during the follicular phase and at midcycle. However, during the luteal phase these athletes had significantly impaired estradiol and progesterone production. Caloric intake, as assessed by nutritional diaries, correlated positively with area under the progesterone curve during the luteal phase. Ratings of subjective stress in the area "partner, family, friends" correlated negatively with the luteal progesterone area.

These data suggest that low caloric intake and high stress may contribute to the development of menstrual disturbances in athletes.

▶ These authors recognize that secondary amenorrhea among women athletes is not caused by loss of body fat alone, and that stress may well play a role. Here at West Point we are certain that it is more than low percent body fat that causes amenorrhea. We have found that the incidence of exercise-induced amenorrhea is as prevalent among young women in the 25% to 27% body fat range as it is among young women with body fat below 20%.— Col. J.L. Anderson, PE.D.

Abnormal Eating Attitude Test Scores Predict Menstrual Dysfunction in Lean Females
Rippon C, Nash J, Myburgh KH, Noakes TD (Univ of Cape Town, South Africa)
Int J Eating Disorders 7:617–624, September 1988   2–26

The incidence of menstrual dysfunction, including amenorrhea and oligomenorrhea, is increased in ballet dancers, runners, and gymnasts. The reasons for this are unclear. The possible contribution of abnormal eating attitudes to menstrual dysfunction was investigated.

The Eating Attitudes Test (EAT), Eating Disorders Inventory (EDI), and a habitual exercise questionnaire were given to 88 lean marathon runners, ballet dancers, and fashion models. A menstrual history for each was obtained. The women were classified according to weight and exercise status into low-mass nonexercisers, low-mass exercisers, and moderate-mass exercisers. Menstrual dysfunction was equally common in all groups. The incidence of increased EAT and EDI scores was high in all groups at 15% to 65%. Elevated EAT scores, but not body mass or exercise, were associated with menstrual dysfunction.

These data, as well as those of other studies, indicate that a high percentage of lean athletic women have elevated EAT scores, suggesting that successful self-imposed starvation, rather than genetic endowment or physical activity, is responsible for their leanness. Conversely, elevated EAT scores are also found in females with moderate-to-high body weights. Thus nutritional habits cannot be predicted from body composition analysis, and increased body mass does not exclude the possibility of chronic self-imposed dietary restriction. Subnormal nutrition may be the critical yet unrecognized factor explaining menstrual dysfunction in lean women.

▶ Self-imposed starvation is not primarily an athlete's problem. Rather, it is a woman's problem. However, I doubt that subnormal nutrition will be found to be the critical yet unrecognized factor explaining menstrual dysfunction in women. Our studies show that secondary amenorrhea develops even when a controlled and balanced diet is followed. The only environmental variable that I have been able to isolate that may cause the amenorrhea is stress.— Col. J.L. Anderson, PE.D.

3 Athletic Training

Introduction

This is the eleventh time I have written an introduction to this chapter. Seven of the 11 introductions have concerned the need for certified athletic trainers on the high school level. I must feel strongly that this is an important issue. There has been some slow progress made these past 11 years, and each year more high schools are employing the services of an athletic trainer. I still believe a faculty trainer is the best solution to the problem. In recent years many schools have hired clinic- or hospital-based athletic trainers to provide what services they can. For many of these schools this has been a satisfactory solution to the problem. There is still a long way to go, however, to provide proper health care for our nation's high school athletes, a group that should not be neglected. School departments cannot afford to be without the services of a certified athletic trainer to improve the health care of their athletes.

F.J. George, ATC, PT

Certified Athletic Trainers in Our Secondary Schools: The Need and the Solution
Stopka C, Kaiser D (Univ of Florida; Central Michigan Univ, Mt Pleasant)
Athletic Training 23:322–324, Winter 1988   3–1

High school athletes have less access to health care professionals than do collegiate and professional athletes. The need for certified athletic trainers in secondary schools is great because high school athletes are younger and less mature physiologically and athletically than their collegiate counterparts.

Despite the fact that more than 636,000 injuries occur annually among high school football players, less than 10% of the nation's high schools currently employ certified athletic trainers. There is only 1 certified athletic trainer for every 5,500 high school athletes. There are at least 8 viable solutions to hiring a certified athletic trainer: the trainer could be full-time, a district athletic trainer, a permanent substitute teacher/athletic trainer, an assistant director/athletic trainer, a part-time athletic trainer, a contracted athletic trainer from a sports medicine center, a graduate assistant athletic trainer, or a teacher/athletic trainer. Hiring a full-time teacher/athletic trainer is probably most economically feasible, with concomitant medical, legal, and educational benefits.

Coaches, administrators, parents, school board personnel, and state legislators must work more aggressively to increase the number of certified athletic trainers working in high schools in the United States.

▶ I have discussed this problem many times with many people. The discussions have included high school athletes and their parents, coaches and school administrators, school boards, city, town, and federal legislators, and executives of the National Federation of State High School Associations. Everyone seems to want a certified athletic trainer in their high school. The major problem is that high school administrators say they cannot afford to pay for an athletic trainer. My answer to that statement is, "You can't afford *not* to have one."

There are many solutions to the problem; the author has presented 8 different ones. I have always favored having a faculty-athletic trainer at every high school. I believe it is method that is most beneficial to the high school athlete.—F.J. George, ATC, PT

Rehabilitation of Football Players With Lumbar Spine Injury
Saal JA (Portola Valley, Calif)
Physician Sportsmed 16:61–67, September 1988   3–2

Rehabilitating a football player with a lumbar spine injury is a significant challenge to sports medicine physicians. Accurate diagnosis followed by early intervention is essential. Once the injury is diagnosed, rehabilitation can be divided into 2 phases: the pain-control phase and the training phase.

The initial aspect of the pain-control phase, back first aid, includes ice application, placement of the patient in a comfortable position, and provision of basic instruction in body mechanics to facilitate movement. Rest is specifically prescribed in this phase, but total bed rest is not necessary. Transcutaneous nerve stimulation or electrical muscle stimulation with ice can also decrease acute pain.

Extension exercises are effective for reducing pain from disk injury. No one should continue with a single type of exercise regimen during the entire treatment program, however. Flexion exercises are most useful in management of injury to the posterior elements of the lumbar spine. Spine immobilization is rarely needed in sports-related injuries. Mobilization techniques can be useful in attaining articular and soft tissue range of motion. Traction may be used to relieve symptoms of disk injury subtypes, such as disk protrusion, herniation, and annular tears. Selective injections (precise localization with precise center) is one of the most powerful tools for pain relief.

It is important to understand the anatomy and biomechanics of the lumbar spine, referred pain, and potential pain generators, the stages of the degenerative process, and lumbar spine injuries when planning rehabilitation.

▶ This is a comprehensive program for the relief of acute low back pain. The author states that total bed rest is ". . .the most abused and overprescribed treatment modality in lumbar spine care. . ." He goes on to quote Deline and Kriz: ". . .excessive bed rest will lead to hypomobile lumbar motion segments, tightened soft tissues, loss of muscle strength, blunting of motivation, and loss of mineral matrix from bone."

Exercise is an important modality in the relief of low back pain.—F.J. George, ATC, PT

Snapping Scapula: A Review of the Literature and Presentation of 14 Patients
Percy EC, Birbrager D, Pitt MJ (Univ of Arizona, Tucson; Bobby Orr Sports Medicine Clinic, Downsview, Ont)
Can J Surg 31:248–250, July 1988   3–3

The scapulothoracic syndrome or "snapping scapula" associated with movement of the shoulder may develop spontaneously as the result of altered shoulder biomechanics after trauma or surgery to the shoulder girdle. The pain of a snapping scapula is caused by microtrauma or tendinitis of the muscles inserting into the scapula. The syndrome sometimes occurs in teenage girls just after skeletal maturity and then is presumed to be postural in origin. Because the snapping scapula has not been widely studied, 14 patients who had previously received treatment for this syndrome were evaluated retrospectively.

Five men aged 30–59 years and 9 girls and women aged 16–39 years with snapping scapula were recalled for clinical and radiologic reassessment of the treatment method. All patients had pain or were experiencing snapping, often audible to others, near or at the vertebral border of the scapula. Symptoms persisted for 1 month to 3 years, and activities that precipitated them in 10 patients included swimming, weight training, gymnastics, football, and softball. Symptoms in the other 4 patients were idiopathic. Tenderness was localized at the levator scapulae in 9 patients, at the trapezius in 5, and at the rhomboid muscles in 4. Three patients complained of subjective tingling in the involved hand.

Ultrasonic treatment, nonsteroidal anti-inflammatory drugs, and transcutaneous nerve stimulation helped to reduce pain, but posture and strengthening exercises appeared to be more effective in eliminating the snapping. Exercises established a more normal scapulothoracic rhythm, which reduced the shearing forces on the undersurface of the scapula. No exostosis was seen in 1 patient who underwent operation.

Nonsteroidal anti-inflammatory drugs and other treatment modalities may offer some immediate pain relief for a snapping scapula, but physical therapy plays an important role in the long-term resolution of this condition.

▶ We have been perplexed by the few cases of snapping scapula that we have evaluated and treated. The authors have presented different treatment options. We will certainly increase our efforts to restore a more normal scapula-thoracic rhythm through strengthening and postural exercises. The authors explain that these exercises may reduce the shearing forces on the undersurface of the scapula.—F.J. George, ATC, PT

Prescription of External Rotation Exercise for the Shoulder
Katz G (Univ of Connecticut, Storrs)
Natl Strength Conditioning Assoc J 10:56–57, June–July 1988   3–4

As resistance training becomes an integral part of sports conditioning, an understanding of injury prevention and management will play an essential role in the success of exercise prescriptions. Injury usually results from overtraining, poor technique, or musculature imbalance.

For normal arthrokinematic motion to occur, specifically shoulder elevation, the supraspinatus, infraspinatus, and teres minor each plays an important role in avoiding pathologic motion. Under normal conditions the deltoids and supraspinatus roll the humeral head upward. To counteract the upward roll, the infraspinatus and teres minor depress the humeral head. This depression enables the humeral head to clear the subacromial structures and avoid impact with the acromion process.

Normal arthrokinematic shoulder motion relies on specific forces of the muscles to ensure proper motion. When athletes concentrate on anterior muscles, the deltoids may become too strong or out of proportion for the infraspinatus and teres minor to function efficiently. This causes an imbalance in the force-coupling pattern, resulting in injury. External rotation exercises are very important in maintaining normal shoulder function.

Regular exercise of the external rotators, the infraspinatus and teres minor, will enable the athlete to progress with a reduced predisposition to injury. Further research in exercise application, muscle function, and mechanism of injury is needed if resistance training is to be effective.

▶ A following study (Abstract 3–14) will explain the problems that muscle imbalance around the knee can produce. The present review (Abstract 3–4) as well as Abstract 3–6 discuss similar problems in the shoulder. The author here stresses the need for external rotation exercises to balance the strong deltoid and anterior shoulder musculature.—F.J. George, ATC, PT

▶ ↓ The following abstracts (3–5 and 3–6) describe the best position in which to exercise the shoulder muscles. Abstract 3–7 discusses the use of concentric vs. eccentric strengthening of the rotator cuff.

A Comparative Study of the Torque Generated by the Shoulder Internal and External Rotator Muscles in Different Positions and at Varying Speeds

Walmsley RP, Szybbo C (Queen's Univ, Kingston, Ont)
J Orthop Sports Phys Ther 9:217–222, December 1987   3–5

A growing number of clinicians have used progressive strength training of the muscles surrounding a musculoskeletal injury to the shoulder complex. To gain insight on the most efficient positions of the shoulder joint complex to use in rehabilitating these muscles, recordings were made of the maximum concentric isokinetic loading on the internal and external rotator muscles of the shoulder at various positions of the shoulder joint complex.

Twelve healthy women aged 19–25 years were tested with the Cybex II Isokinetic Dynamometer and the Cybex Dual-Channel Recorder. None had a history of recent injury or previous surgery to the tested shoulder complex. Torque generated by the shoulder's internal and external muscle groups was measured and recorded when the shoulder was in the neutral position, at 90 degrees of abduction, and at 90 degrees of flexion, with each position tested at speeds of 60, 120, and 180 degrees per second. Each patient performed 3 test contractions per position and per speed to assure a certain amount of reliability. A graphic printout, obtained of the generated torque and the utilized joint range, was used for data analysis.

No interaction between speed and position was observed for either the internal or the external rotator muscles. However, a significant difference was noted across the 3 positions tested. For the internal rotators the difference was significant between neutral position and abduction to 90 degrees, but not between neutral and flexion to 90 degrees, with the greatest torque values achieved in the neutral position. For the external rotator muscles, the difference was significant between the flexion and neutral positions, and between flexion and abduction, but not between neutral and abduction, with the greatest torque values achieved at 90 degrees of shoulder flexion.

Considering the anatomical morphology of the internal rotator muscles, it would seem that the line of pull for these muscles would be most effective when the arm is in the neutral position, whereas placing the arm into abduction or flexion would decrease this mechanical advantage. Although the external rotator muscles are subject to the same mechanical and physiologic factors, the line of most effective pull for these muscles would be different because of their different anatomical orientation. The finding of greater torque values at 90 degrees of flexion supports this assumption.

Knowledge of these most efficient positions should benefit therapists who are using muscle strength training isokinetically as part of a treatment program for patients with shoulder girdle dysfunction.

▶ What is the best position of the shoulder to increase the strength of the rotator muscles? The authors present data indicating that the internal rotators are best strengthened with the shoulder in the neutral position and the external rotators with the shoulder at 90 degrees of flexion.—F.J. George, ATC, PT

Isokinetic Evaluation of Shoulder Rotational Strength in High School Baseball Pitchers

Hinton RY (Children's Hosp and Ctr for Reconstructive Surgery, Baltimore)
Am J Sports Med 16:274–279, May–June 1988   3–6

Pitching is a sequential, total body mechanism that places extraordinary stresses on the shoulder. When throwing, balanced and coordinated action of the rotator cuff is essential to provide glenohumeral stability and protection for the glenoid labrum, capsule, and joint surfaces. Objective testing of the shoulder girdle musculature to establish normative data and to track activity-induced changes in function has lagged behind such investigation of the musculature around the knee. Isokinetic shoulder rotational strength was assessed in 26 high school baseball pitchers before the beginning of spring practice.

Using the Cybex II, data were gathered on the dominant and nondominant shoulders in the supine 90 degrees abducted test position and the standing neutral test position. Tests were performed at 90 and 240 degrees per second. Means and standard deviations for peak torque, total work, peak torque to body weight ratios, and agonist/antagonist ratios were computed.

Peak torque and total work values for the throwing side internal rotators were significantly higher than the nonthrowing side in all tests. Pitching side external rotators did not show this dominance. External/internal rotation ratios for peak torque and total work were significantly lower on the pitching side, which suggests an imbalance of cuff musculature compared with the nonpitching arm. In the 90-degree abducted test position, external rotation peak torque and total work values and external/internal rotation peak torque and total work ratios were higher than those in the neutral test position. Internal rotation peak torque and total work values tended to be higher in the neutral test position.

The rotator cuff imbalances noted in the pitching shoulders in this study draw attention to the need for structured exercise to prevent and correct this deficit, which can be a predisposing factor to injury. Significant differences in torque data suggest the need for multiple position testing for complete assessment and the requirement of specifying test position when comparing shoulder-rotational torque values clinically or experimentally.

▶ This study agrees with the finding in Abstract 3–5 that the neutral position is the best position in which to increase the strength of the shoulder internal rotators. However, in this study external rotation results were higher in the 90-degree abducted test position. The authors did not test in the 90 degrees of flexion position.

This study also stresses the importance of proper muscle strength ratios and the problems of rotator cuff imbalances, as does Abstract 3–4.—F.J. George, ATC, PT

Concentric Versus Eccentric Isokinetic Strengthening of the Rotator Cuff: Objective Data Versus Functional Test
Ellenbecker TS, Davies GJ, Rowinski MJ (Univ of Wisconsin, La Crosse)
Am J Sports Med 16:64–69, January–February 1988   3–7

Eccentric muscular contractions have a role in functional activities and athletics equally significant to concentric muscular contractions. During the follow-through phase of the tennis serve or throwing motion, the infraspinatus and teres minor of the shoulder must undergo high decelerative eccentric contractions to preserve healthy joint arthrokinematics. The rotator cuff is essential in preventing overhead overuse injuries. The dynamic caudal glide, executed by the infraspinatus and teres minor posteriorly and the subscapularis anteriorly, keep the suprahumeral structures from becoming impinged on the coracoacromial arch. A study was conducted to determine whether eccentric or concentric isokinetic training of the rotator cuff is more efficient in increasing power.

Twenty-two female and male college varsity tennis players trained for 6 weeks, the first group using eccentric isokinetic internal and external shoulder rotation and the second group using concentric isokinetic internal and external shoulder rotation. The participants pretested and posttested both concentrically and eccentrically. Three maximally hit tennis serves made before and after training were analyzed by high-speed cinematography to obtain ball velocity.

Analysis of peak torque and peak torque to body weight ratio revealed significant concentric strength gains in the concentric as well as the eccentric training groups. Eccentric strength gains were shown by the concentric training group at selected speeds but were not significantly generated in the eccentric group. Functional test analysis showed an increase in maximal serve velocity in the concentric training group but not in the eccentric group.

These data indicate that significant power gains, especially at fast functional velocities, and increases in muscle explosiveness of the rotator cuff occur through concentric and eccentric isokinetic training. When designing a preventive conditioning or rehabilitation program, the concept of specificity of muscular contraction may be important.

▶ The results of this study indicate that, "Eccentric isokinetic training produced the greatest increases in concentric strength." The authors go on to state that, "Although both experimental groups increased rotator cuff torque acceleration energy work, the transfer to functional skill improvement occurred only in the concentrically trained group." I agree with the findings that lead the authors to conclude: ". . .when designing a preventive conditioning or rehabilitation program, the concept of specificity of muscular contraction appears to be important."

As more of these shoulder studies are completed, we hope to catch up to the information we have gathered from the numerous knee studies that have been done.—F.J. George, ATC, PT

Isokinetic Torque Production of the Shoulder in a Functional Movement Pattern

Day RW, Moore RJ, Patterson P (Orthopaedic and Arthroscopic Sports Injury Specialists, San Diego; San Diego State Univ)
Athletic Training 23:333–338, Winter 1988

3–8

Isokinetic exercise devices have been used to measure peak torque production of various joints in the body. The knee has been the most commonly studied joint. The literature contains no such information on shoulder torque production of any joint at a specific point in the range of motion. Also, previous research has not made allowances for the effect of gravity on torque production in the shoulder. The power production of the shoulder across a spectrum of speeds in function movement patterns was assessed.

Thirty-four men aged 18–29 volunteered for the study. They had not been involved in a throwing sport since their second year of high school, were free of arm and shoulder injuries, and had no cardiac pathology. Each person did reciprocal contractions of both shoulders in patterns of F/Ab/ER and E/Ad/IR at 60, 120, 180, 240, and 300 degrees per second on a dynamometer (Figs 3–1 and 3–2).

Significant differences in mean torque production were noted between the movements for both arms. Mean torque production dropped significantly as the contraction speed rose for both arms and movements. Mean

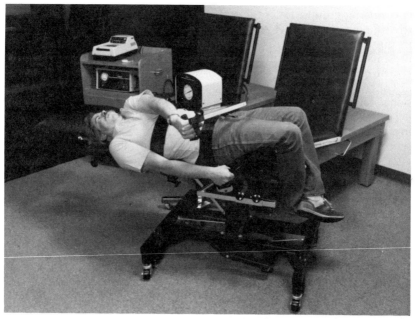

Fig 3–1.—Correct position for full extension/adduction/internal rotation of the arm. (Courtesy of Day RW, Moore RJ, Patterson P: *Athletic Training* 23:333–338, Winter 1988.)

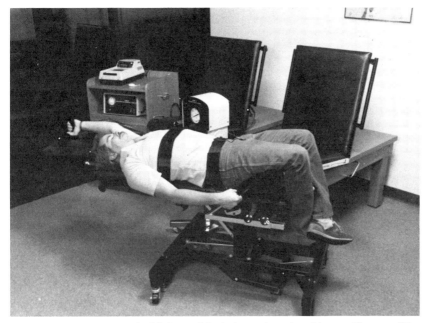

Fig 3–2.—Correct position for full flexion/abduction/external rotation of the arm. (Courtesy of Day RW, Moore RJ, Patterson P: *Athletic Training* 23:333–338, Winter 1988.)

torques of F/Ab/ER and E/Ad/IR were not significantly different between dominant and nondominant arms. The ratios of F/Ab/ER to E/Ad/IR were not significantly different between arms. As the testing velocity increased, the ratios did not change.

The results cast doubt on the assumption that the dominant limb is always stronger than the nondominant in the major muscle groups of the shoulder.

▶ The authors tested subjects in traditional upper extremity proprioceptive neuromuscular facilitation patterns with a Cybex Dynamometer and had some very interesting results. Most notable were their findings concerning limb dominance and the effects of speed on the torque generated in the different patterns.—F.J. George, ATC, PT

Isokinetic Peak Torque and Work Values for the Shoulder
Maddux REC, Kibler WB, Uhl T (Lexington Clinic East, Lexington, Ky)
J Orthop Sports Phys Ther 10:264–269, January 1989   3–9

Relative peak torque has been proposed to be an important consideration when comparing muscular performance in males and females and in athletes in different sports. Peak torque (PKT) was measured at 60 degrees and 180 degrees/second of angular velocity and work data at 180

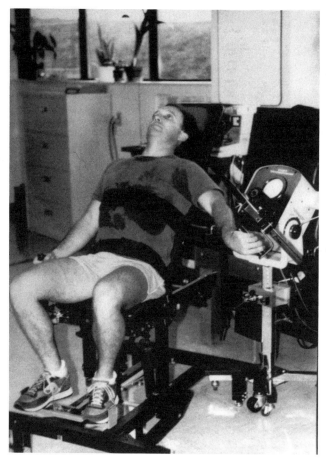

Fig 3–3.—Testing position for the supraspinatus. MOD-AB/AD. (Courtesy of Maddux REC, Kibler WB, Uhl T: *J Orthop Sports Phys Ther* 10:264–269, January 1989.)

degrees/second of angular velocity for isokinetic muscular performance during external and internal rotation (ER/IR) and modified abduction and adduction (MOD-AB/AD) tests. The dominant and nondominant upper extremity data were compared, as was the relative peak torque between sexes.

Twenty-one men and 20 women had isokinetic testing at 60 degrees and 180 degrees/second in MOD-AB/AD and ER/IR (Fig 3–3). No significant differences were found between the dominant and nondominant shoulders for the PKT. However, a significant difference was found between men and women when comparing PKT, total work, and power. No significant differences were found between sexes when comparing endurance and agonist/antagonist PKT and work ratios. Large standard deviations were observed, suggesting the need for specific categorization of persons in establishing normative values.

Differences in absolute muscular performance between men and women did not change when the peak torque was normalized by body weight or lean body mass, a finding at variance with previous reports. The MOD-AB/AD position used does not appear to be a feasible way to test supraspinatus muscular performance because of the inherent discomfort from possible supraspinatus muscle impingement.

▶ The authors agree with previous study (Abstract 3–8) that there is no significant difference in peak torque generated by the dominant or nondominant limb. They also express the difficulties that arise when attempting to do an objective strength test of the supraspinatus muscle. To date, our testing of this muscle has been purely subjective.—F.J. George, ATC, PT

Upper Extremity Range of Motion and Isokinetic Strength of the Internal and External Shoulder Rotators in Major League Baseball Players
Brown LP, Niehues SL, Harrah A, Yavorsky P, Hirshman HP (Scripps Clinic and Research Found, La Jolla, Calif)
Am J Sports Med 16:577–585, November–December 1988   3–10

Adaptive changes can result from the extreme stresses placed on the shoulder joint by athletes when throwing. In a study of professional baseball players designed to determine the relationship of upper extremity strength to throwing speed, no significant difference was found between the dominant and nondominant arm for external shoulder rotation. However, evidence suggested a difference in internal shoulder rotation between arms. Descriptive statistics were determined for upper extremity range of motion and isokinetic strength of the internal and external shoulder rotators of 41 professional baseball players.

Pitchers had 9 degrees more external shoulder rotation with the arm abducted, 5 degrees more forearm pronation, and 9 degrees less shoulder extension on the dominant side than the dominant side of position players. Pitchers also had 9 degrees more external rotation in abduction, 5 degrees less shoulder flexion, 11 degrees less horizontal extension, 15 degrees less internal rotation in abduction, 6 degrees less elbow extension, 4 degrees less elbow flexion, and 5 degrees less forearm supination on the dominant side than on their nondominant side. Position players had 8 degrees more external rotation in abduction, 14 degrees less horizontal extension, and 8 degrees less elbow extension on the dominant side than on their nondominant side.

Pitchers produced greater torque than position players for the dominant and nondominant arm at all test speeds for both mean peak and mean average torque. Greater torque was noted in the dominant arm compared with the nondominant arm at all test speeds for both measures. There was no difference between the rotation ratios for either arm for pitchers or position players at any speed (Tables 1 and 2).

Significant differences were found in range of motion between pitchers and position players and between dominant and nondominant arms. This

TABLE 1.—Dominant Versus Nondominant Range of Motion

Motion	Position players		Pitchers	
	Means	SD	Means	SD
Shoulder flexion				
Dominant	164	10.2	163[a]	7.9
Nondominant	168	8.7	168	6.3
Shoulder extension				
Dominant	81	11.3	72	15.5
Nondominant	81	11.8	78	13.3
Horizontal flexion				
Dominant	98	6.9	100	9.5
Nondominant	96	8.2	99	7.4
Horizontal extension				
Dominant	83[b]	15.2	83[a]	11.7
Nondominant	97[b]	15.9	94[a]	19.5
Glenohumeral abduction				
Dominant	100	11.0	98	10.8
Nondominant	101	8.0	105	10.3
Full range abduction				
Dominant	170	10.8	168	8.4
Nondominant	172	11.3	172	11.6
Internal rotation in neutral				
Dominant	86	4.6	86	4.9
Nondominant	86	4.2	88	5.0
External rotation in neutral				
Dominant	67	11.3	71	6.9
Nondominant	69	9.7	71	9.4
Internal rotation at 90° abduction				
Dominant	85	11.9	83[b]	13.9
Nondominant	91	13.0	98	13.2
External rotation at 90° abduction				
Dominant	132[a]	9.8	141[a]	14.7
Nondominant	124	12.7	132	14.6
Elbow extension				
Dominant	8[b]	8.9	4[b]	7.1
Nondominant	0	6.2	−2[b]	6.9
Elbow flexion				
Dominant	145	5.7	144[a]	7.0
Nondominant	145	7.0	148	4.9
Forearm pronation				
Dominant	82	6.8	87	6.3
Nondominant	86	10.6	91	9.7
Forearm supination				
Dominant	97	8.7	100[a]	8.6
Nondominant	101	9.5	105	9.5

[a]Significant at $P < .05$.
[b]Significant at $P < .001$.
(Courtesy of Brown LP, Niehues SL, Harrah A, et al: *Am J Sports Med* 16:577–585, November–December 1988.)

TABLE 2.—Range of Motion: Pitchers Versus Position Players[a]

Motion	Dominant		Nondominant	
	Means	SD	Means	SD
Shoulder flexion	163 (p)	7.9 (p)	168 (p)	6.3 (p)
	164 (pp)	10.2 (pp)	168 (pp)	8.8 (pp)
Shoulder extension	72 (p)[b]	15.5 (p)	78 (p)	13.3 (p)
	81 (pp)	11.3 (pp)	81 (pp)	11.8 (pp)
Horizontal flexion	55 (p)	9.5 (p)	54 (p)	7.4 (p)
	53 (pp)	6.9 (pp)	51 (pp)	8.2 (pp)
Horizontal exten-sion	128 (p)	11.7 (p)	139 (p)	19.5 (p)
	128 (pp)	15.2 (pp)	142 (pp)	15.9 (pp)
Glenohumeral ab-duction	98 (p)	10.8 (p)	105 (p)	10.3 (p)
	100 (pp)	11.0 (pp)	101 (pp)	8.0 (pp)
Full range abduc-tion	168 (p)	8.4 (p)	172 (p)	11.6 (p)
	169 (pp)	10.8 (pp)	172 (pp)	11.3 (pp)
Internal rotation in neutral	86 (p)	4.9 (p)	88 (p)	5.0 (p)
	86 (pp)	4.6 (pp)	86 (pp)	4.2 (pp)
External rotation in neutral	71 (p)	6.9 (p)	71 (p)	9.4 (p)
	67 (pp)	11.3 (pp)	68 (pp)	9.7 (pp)
Internal rotation at 90° abduction	83 (p)	13.9 (p)	98 (p)	13.2 (p)
	85 (pp)	11.9 (pp)	91 (pp)	13.0 (pp)
External rotation at 90° abduction	141 (p)[b]	14.7 (p)	132 (p)	14.6 (p)
	132 (pp)	9.8 (pp)	124 (pp)	12.7 (pp)
Elbow extension	4 (p)	7.1 (p)	−2 (p)	6.9 (p)
	8 (pp)	8.9 (pp)	0 (pp)	6.2 (pp)
Elbow flexion	144 (p)	7.0 (p)	148 (p)	4.9 (p)
	145 (pp)	5.7 (pp)	145 (pp)	7.0 (pp)
Forearm pronation	87 (p)[b]	6.3 (p)	91 (p)	9.7 (p)
	82 (pp)	6.8 (pp)	86 (pp)	10.6 (pp)
Forearm supination	100 (p)	8.6 (p)	105 (p)	9.5 (p)
	100 (pp)	8.7 (pp)	101 (pp)	9.5 (pp)

[a]Legend to letters in parentheses: *p*, pitchers; *pp*, position players.
[b]Significant at $P < .05$.
(Courtesy of Brown LP, Niehues SL, Harrah A, et al: *Am J Sports Med* 16:577–585, November–December 1988.)

has implications for rehabilitation of the upper extremity after injury and in the prevention of injury for professional baseball pitchers and position players.

▶ In this study the subjects tested were baseball players, and, as expected, the results of their tests are different from those reported in the previous 2 studies (Abstracts 3–8 and 3–9) when nonthrowing subjects were tested. This reminds us how important it is to consider the subjects tested when comparing test results.

This study has many findings that must be considered in our rehabilitation programs of baseball players, especially pitchers.— F.J. George, ATC, PT

Piriformis Syndrome: A Hidden Cause of Sciatic Pain
Carter AT (Butler County Community College, El Dorado, Kan)
Athletic Training 23:243–245, Fall 1988

3–11

The piriformis syndrome consists of pain or disability in the low back, buttocks, or posterior upper thigh and is caused by hyperirritability of the piriformis muscle, which pressures the sciatic nerve. Anatomically, the piriformis muscle arises from the anterior surface of the sacrum, the gluteal surface of the ilium near the posterior iliac spine, and the capsule of the sacroiliac joint. It passes through and greater sciatic foramen and attaches by a rounded tendon to the upper border of the greater trochanter (Fig 3–4).

Initial evaluation includes history, observation, and palpation. Stress tests are then done. The Laseque test, usually positive on the affected side, is done with the athlete in the supine position. The examiner flexes the involved side's hip and knee. Pain along the back of the thigh or over the sciatic notch as the knee is passively extended is a positive finding. Resistance to abduction-external rotation of the hip is a more consistent stress test in the diagnosis of piriformis syndrome. The patient sits with knees together and feet hanging over the edge of a table. The examiner then resists as the patient tries to push the knees apart.

Piriformis syndrome is likely when weakness or pain occurs and the patient complains of point tenderness over the sciatic notch area. Surgery is no longer the treatment of choice for this syndrome; rather, the deep muscle is directly injected with an anesthetic and steroid mixture.

Piriformis syndrome is relatively uncommon and often undiagnosed. Athletic trainers should be able to differentiate piriformis syndrome from other common low back pain problems so that appropriate treatment can begin.

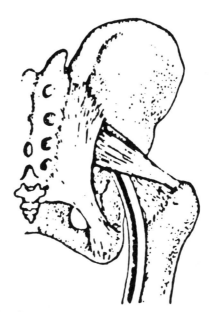

Fig 3–4.—Relationship of the sciatic nerve to the piriformis muscle. (From Hallin R: *Postgrad Med* 73:102, 1983. Courtesy of Carter AT: *Athletic Training* 23:243–245, Fall 1988.)

▶ Conservative measures such as cryokinetics, ultrasound, EMS, TENS, flexibility exercises, or heel lifts if there is a leg length discrepancy are usually attempted before an injection or surgical procedure is considered. We have also had some success with a combination of the above approaches and nonsteroidal anti-inflammatory medications and rest.

As the author states, this is a difficult diagnosis to make and a difficult problem to treat. We have tried just about every conservative approach, including analysis of the running gait, which proved beneficial in 1 case.—F.J. George, ATC, PT

Prophylactic Knee Braces and Injury to the Lower Extremity
Grace TG, Skipper BJ, Newberry JC, Nelson MA, Sweetser ER, Rothman ML
(Greater Albuquerque Med Society Sports Medicine Committee, Albuquerque and Santa Fe)
J Bone Joint Surg [Am] 70-A:422–427, March 1988   3–12

The incidence of knee ligament injuries among high school football players is high. This has led to the development and marketing of a number of orthotic knee supports that have rapidly gained popularity. However, scientific documentation on the efficacy or potential deleterious effects of prophylactic knee braces among high school football players is sparse, and the use of prophylactic knee braces in this age group remains controversial. To determine whether high school football players should wear prophylactic knee braces, a study was designed to identify and match pairs of athletes according to size, weight, and the position that each played. One athlete in each matched pair wore knee braces, the other did not. The study extended over 2 football seasons.

Of 580 high school football players, 247 wore single-hinged knee braces, 83 wore double-hinged braces, and 250 matched players did not wear braces. Only players who participated for at least 10 weeks during the regular playing season were included in the analysis, unless nonattendance was related to an injury of the lower extremity. Athletes with rehabilitative knee braces worn to protect an injured knee, or functional knee braces worn to stabilize an unstable knee were excluded from the study.

There were 53 knee injuries ranging from grade 0 to grade III during the 2-season study period. Knee injuries occurred in 37 (15%) of the 247 players who wore single-hinged braces, in 5 (6%) of the 83 players who wore double-hinged braces, and in 11 (4%) of the 250 controls who did not wear knee braces (table). The incidence of knee injuries among players who wore single-hinged braces was 3.7 higher than that among players who did not use any knee braces. The difference in the incidence of knee injuries between players who wore double-hinged braces and that in their nonbraced matched controls was not statistically significant. The number of foot and ankle injuries among football players who wore braces was also dramatically increased compared to that among nonbraced control persons.

Athletes Who Had Injuries of the Knee and Other Areas of the Lower Extremity

Site of Injury	Single-Hinged Braces (N = 247)			Double-Hinged Braces (N = 83)			No Braces (N = 250)		
	First Season	Second Season	Total	First Season	Second Season	Total	First Season	Second Season	Total
No injury	131	54	185	72	1	73	152	79	231
Knee	21	14	35	4	1	5	5	5	10
Lower extremity other than the knee*	7	18	25	4	1	5	2	6	8
Knee and other area of the lower extremity*	0	2	2	0	0	0	0	1	1

*These figures include only grade III injuries in players who completed less than 10 weeks of practice and play during the preseason and season.
(Courtesy of Grace TG, Skipper BJ, Newberry JC, et al: J Bone Joint Surg [Am] 70-A:422–427, March 1988.)

These results indicate that the use of single-hinged prophylactic knee braces increases the knee injury rate in high school football players. Such braces should therefore not be used in this age group.

▶ Many studies have been done on this subject in the past few years. Some indicate that bracing may help to prevent knee injuries. Most indicate that bracing does not reduce the incidence or severity of knee injuries. A number of these studies were reviewed in the 1987 and 1988 editions of the YEAR BOOK OF SPORTS MEDICINE.— F.J. George, ATC, PT

Assessment of Quadriceps/Hamstring Strength, Knee Ligament Stability, Functional and Sports Activity Levels Five Years After Anterior Cruciate Ligament Reconstruction
Seto JL, Orofino AS, Morrissey MC, Medeiros JM, Mason WJ (Kerlan-Jobe Orthopaedic Clinic, Inglewood, Calif; Stanford Univ)
Am J Sports Med 16:170–180, March–April 1988   3–13

Surgical reconstruction of a damaged anterior cruciate ligament (ACL) is intended to prevent progressive deterioration of the knee and to compensate structurally for decreased knee stability. Studies in patients with surgically reconstructed ACLs have shown that increased knee stability and thigh muscle strength are associated with a satisfactory return to preinjury sports activity. Patients who had undergone ACL reconstruction were reexamined 5 years later to measure strength, function, and stability of the treated knee and to assess the level of current participation in sports activities.

Of 25 study participants aged 22–48 years, 15 had undergone extra-articular ACL reconstructions and 10 had intra-articular ACL operations. Twenty-three patients had sustained knee injuries during sports activities; the other 2 were involved in motor vehicle accidents. All patients completed a functional activity questionnaire and a sports participation survey. Knee ligament stability was assessed by objective knee examination. Isokinetic quadriceps and hamstring muscle strength also were measured.

In neither surgical group was there a significant difference for symptoms of effusion, crepitus, or joint line tenderness between the treated and the control leg. Only the knee flexion range of motion (ROM) in patients who had undergone intra-articular ACL operations was significantly less than that in the control leg. Anterolateral rotatory instability and a positive Lachman sign were elicited on the treated leg in 80% of the patients, but there was no significant association between objective instability and functional activity scores. However, there was a significant association between increased quadriceps and hamstring strength of the operated-on leg and functional activity scores. The ability to return to preinjury activities was positively associated with functional activity scores. Persons who had participated in cutting sports such as football, downhill skiing, and tennis were less successful in returning to preinjury

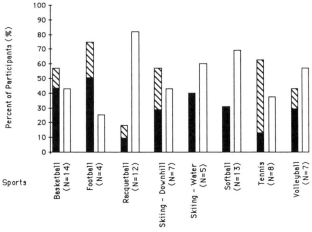

Fig 3–5.—Percent of participants (%) vs. level of cutting sports. *Black column,* individuals who quit participating in a sport because of knee problems. *Diagonal lines,* individuals who decreased their preinjury participation level. *White column,* individuals who returned to or improved their preinjury participation level. (Courtesy of Seto JL, Orofino AS, Morrissey MC, et al: *Am J Sports Med* 16:170–180, March–April 1988.)

participation levels than those involved in noncutting sports such as golf, swimming, and weight-lifting (Fig 3–5).

Because a previous study showed that functional return is not related to the hamstrings' strength but, rather, to the ability to contract reflexively, rehabilitation of the knee after ACL reconstruction should include reflex training of the medial and lateral hamstrings to reduce anteromedial and anterolateral rotary instability.

▶ Strengthening the hamstrings of ACL patients with just straight plane exercises is not sufficient. To improve function, the tibial internal and external rotators must be strengthened and reflex or functional training must be done. Proprioceptive neuromuscular facilitation types of exercises and patterns may be used to strengthen the rotators. Functional exercises must be done under supervision in the initial stages. With improvement, the intensity and duration of these exercises should be generally increased. After straight line running is performed satisfactorily, graduated curves and circles may be increased to sharper cutting maneuvers. The athlete is never advanced to a more difficult exercise before the previous step is completed satisfactorily.—F.J. George, ATC, PT

Muscular Coactivation: The Role of the Antagonist Musculature in Maintaining Knee Stability
Baratta R, Solomonow M, Zhou BH, Letson D, Chuinard R, D'Ambrosia R (Louisiana State Univ)
Am J Sports Med 16:113–122, March–April 1988   3–14

Whereas the ligaments associated with a given limb joint are widely regarded as responsible for the joint's stability, the role of the associated muscles in limb joint stability has received less attention. A study was conducted to quantify the coactivation patterns of the knee flexor and extensor muscles.

The study population included 7 nonathletic, normal control persons aged 20–42 years; 7 high-performance athletes aged 18–27 years involved in volleyball, basketball, or high/long jumping who had not performed any hamstring exercises before testing; and 10 high-performance athletes aged 18–34 years involved in the same sports who had routinely engaged in hamstring exercises. None of the study participants had previously experienced any knee problems. All 24 underwent simultaneous electromyographic recording from the flexor and extensor muscles of the knee during maximal-effort slow isokinetic contractions over the range of motion of each knee.

The hamstring coactivation patterns of athletes who did not exercise the hamstrings were substantially depressed compared with the patterns of controls and of athletes who regularly exercised the hamstrings. Suppression of antagonist coactivation patterns of the hamstrings probably resulted from hypertrophied quadriceps, developed by jumping activities, which exerted a strong inhibitory effect on hamstring coactivation. However, antagonist activity is vital to safe pressure distribution over the articular interface. Because reduced antagonist activity diminishes the total

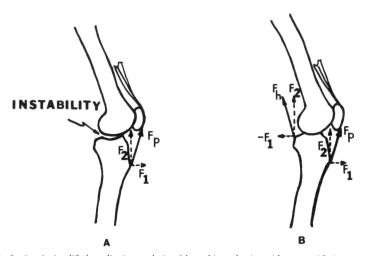

A　　　　　　　　　　　　**B**

Fig 3–6.—A simplified qualitative analysis of knee biomechanics without considering antagonist forces (**A**), and when including antagonist forces (**B**). The patellar tendon force (F_p) is decomposed to its constituent components perpendicular to the tibia (F_1) and along the tibia (F_2). Whereas F_1 tends to displace the tibia anteriorly, causing instability (articular surface separation), F_2 causes a single contact point between femur and tibia to absorb all the articular pressure. In **B**, the hamstring force (F_h) is shown with its components, F_1 and F_2. The F_1 components from each muscle are in opposing directions and probably cancel out, whereas the F_2 components are applied each at a different end of the articular surface, allowing pressure distribution over a bigger area (or reduction in articular surface pressure). (Courtesy of Baratta R, Solomonow M, Zhou BH, et al: *Am J Sports Med* 16:113–122, March–April 1988.)

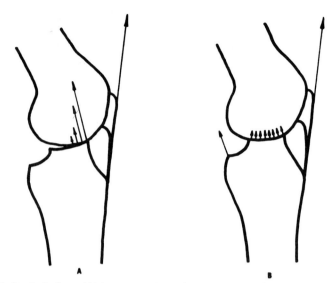

Fig 3−7.—**A**, the focused high-pressure point at the anterior aspect of the articular surface that results from the absence of opposing hamstring antagonist coactivation. **B**, the low, evenly distributed, articular surface pressure, the configuration in which the hamstring coactivation is fully active. (Courtesy of Baratta R, Solomonow M, Zhou BH, et al: *Am J Sports Med* 16:113−122, March−April 1988.)

stabilizing force available to the joint during extension loading, thus exposing the ligaments to most of the loading force, high-performance athletes with overdeveloped quadriceps are susceptible to an increased risk of anterior cruciate injuries (Figs 3−6 and 3−7).

These data indicate that significant muscle hypertrophy associated with a given joint should be avoided. Sports that inherently emphasize 1 muscle over its antagonist should be complemented with resistive exercises aimed at increasing antagonist tone to the extent that imbalance is prevented.

▶ This is a very interesting study that indicates the importance of avoiding muscle imbalances in our conditioning programs. It has generally been accepted that an imbalance in the quadriceps/hamstring strength ratio may cause hamstring injuries. The authors indicate that such an imbalance may also lead to anterior cruciate stress and injury to the ACL. If enough athletes could be found who were tested before an ACL injury occurred, it would be very educational to compare their quadricep/hamstring strength ratios to those in a control group. I don't believe I have ever read a study of this type.—F.J. George, ATC, PT

Manual Therapy: Mobilization of the Motion-Restricted Knee
Quillen WS, Gieck JH (Univ of Virginia)
Athletic Training 23:123−130, Summer 1988   3−15

Despite aggressive rehabilitation, advances in arthroscopic surgery, use of constant passive motion (CPM) devices, and functional postoperative bracing, athletes occasionally have difficulty in regaining normal joint motion after inflammation or prolonged immobilization of a joint. The traditional approach to a stiff joint has been to apply a passive sustained stretch without analyzing what is causing the stiffness. However, if motion limitation is caused by contracture of the joint capsule or the ligament, full restoration of function may not happen because muscular resistance interferes before connective tissue can be effectively stretched.

Manual mobilization techniques were divided into 4 grade levels of force, based on the available range of motion (ROM), ranging from grade I for mobilizations of small amplitude that are used at the beginning of the available ROM, to grade IV small-amplitude motions used at the end of the available ROM. Manual mobilization involves elongating the joint structure in the direction of the motion restriction, then oscillating the joint structures for a period of 20–60 seconds 4 or 5 times within a treatment session. Manual mobilization should be done every other day to allow connective tissue structures to recover.

The direction of application of the mobilization force depends on the joint surface contour of the limb that is to be mobilized. The Concave-Convex Rule states that if the joint surface of the limb to be moved is concave, a mobilization force should be applied in the direction of the restriction, whereas if the joint surface is convex, the limb should be moved opposite to the direction of the restriction (Fig 3–8). To restore accessory motions through lengthening connective tissue structures, the mobilization force must be of sufficient duration and applied in a biomechanically correct manner.

Manual mobilization is a highly effective addition to the standard therapeutic regimen in restoration of motion to a stiff or contracted joint. The technique safely lengthens connective tissue adhesions that restrict accessory motion and joint play and that eventually limit the normal ROM of the joint if left untreated.

▶ Different techniques have been used by athletic trainers and physical therapists to reduce joint contractures. The authors have described methods of joint mobilization to increase motion of contracted knees. We have used joint mobi-

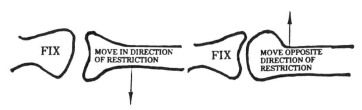

Fig 3–8.—Concave-Convex Rule. If the joint surface of the limb to be moved is concave, move it in the direction of restriction. If joint surface is convex, mobilize opposite the direction of restriction. (Adapted from Barak T, Rosen ER, Sofa R: *Orthopaedic and Sports Physical Therapy.* 1985, pp 212–227. Courtesy of Quillen WS, Gieck JH: *Athletic Training* 23:123–130, Summer 1988.)

lization with varying degrees of success. The more skilled the clinician and the more experience the clinician has with joint mobilization, the better the results. With practice, the clinician can develop a real "feel" for these joint contractures and which procedures will provide the best results. We have also used many of these techniques when evaluating knee injuries. I have found many of the "gentle" movements used in joint mobilization help the patient to relax and allow for a better evaluation.—F.J. George, ATC, PT

Electrical Stimulation Versus Voluntary Exercise in Strengthening Thigh Musculature After Anterior Cruciate Ligament Surgery
Delitto A, Rose SJ, McKowen JM, Lehman RC, Thomas JA, Shively RA (Washington Univ; Irene Walter Johnson Rehabilitation Inst, St Louis; Sports Medicine Physical Performance and Rehabilitation Ctr, St Louis)
Phys Ther 68:660–663, May 1988   3–16

Patients who have undergone anterior cruciate ligament (ACL) reconstruction have experienced a disproportionate loss of quadriceps femoris muscle strength. However, the common terminal knee extension exercises used for rehabilitating and strengthening these weakened muscles after traditional intra-articular repairs and reconstructions are considered detrimental to ACL reconstruction and are therefore contraindicated. Rehabilitation techniques that use the concept of co-contraction of the hamstring muscles to strengthen the quadriceps femoris muscles in patients with ACL deficiencies are now believed to be safe.

A comparison study was made on the effectiveness of voluntary exercise (VE) and electrical stimulation (ES), both commonly used in the immediate postoperative phase of ACL reconstruction, involving 20 patients aged 19–44 years who had undergone ACL reconstructions, with 10 patients assigned to either VE or ES. Each protocol called for a 3-week period of exercise, performed 5 days a week, within the first 6 postoperative weeks. All patients used a training regimen consisting of exercises that simultaneously contracted the quadriceps femoris and the hamstring muscles.

Patients assigned to the ES protocol finished the 3-week training regimen with significantly greater isometric strength gains of both knee extensor and flexor muscles than did patients in the VE group. Because the latter patients did not come to the clinic for every treatment but exercised at home, and patients in the ES group attended the rehabilitation clinic on a daily basis, it is possible that noncompliance with the prescribed exercise regimen among VE-treated patients played a role in the outcome.

Indications are that patients enrolled in an ES treatment program after ACL reconstruction can achieve greater individual thigh musculature strength than can patients instructed to use VE at home.

▶ There have been many studies done on the use of electrical muscle stimulation (EMS) vs. VE to improve muscle strength. Of course not all of the protocols were the same in all of the studies, which makes comparison of results difficult. Some studies indicate that EMS is beneficial and others that it is not. Some studies indicate it to be beneficial in the initial stages of rehabilitation but not in the final results. Some treatment guidelines for ACL repairs indicate that EMS should not be used on the quadriceps because of the anterior shear it may cause to the knee. This study indicates that the use of EMS is beneficial.

I agree wholeheartedly with the concept of co-contraction of the hamstrings and quadriceps in all ACL rehabilitation programs.—F.J. George, ATC, PT

A Biomechanical Evaluation of Tibiofemoral Rotation in Anterior Cruciate Deficient Knees During Walking and Running
Czerniecki JM, Lippert F, Olerud JE (Univ of Washington)
Am J Sports Med 16:327–331, July–August 1988   3–17

Anterior cruciate ligament (ACL) injuries have been associated with increased knee instability in in vitro and in vivo studies using passively applied forces. Tibiofemoral rotation after ACL injury during the functional activity of treadmill ambulation was studied using a triaxial electrogoniometer.

Eleven patients with ACL injuries involving 1 knee and 9 uninjured persons participated in the study. The Cybex II isokinetic dynamometer was used to obtain isometric and isokinetic peak torques of the quadriceps and hamstrings. Significant increases occurred in tibiofemoral rotation with increased running speed in both injured and normal knees. The degree of rotation in the injured leg did not significantly exceed that in the uninjured leg. Isokinetic strength of the quadriceps and hamstrings correlated significantly with extent of rotation.

The greater the isokinetic peak torque of the hamstrings or quadriceps, the smaller the relative tibiofemoral rotation. Isokinetic muscle strength may therefore play a role in stabilizing rotational motion at the knee. The significant inverse correlation between rotation and isokinetic peak torque and the absence of a correlation between rotation and isometric peak torque suggest that stability of the knee during dynamic activity might depend more on isokinetic muscle power than on isometric muscle power.

▶ Here is a strong case for including isokinetic exercises in the rehabilitation programs of ACL patients. We use the Johnson Anti-Shear device when doing isokinetic quadriceps exercises with our ACL patients. We do not use the device when exercising the hamstrings. I wonder if the use of this device in a rehabilitation program would produce results similar to those found in this study.—F.J. George, ATC, PT

Does a Torn Anterior Cruciate Ligament Lead to Change in the Central Nervous Drive of the Knee Extensors?

Elmqvist L-G, Lorentzon R, Johansson C, Fugl-Meyer AR (Univ Hosp of Umeå, Sweden)
Eur J Appl Physiol 58:203–207, October 1988   3–18

A recent investigation of patients with anterior cruciate ligament (ACL) tears disclosed a 5% shrinkage of quadriceps on computed tomography. The isokinetic mechanical output of the knee extensors was 71% to 87% of that of the uninjured knee. Mechanical output corrected for differences in quadriceps cross-sectional area was significantly lower in the injured limb. Because there were no correlations between isokinetic performance and muscle size or qualitative morphology or morphometric data, it was hypothesized that the significant decrease in the quadriceps' mechanical output was caused by reduced or changed motor unit activation.

Integrated surface electromyograms of the 3 superficial portions of the quadriceps and isokinetic knee extensor maximum torque and power production were recorded at the same time and at different angular velocities in both legs in 11 men with unilateral tear of the ACL. Computed tomography was used to measure the cross-sectional area of the thigh and its muscular components. A small but significant reduction in the quadriceps cross-sectional area on the affected side was found. A lessened active but not passive range of motion, decreased mechanical output, and reduced electromyographic activity, especially in rectus femoris, occurred on the affected side.

The reason for the decreased maximum and total knee extensor performance observed in these patients is a change in knee receptor afferent inflow. Because the morphological changes in this series were minor, changes in joint receptor afferent inflow caused by ACL rupture lead to deficits in motor unit activation and synchronous function, resulting in reduced mechanical output.

▶ We will continue to require our ACL-deficient knees to regain 100% of quadriceps strength. If the athlete was not tested before the injury, we use the opposite knee as our norm. Our minimum goal for hamstring strength is 70% of the quadriceps at 60 degrees per second. We strongly encourage these athletes to increase hamstring strength beyond this goal and have had many surpass a ratio of 80%.—F.J. George, ATC, PT

Peak Torque and Total Work Relationship in the Thigh Muscles After Anterior Cruciate Ligament Injury

Kannus P (Univ of Tampere, Finland)
J Orthop Sports Phys Ther 10:97–101, September 1988   3–19

The development of commercial versions of isokinetic strength testing devices has increased routine isokinetic testing of patients who are recovering from knee injuries. The peak torque corresponding to the single highest torque output of the joint produced by muscular contraction as the limb moves through the range of motion has been the most commonly measured parameter, but new computer-linked isokinetic dynamometers now allow readily available measurement of other parameters.

Assessment was made of the relationship between isometric and isokinetic peak torques and total work output of multiple contractions of the quadriceps and hamstrings in patients with an anteriorly unstable knee resulting from total loss of the anterior cruciate ligament (ACL). The association between muscle function parameters and subjective and functional outcome also was analyzed.

The study group included 36 patients aged 16–59 years who had a confirmed chronic ACL-insufficient knee. All of them had 1 healthy knee. A microcomputer-linked Cybex II isokinetic dynamometer was used to measure isokinetic quadriceps and hamstrings peak torques at 60 degrees and 180 degrees per second. Each test was done 6 times, and recordings were made of the best peak torque value of each knee extension and flexion. Total work was recorded as the work produced by 6 repetitions at 180 degrees per second. One minute after the isokinetic tests, maximal isometric extension and flexion strength was measured with the knee at a flexion angle of 60 degrees from full extension.

At all test speeds, coefficients between peak torque and total work correlated significantly for the quadriceps and hamstrings of both the uninjured and the ACL-insufficient knees. The peak torque and the total work parameters of quadriceps and hamstrings both correlated significantly with subjective and functional outcome of the ACL-insufficient knees. The nearer the muscular performance of the ACL-insufficient knee was to that of the uninjured knee, the better the outcome achieved. No determination was made as to whether good muscle function of the ACL-insufficient knee is a cause or a result of good subjective and functional outcome, or if poor muscle function is a cause or a result of poor recovery. Measurement of total work contributes little additional information to that obtained from peak torque measurements. Because peak torques of the quadriceps and hamstring muscles correlate significantly with subjective and functional results in the ACL insufficient knee, undisturbed muscle function may be crucial for a patient's optimal recovery after a knee ligament injury.

▶ This study strongly supports what knee rehabilitation is all about. Anterior cruciate ligament-deficient knee patients must build the strength of the hamstrings and quadriceps to equal or even surpass the strength of the uninvolved knee. I would recommend that the calf and hip muscles also be included in this rehabilitation regimen.—F.J. George, ATC, PT

Knee Extension Torque Joint Position Relationships Following Isotonic Fixed Resistance and Hydraulic Resistance Training
Hunter GR, Culpepper MI (Univ of Alabama)
Athletic Training 23:16–20, Spring 1988   3–20

With fixed resistance isotonic strength training, the attained increases in force at the strongest positions in the torque, or force-position curve, are relatively small. Although resistive exercise equipment, or variable resistance equipment, was developed for the purpose of fitting exercise equipment to the force-position curve, whether it actually does this for different individuals using these machines is questionable.

Isokinetic or fixed velocity exercise equipment, thought to supply maximal force production throughout the entire force-position curve, is made by several companies. One of them manufactures omnikinetic equipment that provides modified isokinetic exercises by retarding movement through the use of either hydraulics or friction. The effects were investigated of isotonic fixed resistance (FR) and hydraulic resistance (HR) strength training on the maximal torque-position curve of the knee.

A study group included 6 men (mean age, 21 years) and 4 women (mean age, 21 years) who were tested before and after an 8-week training program. Each patient exercised 3 times per week with at least 48 hours between sessions, training 1 leg on an FR knee extension device and the contralateral leg on an HR knee extension device.

Both training modalities produced significant increases in isotonic and isokinetic strength. The FR-trained leg showed greater strength gains when tested isotonically and isokinetically than the HR-trained leg did, but the difference was not statistically significant. Increases in torque throughout the 7 joint positions on the force-position curve were uniform for both legs. Although strength gains attained with FR training can be similar throughout the torque-position curve, some kinds of strength may be developed more with FR training than with HR training.

▶ Isokinetic training has become very popular because of the different speeds that can be used in rehabilitation programs. I agree with the authors that fixed resistance isotonic exercises will produce results similar to exercising isokinetically at 60 degrees per second. The advantage that isokinetic devices have is that high-speed exercises can be controlled. Many of our rehabilitation programs use high-speed muscle contractions to avoid excessive torque on injured or postsurgical joints.— F.J. George, ATC, PT

Effects of Speed and Limb Dominance on Eccentric and Concentric Isokinetic Testing of the Knee
Hageman PA, Gillaspie DM, Hill LD (Univ of Nebraska)
J Orthop Sports Phys Ther 10:59–65, August 1988   3–21

Current isokinetic rehabilitation techniques for increasing muscle strength primarily involve the use of concentric exercise. Despite the availability of isokinetic devices capable of eccentric exercise, documentation of appropriate isokinetic rehabilitation using eccentric muscle training for the knee is limited. The effects of speed and limb dominance on torque values and ratios of the quadriceps and hamstrings during eccentric and concentric exercise were studied.

Both knees of 13 women and 12 men aged 21–33 years were tested at 30 and 180 degrees per second with a computer-controlled dynamometer. Concentric quadriceps torque values and torque/body weight ratios decreased significantly at the higher speed. No significant changes in eccentric quadriceps or eccentric hamstrings torque were noted at the 2 speeds. There were no significant differences in torque values or torque/body weight ratios between dominant and nondominant knees during both concentric and eccentric exercise at both speeds. Hamstring/quadricep torque ratios increased significantly at the higher speed during concentric exercise. In men the hamstring/quadricep ratios were significantly greater in the nondominant limb during both concentric and eccentric exercise at both speeds.

These results are useful in providing additional information about hamstrings and quadriceps activity in healthy young men and women during eccentric and concentric activity during 2 speeds. These findings should be considered when establishing rehabilitation goals during isokinetic eccentric activity.

▶ A finding in this study surprising to me is that, "No significant changes in eccentric quadriceps or eccentric hamstrings torque were noted at the 2 speeds." Another finding that I have not observed or read about is that, "In men the hamstring/quadriceps ratios were significantly greater in the nondominant limb during both concentric and eccentric exercises at both speeds."—F.J. George, ATC, PT

Effects of Speed, Hip and Knee Angle, and Gravity on Hamstring to Quadriceps Torque Ratios
Figoni SF, Christ CB, Massey BH (Wright State Univ, Dayton, Ohio)
J Orthopaed Sports Phys Ther 9:287–291, February 1988   3–22

The hamstring-to-quadriceps torque ratio (H/Q) measures the relationship between strengths of the hamstring and quadriceps muscle groups around the knee. It has traditionally been based on the peak isometric or isokinetic torque values obtained with the knee flexor and extensor muscle groups without regard for the hip and knee angles at which peak torques occurred or the effects of gravity on these measurements. A study was conducted to determine the effect of speed, hip angle, knee angle, and gravity on H/Q torque ratios.

Eighteen healthy college-aged men performed 3 maximal-effort knee extension and flexion repetitions on a Cybex II isokinetic dynamometer at 15 and 90 degrees per second. Hamstring and quadriceps torques were measured at various knee flexions and at the angles at which peak torque occurred. Torques were also measured at 5 and 120 degrees of hip flexion. Gravity-corrected ratios decreased with increased knee angles from 15 to 60 degrees. The higher hip angle at each speed resulted in higher ratios at knee angles between 30 and 90 degrees. The effect of speed on ratios varied and interacted with hip and knee angle. Correction for gravity decreased the ratios at all knee angles except 90 degrees. The H/Q torque ratios at selected knee angles ranged from 0.20 to 2.00, differed from H/Q peak torque ratios 40% of the time, and did not always correlate highly with H/Q peak torque ratios.

The H/Q peak torque ratios did not indicate H/Q torque ratios at selected knee angles. Knee angle-specific H/Q torque ratios may provide different and possibly more useful information on hamstring and quadriceps function than do H/Q peak torque ratios.

▶ The effect of gravity on peak torque has been a controversial subject, especially if results are to be compared to an opposite limb. The authors state that elimination of gravitational torques is very important at the lowest knee angles or if subjects are able to generate only low torque because of weakness, injury, or fatigue. The effects of gravity become even more important when testing weaker joints such as the shoulder, elbow, or wrist.—F.J. George, ATC, PT

The Diagonal Medial Plica: An Underestimated Clinical Entity
Kegerreis S, Malone T, Johnson F (Univ of Indianapolis; Methodist Sports Medicine Ctr, Indianapolis)
J Orthop Sports Phys Ther 9:305–309, March 1988   3–23

Patella plica syndrome (PPS) is a commonly reported entity, but the specific diagnoses of PPS remain controversial. The condition is usually associated with macro- or microtrauma to the synovial fold, particularly with repetitive knee-bending activities. Patients with PPS complain of a dull, chronic ache that increases with activity, and some experience pseudolocking and a "giving way" that can be attributed to neurologic inhibition. The occasionally observed "clicking," "catching," and "stuttering" of the patella can be attributed to the more traditionally recognized PPS, or to dysfunction of other accompanying extensor mechanisms.

It has been advocated that the knee be examined for suprapatellar plicas by passively flexing and extending the knee with the tibia held in internal rotation and the patella slightly displaced medially. The medial patellar border should then be palpated for a pop or tenderness. Various additional palpating positions have been suggested, and when the medial plica as a readily palpable entity could not be identified, a palpable plica-like band over the superior aspect of the medial femoral condyle was found at once. This plica-like band often could be rolled and followed in a medial diagonal direction to the medial joint line and was commonly thickened when pathologic.

Conservative treatment for PPS should be tailored to its underlying etiology. If a plical band has become fibrous and lost its elasticity, conservative treatment will probably be ineffective and may ultimately require operation. The use of phonophoresis with 10% hydrocortisone cream, ice packs, and aspirin is effective in decreasing the acute inflammatory reaction. Repetitive flexion/extension exercises should not be prescribed during this early phase of treatment; only isometrics performed submaximally and progressing to maximal efforts as tolerated are recommended. Once the inflammatory process is under control, the exercise program may be increased to include carefully introduced isotonic/isokinetic activities, performed in addition to continued multiple angle isometrics at maximal levels. However, patients should not do flexion/extension activities through the painful range. If patients with microtraumatically produced PPS do not respond to conservative management, surgery may be the only option. Postoperative rehabilitation is similar to that used in conservative management.

Although the diagnosis and management of patella plical syndrome may be controversial, conservative techniques should be used as a first-line approach to its treatment.

▶ The authors present good advice for exercising patients with patella plica syndrome. They suggest the use of multiple angle submaximal isometrics. This type of exercise is considered safe for the knee and patellofemoral joints and an effective means of increasing strength.

We have also included flexibility exercises for the hamstrings and quadriceps within pain-free ranges for these patients.—F.J. George, ATC, PT

Anterior Knee Pain
Bourne MH, Hazel WA Jr, Scott SG, Sim FH (Mayo Clinic and Found, Rochester, Minn)
Mayo Clin Proc 63:482–491, May 1988   3–24

Anterior knee pain is often a source of impairment. The cause of such pain frequently remains unknown and the condition may be self-limited, but a specific diagnosis should be sought and therapy instituted.

The patellar retinaculum is especially important laterally, where it also inserts into the hamstring musculature. Tightened hamstrings can, therefore, result in patellofemoral symptoms. Maximal patellofemoral forces are 35–40 degrees of flexion when the knee is moved through a range of motion against resistance. Rehabilitation for patients with a patellofemoral pain syndrome consists of 4 stages—acute, subacute, chronic, and maintenance.

In the acute stage specific exercises should be prescribed. Isometric exercises for the quadriceps and hip adductors and prolonged stretching for the hamstring and iliotibial band muscle groups should be included. Also, in this stage, toe raises and general range-of-motion exercises for the knee are begun. When ice application does not alleviate pain, transcutaneous electrical nerve stimulation or high-intensity galvanic stimulation may be tried.

The goals of subacute rehabilitation are to increase strength and flexibility, protect the patellar surface, and do 30 minutes of exercise 2–3 times daily. Patients are usually advanced to this phase of treatment when they have minimal swelling, pain, and inflammation. The use of anti-inflammatory measures is continued, and low-resistance strengthening exercises are begun. Patients should be taught to avoid knee hyperextension, which often aggravates symptoms. Flexibility exercises are increased, including prolonged pain-free static stretching of the hamstrings, quadriceps, heel cords, and lateral retinaculum.

For patients with anterior knee pain, careful physical and radiographic examination followed by first-line, nonoperative intervention are recommended. Rehabilitation should include strengthening, nonsteroidal anti-inflammatory medications, ice, and bracing. If this strategy fails, cautious surgical intervention should focus on the area of anatomical abnormality.

Case Study: Rehabilitation of a Collegiate Football Placekicker With Patellofemoral Arthritis
Murray PB (Northern Virginia Ctr for Orthopaedic and Sports Rehabilitation, Alexandria)
J Orthop Sports Phys Therapy 10:224–227, December 1988   3–25

Patellofemoral pain syndromes are a major cause of knee pain.

Man, 24, a National Collegiate Athletic Association Division I placekicker, complained of pain and stiffness in his knee 4 months after the season ended. He described subsequent loss of power and distance with his kicks toward the end of the previous season. The rehabilitation program for his patellofemoral arthritis consisted of end-range isotonics for the quadriceps, short-arc isokinetics at intermediate speeds, and full range isokinetics at high contractile speeds for knee extension and flexion, lower extremity stretching, electrical stimulation to the quadricep musculature, and underwater kicking workouts along with placekicking and kickoff workouts. He was treated in the clinic 3 times a week for 8 weeks. On discharge he said he had regained distance and power with his kicks. An increase in peak torque at 60 and 180 degrees per seconds of 14% and 15%, respectively, of the quadriceps in the affected leg was noted on Cybex testing.

This patient was successfully rehabilitated with a combination of proper exercises and education. He was better able to deal with his condition once he understood the mechanism involved and what he should do to prevent it. He reported relief both physically and psychologically.

► The preceding 2 studies (Abstracts 3–24 and 3–25) describe patellofemoral joint problems, their causes, and conservative treatment approaches. When our patients have this problem, we have them do stretching of the hamstrings, the hip musculature, and the lateral retinaculum if those areas are found to be tight. If a patient has been immobilized in a cast or cast brace, we always carry out patellofemoral mobilization techniques before vigorous range-of-motion exercises are attempted.—F.J. George, ATC, PT

Effects of Ankle Taping on the Motion and Loading Pattern of the Foot for Walking Subjects
Carmines DV, Nunley JA, McElhaney JH (Duke Univ)
J Orthop Res 6:223–229, 1988   3–26

Prophylactic ankle taping is widely used by trainers to reduce ankle injury potential in athletes. Some clinicians also use ankle taping in the rehabilitation treatment of patients with severely sprained ankles. The purpose of ankle taping is to limit the ankle's range of rotation to reduce the strain on the ligaments around the joint. Gait analysis was used to compare motions and dynamic loading patterns of taped and untaped normal ankles during level walking.

The study group included 7 patients with normal ankles, 3 women and 4 men, aged 21–25 years, who were tested with and without their right ankles taped in the neutral position. All tests were carried out while the patients were walking barefoot, each at his or her normal cadence. Gait analysis was performed with a Gola-type custom built suspension force plate, an ankle goniometer, and 2 accelerometers mounted on the top of the foot that measured the rotations of both the ankle and the foot around the metatarsal heads.

The ground reaction forces showed no changes between the same ankle, taped and untaped. The primary variations observed with ankle taping occurred in the ankle and toe rotations measured in the sagittal plane. Taping caused a mean total reduction in rotation of 20%, a mean reduction in plantar flexion of 22%, and a mean reduction in dorsiflexion of 18.6%. Reduced dorsiflexion of the taped ankle caused the heel to come up sooner in stance. The mean degree of heel–up occurred at 71.5% of stance without taping and at 67.1% with taping. The difference was statistically significant. Each taped ankle caused a greater degree of rotation around the metatarsal heads during heel–up than the same ankle did when it was not taped.

Indications are that the restricted rotation of a taped ankle may adversely affect the metatarsophalangeal joint by increasing stress on the phalangeal ligaments. This finding is important for patients experiencing a tender forefoot caused by a stress fracture of the metatarsals, metatarsalgia, or Morton's neuroma. For them ankle taping would have an adverse effect.

▶ The authors have indicated that athletes with certain forefoot problems should not have their ankles taped because of the stress it may put on the forefoot. I would add "Turf Toe" or sprained first metatarsal phalangeal joint to their list of problems.—F.J. George, ATC, PT

Retrospective Comparison of Taping and Ankle Stabilizers in Preventing Ankle Injuries
Rovere GD, Clarke TJ, Yates CS, Burley K (Wake Forest Univ)
Am J Sports Med 16:228–233, May–June 1988   3–27

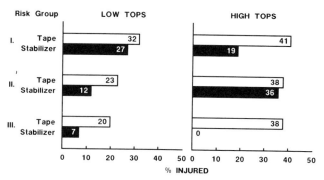

Fig 3–9.—Assessment of relative risk from shoe type and ankle support on the basis of frequencies of annual injuries (*numbers on bars*). *OL*, offensive lineman; *DL*, defensive lineman; *LB*, linebacker; *RB*, running back; *DB*, defensive back; *WR*, wide receiver; *QB*, quarterback. (Courtesy of Rovere GD, Clarke TJ, Yates CS, et al: *Am J Sports Med* 16:228–233, May–June 1988.)

Controversy exists over the use of prophylactic ankle taping and other ankle stabilizers in the prevention of football injuries. A retrospective study assessed the effectiveness of ankle taping and laced stabilizers in the prevention of ankle injuries and ankle reinjuries among collegiate football players.

During a 6-season study period, 297 football players attended 536 practices (for a total of 46,789 practice exposures) and played 77 games (for a total of 5,142 game exposures). During the first 2 seasons each player had his ankles taped for all practice sessions and games. Thereafter, players were given a choice between ankle taping and wearing laced ankle stabilizers. In all, 233 athletes with taped ankles were involved in 38,658 exposures, and 127 athletes who wore self-applied stabilizers were involved in 13,273 exposures, or a total of 51,931 exposures. Player or coach preference determined whether high-top or low-top shoes were worn. The team physician evaluated injured players on the day of injury. For this study, an injury was defined as a ligamentous or bone insult that caused an athlete to miss at least 1 game or 1 practice.

During 51,931 exposures to injury, 224 ankle injuries and 24 ankle reinjuries occurred. Tape had been worn when 159 of the 224 ankle injuries and 23 of the 24 reinjuries occurred; an ankle stabilizer had been worn when 37 injuries and 1 reinjury occurred. When the players were classified as being at high, moderate, or low risk for ankle injury by player position, an analysis of the injury data showed that in the high-risk group, the ankle injury rate was 41% for the combination of high-top shoes and ankle taping, compared to 27% for the combination of low-top shoes and ankle stabilizers (Fig 3–9).

A comparison of the relative safety of combinations of ankle support and shoe type showed that low-top shoes with ankle stabilizers provided the most protection, and high-top shoes with tape were the least safe.

▶ The results of this study were most surprising to me. I would subjectively have selected the combination of taped ankle with high-top shoe as being associated with the lowest injury risk. The authors report that the lowest injury risk group was that in which the low-top shoe and ankle stabilizer were used. The authors explain that the combination of low-top shoe and ankle stabilizer may be the most effective because during breaks in a practice or game the athlete has a better opportunity to get to and retighten the stabilizer. We have used ankle braces on a fairly wide scale for the past 2 years. We have found them to be effective in preventing injuries and to be cost effective.—F.J. George, ATC, PT

Ice and High Voltage Pulsed Stimulation in Treatment of Acute Lateral Ankle Sprains
Michlovitz S, Smith W, Watkins M (Hahnemann Univ, Philadelphia; USCG Training Ctr, Cape May, NJ)
J Orthop Sports Phys Therapy 9:301–304, March 1988   3–28

Conventional management of ankle sprains includes application of ice and compression, as well as elevation. High-voltage pulsed stimulation (HVPS) decreases edema and pain in patients with acute injuries. A study was conducted to compare the effects of ice vs. ice and HVPS in the treatment of acute ankle sprains. Thirty young adults with grade I or II lateral ankle sprain were randomly assigned to receive either an ice pack for 30 minutes (group I, 10 patients), an ice pack combined with HVPS using negative polarity continuous modulation at 28 pulses per second (pps) (group II, 10 patients), or ice pack plus HVPS at 80 pps (group III, 10 patients). Treatment was given once daily for 3 days and the effects on ankle edema, range of motion, and pain were evaluated.

Both ice and HVPS at 28 and 80 pps produced a decrease in foot and ankle volume, an increase in ankle dorsiflexion, and a decrease in pain. One-way analysis of variance for edema and dorsiflexion changes, however, showed no significant differences in treatment effects among those who received ice alone and those who had ice and HVPS. The latter does not appear to enhance the treatment effects of conventional methods on acute lateral ankle sprains.

▶ There have been many statements made in the literature and claims made by manufacturers and respected clinicians that high-voltage electrical stimulation reduces edema in acutely sprained ankles. I have never seen a scientific study that proved that statement to be true. In my own experience, trying many different pulse settings, I never observed a reduction in swelling using high-voltage electrical muscle stimulation on acutely sprained ankles. I have followed the manufacturers' recommendations and many different treatment protocols used by those claiming success with this treatment. I agree with the authors' findings in this study.—F.J. George, ATC, PT

Hydrocolloid Dressings in the Treatment of Turf Burns and Other Athletic Abrasions
Mellion MB, Fandel DM, Wagner WF, Kwikkel MA (Univ of Nebraska; Creighton Univ, Omaha)
Athletic Training 23:341–346, Winter 1988   3–29

"Turf burns" and other abrasions acquired while playing a sport present a special challenge for health care professionals who treat athletes. These lesions can limit performance in practice and competition. A wound care regimen using DuoDerm hydrocolloid dressing in athletic abrasions was evaluated.

Thirty-two college football players with partial-thickness skin abrasions were treated with a hydrocolloid dressing. All abrasions healed in 4–8 days. Athletic trainers rated skin appearance at the end of therapy as good to excellent in 83.9% and average in 16.1%.

Procedure.—Clinicians first cleanse the wound with povidone iodine and remove residual scrub with water or saline lavage. Any visible foreign body particles are then scrubbed out or débrided. A wound margin of at least 1 in. is shaved, and the surrounding skin is dried. The hydrocolloid dressing is cut to extend at least 0.75 in. beyond the wound margin. The dressing is then applied directly over the wound and smoothed in place. Abrasions on extremities should be covered with taping underwrap held in place with elastic tape. An additional layer of combined dressing or other padding may be added, secured with taping underwrap and an elastic bandage, for patients participating in contact and collision sports. The dressing should be changed at 24 hours on all but very small or superficial abrasions. At this time the wound may be rinsed but should not be scrubbed of residual gel. Subsequent dressing changes are indicated if there is leakage of wound exudate or the hydrated gel formation visible under the dressing reaches to within 0.25 in. of the border. At 6–7 days after injury, the dressing is removed for wound assessment. A fresh dressing is applied if healing is not complete. No hydrocolloid dressing should be left in place for more than 7 days.

The use of hydrocolloid dressings in the treatment of abrasions in athletes was effective.

▶ We have used this treatment with a good deal of success. It's natural to want to remove the dressing to check on infection or healing, but it works much better if the dressing is left in place undisturbed.—F.J. George, ATC, PT

The Role of Warmup in Muscular Injury Prevention
Safran MR, Garrett WE Jr, Seaber AV, Glisson RR, Ribbeck BM (Duke Univ)
Am J Sports Med 16:123–128, March–April 1988   3–30

Athletes commonly warm up before exercising, but the performance benefits of this practice are uncertain. Both stretching exercises and active muscle contraction or exercise frequently are included in the warmup period. The biomechanical properties were examined of control and stimulated rabbit muscles that were torn. Study animals had their muscles isometrically preconditioned (stimulated before stretching). Tibialis anterior, extensor digitorum longus, and flexor digitorum longus muscles were used in the experimental model.

Preconditioned muscles required more force to fail than did control (unconditioned) muscles and they stretched to a greater length from rest before failing. All muscles failed at the musculotendinous junction. Length-tension deformation recordings showed that preconditioned muscles attained less force at a given increase in length before failing, indicating a relative increase in elasticity. The difference was significant only for the extensor digitorum longus muscle.

Apparently, the warmup process stretches the musculotendinous unit and leads to increased muscle length at a given load. As a result, less tension is put on the musculotendinous junction, thus decreasing the risk of injury.

▶ A good deal of controversy has surrounded the warmup issue and a number of questions remain unanswered. How much energy should be expended in the warmup? How much of a rest (if any) should there be between warmup and actual performance? What are the best exercises to include in a warmup? What equipment or clothing should be worn? Are the benefits of warmup psychological, physical, or both?

This article lends credence to the theory that warmup should be done to prevent injury. Serious athletes usually accept warming up as a part of their routine. Recreational athletes tend to blame lack of time as the reason for not warming up properly. Perhaps recreational athletes should make the first 15 or 20 minutes of their activity light and then gradually increase the intensity. Please read Abstracts 7–31, 7–32, and 7–33, which discuss warmup techniques.—F.J. George, ATC, PT

Warm-Up Techniques and Their Place in Patient Education
Stalker R (Dalhousie Univ Sport Medicine Clinic, Halifax, NS)
Can Fam Physician 34:177–181, January 1988   3–31

A growing body of evidence suggests that, if properly executed, warmup benefits the exerciser both physically and psychologically. Family practitioners and others should be familiar with the principles and phases of warmup to instruct athletic patients properly and prevent musculoskeletal injury.

Many beneficial effects of warmup have been reported, including benefits to the heart. In the general warmup phase, aerobic activity using the large muscles (e.g., light jogging, calisthenics, or bicycling) should be advocated. Such activity is more effective in raising the core temperature than are passive activities such as massage, heating pads, or sitting in a sauna. The core temperature should be raised to make the muscles more elastic and to protect the heart. This period should be followed by a period of flexibility exercises. Flexibility programs must be individualized for each athlete, depending on the demands of that athlete's sport. Static stretching should be done as the initial flexibility technique in warmup. Ballistic stretching should be discouraged. Proprioceptive neuromuscular facilitation flexibility techniques may produce dramatic increases in range of motion.

▶ The heart is a muscle that also benefits from warmup before strenuous activity, and the author explains how and why this should be done. He goes on to describe different types of stretching (see Abstracts 3–30, 3–32, and 3–33) and illustrates methods of stretching certain muscles. Also included are illustrations of stretching exercises *not* to do, such as the "hurdler's stretch" and bending over from the upright position to do "toe touches."—F.J. George, ATC, PT

Muscle Stretching and Motoneuron Excitability
Guissard N, Duchateau J, Hainaut K (Univ of Brussels)
Eur J Appl Physiol 58:47–52, October 1988   3–32

Slow or static muscle stretching now is preferred to repeated rapid joint movements because it avoids the reflex activity of the stretched muscles. Changes in motoneuron excitability were examined during 3 basic methods of slow or static stretching of the soleus muscle in 28 healthy persons aged 19–33 years, most of whom were physical education students. The tendon and Hoffmann reflexes were analyzed during passive muscle stretching, static stretching preceded by a maximal isometric contraction or contraction-relaxation (CR), and stretching by contracting the antagonist muscles (AC).

There was a significant difference between the tendon and Hoffmann reflexes during static stretching with progressive dorsiflexion of the foot, but the amplitude of the direct motor response to maximal stimulation was unchanged. Maximal joint mobilization during static stretching, CR, and AC was closely related to the decrease in the Hoffmann response. The decrease was least in static stretching. With all stretching methods the Hoffmann reflex recovered as soon as the maneuver ceased.

Apparently, changes in excitability of the muscle motoneuron pool control joint mobilization during slow or static stretching. Inhibition of the motoneurons ceases when the stretching maneuver is over. From a practical viewpoint, both AC and CR seem to be more efficient than static stretching.

▶ Another study supporting the claim that flexibility techniques incorporating proprioceptive neuromuscular facilitation type stretching are more effective than static stretching. Many of our teams use the "buddy system" to include these exercises in their warmup and cool-down regimes. They are an important part of every practice session and pregame warmup. We never use ballistic stretching and never stretch cold muscles. A general warmup such as jogging or light activity always precedes our stretching regime. Please read Abstracts 3–30, 3–31, and 3–33.—F.J. George, ATC, PT

Chronic and Acute Flexibility of Men and Women Using Three Different Stretching Techniques
Etnyre BR, Lee EJ (Rice Univ, Houston)
Res Q Exerc Sport 59:222–228, September 1988   3–33

Because most organized physical activities are preceded by some flexibility exercise, it would be beneficial to know the effects of different flexibility methods for increasing range of motion (ROM). The most commonly used methods for increasing ROM are ballistic stretching, static stretching (SS), and variations on proprioceptive neuromuscular facilitation (PNF) techniques.

Chronic and acute ROM changes of hip flexion and shoulder extension in men and women were compared using 3 stretching techniques and a control group. The program lasted for 12 weeks. Treatment groups performed either SS, contract-relax, or contract-relax with agonist-contraction (CRAC) stretching techniques. Range-of-motion measurements were taken before training and once every 3 weeks thereafter.

All treatment groups had significant increases in ROM compared with the control group. Women had greater ROM than men throughout the program, but their comparative increases were not significantly different from the men's.

The PNF techniques (contract-relax and CRAC) were more effective than SS for increasing ROM for both hip flexion and shoulder extension in both sexes. Because the control group lost ROM through the program, it was recommended that some stretching procedures precede physical activity to enhance flexibility. As a result of the latent decreases in ROM for women and only slight gains for men using SS, the use of this method should be discouraged when a PNF method can be used instead. Although women attained similar ROM increases with either PNF method, men had the greatest ROM increases using CRAC.

▶ The 3 previous abstracts (3–30, 3–31, and 3–32) stress the importance of warmup and different flexibility techniques. The above abstract compares the results of SS with 2 PNF methods. The authors strongly recommend that PNF stretching exercises be done whenever possible, because of the superior results attained with this type of exercise. They also recommend that men use the CRAC (contract-relax agonist-contract) method, because better results for men were achieved using that technique.—F.J. George, ATC, PT

Etiologic Factors Associated With Selected Running Injuries
Messier SP, Pittala KA (Wake Forest Univ)
Med Sci Sports Exerc 20:501–505, October 1988   3–34

TABLE 1.—Mean (±SE) Anthropometric Values for the
Control and Injury Groups

Parameter	C	SS	PF	ITBFS
Sit and reach (cm)	44.35 (2.13)	43.66 (1.96)	48.84 (1.93)	48.59 (2.46)
Plantar flexion ROM (degrees)	56.58 (2.09)	60.24 (2.63)	63.67 (1.50)	58.69 (2.37)
Dorsiflexion ROM (degrees)	19.26 (1.27)	16.53 (1.27)	19.07 (1.65)	16.31 (1.09)
Q angle (degrees)	13.58 (1.30)	14.12 (1.07)	13.00 (1.46)	15.92 (1.15)
Foot print	0.31 (0.03)	0.28 (0.03)	0.30 (0.04)	0.24 (0.04)

Groups: C, control; SS, shin splints; PF, plantar fasciitis; ITBFS, iliotibial band friction syndrome.
ROM, range of motion.
(Courtesy of Messier SP, Pittala KA: Med Sci Sports Exerc 20:501–505, October 1988.)

TABLE 2.—Percent of Subjects With Abnormal Flexibility
and Leg Length Differences

Parameter	C	SS	PF	ITBFS
Hamstring flexibility (% abnormal)	47	47	47	31
Lower leg flexibility (% abnormal)	32	29	20	31
Leg length difference (% >0.64 cm)	21	29	53	38

Groups: C, controls; SS, shin splints; PF, plantar fasciitis; ITBFS, iliotibial band friction syndrome.
(Courtesy of Messier SP, Pittala KA: Med Sci Sports Exerc 20:501–505, October 1988.)

Injuries most often associated with running are those classified as overuse syndromes. Many studies have tried to document the etiologic factors associated with certain running injuries, but most are based on expert opinion or are descriptive. Thus there is a need to establish whether a certain combination of biomechanical, anthropometric, and training variables is related to certain injuries. Whether there is a relationship among selected biomechanical, anthropometric, and training variables and iliotibial (IT) band friction syndrome, shin splints, and plantar fasciitis was investigated in competitive and recreational runners. Nineteen individuals comprised an uninjured control group; 13, an IT band friction syndrome injury group; 17, a shin splint injury group; and 15, a plantar fasciitis injury group.

According to discriminant function analysis, there were 2 significant discriminators between the control and shin splint groups—maximum pronation velocity and maximum pronation. Plantar flexion range of motion was a significant discriminator between the control and plantar fasciitis groups (Tables 1 and 2). Nonsignificant trends between the injury and control groups also were identified: Maximum pronation, total rearfoot motion, and maximum velocity of pronation were greater in the injured groups; injured persons had a trend toward a higher arch; dorsiflexion range of motion was decreased in the shin splint group; more injured runners had a leg length difference; more runners in the injury groups ran hills; and more runners in the IT band friction syndrome group ran on crowned roads.

▶ The authors try to help us find which factors may cause a specific injury in runners. There was one significant finding and a number of trends that were discovered. The study points out the need to evaluate runners biomechanically to determine if some of these factors exist. If a problem is found it may possibly be corrected with strengthening and flexibility exercises and, if necessary, the use of orthotics.—F.J. George, ATC, PT

Management of Overuse Injuries
Puffer JC, Zachazewski JE (Univ of California, Los Angeles)
Am Fam Physician 38:225–232, September 1988   3–35

Overuse syndromes are increasingly seen as more Americans exercise regularly. Repeated microtrauma accumulates over time and leads to local tissue destruction and inflammation. The pain and dysfunction that result constitute overuse; its most frequent form is tendinitis. A functional classification of pain (Table 1) can be a useful guide to management. Overuse injury or tendinitis usually responds well to conservative management (Table 2).

Vigorous physical therapy is the key part of treating overuse syndromes involving the muscle-tendon unit. Active rest should be attempted before passive rest. Absolute rest or immobilization is appropriate only for the most severe, chronic cases of tendinitis and only after active rest has failed. Nonsteroidal anti-inflammatory drugs may relieve pain, but

TABLE 1.—Functional Classification of Pain

Classification	Characteristics
Type 1	Pain after activity only
Type 2	Pain during activity, not restricting performance
Type 3	Pain during activity, restricting performance
Type 4	Chronic, unremitting pain

(Courtesy of Puffer JC, Zachazewski JE: *Am Fam Physician* 38:225–232, September 1988.)

TABLE 2.—Management of Overuse Injuries

Type 1 pain
1. Reduction in workload (25 percent)
2. Ice massage after activity
3. Stretching program
4. Physical therapy and rehabilitation

Type 2 pain
1. Reduction in workload (50 percent)
2. Ice massage after activity
3. Stretching program
4. Physical therapy and rehabilitation
5. Nonsteroidal anti-inflammatory agents

Type 3 pain
1. Complete rest
2. Physical therapy and rehabilitation
3. Nonsteroidal anti-inflammatory agents
4. Judicious use of injectable steroids

Type 4 pain
1. Exhaustion of all conservative therapy modalities
2. Consideration of surgical intervention

(Courtesy of Puffer JC, Zachazewski JE: *Am Fam Physician* 38:225–232, September 1988.)

they do not dispel the underlying cause of symptoms. If these drugs are ineffective, topical or injected steroids may be tried. Various physical methods (e.g., application of ice or heat, electrical stimulation, and deep friction massage) may be helpful at various stages of healing.

Strong, flexible tissues are best able to adapt to loads without sustaining structural damage. Starting with isometric exercise in pain-free positions, rehabilitation progresses toward the lengthened position, followed by isotonics based on an eccentric exercise program. The key is a progressive increase in the velocity of exercise. Pain is the best guide to progress. Proper physical therapy not only speeds recovery but also helps to prevent chronicity and recurrence.

▶ The authors repeatedly stress the importance of therapeutic exercise in the management of overuse injuries. Improper training techniques may be the cause of most of these injuries. Training methods must be examined as closely as the treatment regimen to prevent recurrence of the injury. The author states that the key in rehabilitation of these injuries is progressive exercise, and that pain is the best guide to progress.—F.J. George, ATC, PT

The Effect of Differential Training on Isokinetic Muscular Endurance During Acute Thermally Induced Hypohydration
Caterisano A, Camaione DN, Murphy RT, Gonino VJ (Furman Univ, Greenville, SC; Univ of Connecticut, Storrs)
Am J Sports Med 16:269–273, May–June 1988   3–36

Hypohydration, whether a result of exercise, thermal regimens, or both, limits work capacity. Previous studies on muscular endurance and hypohydration yielded conflicting results. The effect of acute thermal hypohydration on muscle endurance performance was investigated in 3 groups of differentially trained persons.

Group I included 6 anaerobically trained athletes, group II included 5 aerobically trained athletes, and group III included 6 sedentary persons. Experimental trials consisted of maximal leg extensions on a Cybex II dynamometer under conditions of euhydration and hypohydration of −3% body weight. Integrated electromyographic data were collected during each trial. The maximum number of leg extension repetitions performed at or above 50% of each person's peak torque output were compared between treatments and among groups.

There was a significant decrease in muscle endurance when euhydration was compared with hypohydration among the anaerobically trained individuals as well as among sedentary individuals. In the aerobically trained athletes no significant decline was noted in muscle endurance when comparing performance under both experimental conditions.

Training adaptations that occur with aerobic conditioning and are associated primarily with increased plasma volume may be the key to explaining these results. These findings suggest that aerobic training in the off-season and preseason training periods may prepare athletes to withstand the effects of hypohydration.

▶ This study proves that we have another good reason to include aerobic training in preseason and off-season conditioning programs. When football practice begins in August, many problems arise that are associated with hypohydration. Aerobic training during the preceding summer months will not only acclimate the athletes to exercising in the heat but, through increases in blood plasma, may also reduce the effects of hypohydration.

If this article is read in conjunction with Abstract 9–2, the reader will see that there is strong evidence that aerobic training in the form of a 2-mile run benefits VO_{2max} and reduces the effects of hypohydration.—F.J. George, ATC, PT

The Influence of High-Velocity Resistance Circuit Training on Aerobic Power
Petersen SR, Miller GD, Quinney HA, Wenger HA (Univ of Alberta, Edmonton; Univ of Victoria, BC)
J Orthop Sports Phys Ther 9:339–343, April 1988   3–37

Many athletes use resistance training to enhance their muscular strength and power, but it has not generally been used to improve aerobic power. The influence of high-velocity resistance circuit training on maximal aerobic power was investigated in 27 trained men, 16 of whom underwent additional training; 11 served as controls.

The training group exercised for two 20-second sets at each of 6 stations of a hydraulic, variable resistance apparatus over 2–3 circuits, maintaining an exercise to relief ratio of 1:2 in each circuit. The men trained 4 times a week for 5 weeks. The resistance at each station was adjusted as needed to maintain consistent angular limb velocities of about 3.2 rad per second.

The maximal oxygen uptake ($\dot{V}O_{2max}$) for the training group was increased by 9.5% when expressed in either absolute or relative terms. No changes were seen in the control group. Oxygen consumption responses measured over 2 circuits for 6 men in the training group averaged 61% and 57% of $\dot{V}O_{2max}$ for exercise and relief intervals, respectively.

This relatively brief program of hydraulic resistance circuit training significantly increased the $\dot{V}O_{2max}$ of previously trained men. The hydraulic circuit resistance program described may elicit a metabolic intensity sufficient to improve aerobic power, even in previously trained persons.

▶ This study proves that if the training regimen is aerobic in nature and of a sufficient intensity, $\dot{V}O_{2max}$ can be improved using high-velocity hydraulic resistance circuit training. We are often looking for "other" methods of increasing $\dot{V}O_{2max}$, not only to prevent training boredom but also to prevent overuse injuries. The authors have outlined a method that may be used as an alternative workout for many sports.—F.J. George, ATC, PT

Residual Muscular Swelling After Repetitive Eccentric Contractions
Fridén J, Sfakianos PN, Hargens AR, Akeson WH (Univ of Umeå, Sweden; VA Med Ctr, San Diego; Univ of California, San Diego)
J Orthopaed Res 6:493–498, 1988   3–38

Much has been written about delayed muscle soreness (DMS), but its exact mechanism is still debated. The most predictable way of pruducing DMS is to subject the muscles to eccentric contractions. The morphological changes that occur after eccentric exercise were differentiated and correlated with intramuscular pressure readings.

Eight healthy men exercised their right lower leg anterior compartment eccentrically and their left concentrically. Four-hundred submaximal contractions were performed in each exercise regimen over a 20-minute period against a load corresponding to 15% of the individual's maximal dorsiflexion torque. Tissue fluid pressures were measured by the slit-catheter method before, during, and after exercise and 48 hours later. Needle biopsy specimens of both anterior tibialis muscles were obtained 48 hours after cessation of exercise.

Overall morphology of the specimens showed a greater cross-sectional fiber area in the eccentrically exercised muscle compared with the concentrically exercised muscle. There was little evidence of inflammation, and no fiber necrosis was observed. Fiber type proportions were equal on both sides; type 1 fiber was biased. Extremely large type 2 fibers were noted in 4 of 8 individuals from the eccentric specimens. This incidence correlated with the length of time to return to resting pressure after eccentric exercise. The percentage of water content was significantly higher in eccentrically exercised muscles.

Muscle fiber swelling is a predominant feature after eccentric exercise and is directly associated with delayed muscle soreness. The eccentric muscle averaged about 3% more water content than the concentric muscle, which supports the belief that muscle fiber swelling as a result of myofibrillar damage is a major component in the development of DMS. Patients with DMS should avoid repetitive contractions of the same magnitude as those that induced the soreness. When muscles are sore after exercise, a moderate exercise level is suggested to dissipate edematous tissue.

▶ There has been some controversy over the causes of DMS. The authors state that swelling of the muscle fibers caused by myofibrillar damage is a major component of this pain. It is generally agreed that more of this soreness accompanies eccentric than concentric exercise. A light workout when the muscles are sore may dissipate some of the swelling and alleviate the soreness.—F.J. George, ATC, PT

The Effects of Constant External Resistance Exercise and Isokinetic Exercise Training on Work-Induced Hypertrophy
Pearson DR, Costill DL (Ball State Univ, Muncie, Ind)
J Appl Sport Sci Res 2:39–41, August–September 1988   3–39

At present, progressive constant external resistance exercise (CERE) is most often used in strength training by coaches and athletes. Isokinetic training with the Cybex device is a relatively new form of training in which limb motion is kept at a preset velocity and increased self-generated exertion receives increased resistance. Training-induced hypertrophy of the knee extensors was compared before and after these 2 training methods in 6 men (mean age, 26 years). Training with CERE was carried out before isokinetic training.

There were nearly twice as many isokinetic contractions as CERE repetitions when exercise sessions were equated by total torque production. The CERE-trained thigh gained significant strength compared with the isokinetically trained thigh when tested on a CERE lifting device. Whereas the thigh trained isokinetically gained significant strength at all test velocities (60, 180, 240 degrees/second), the CERE-trained thigh did not. After correcting for subcutaneous fat, only the CERE-trained thigh enlarged significantly.

Training with the CERE method appears to be superior to isokinetic training in producing thigh hypertrophy. Both muscle hypertrophy and strength change may be training specific.

▶ We have noticed results similar to those indicated in this study regarding "specificity of training" and hypertrophy. The authors explain that, "These results are not surprising in light of the dual mechanism by which a muscle may increase in strength. Initially, muscle strength gains are the results of neurological factors such as fiber recruitment; and later are due to an increased cross-sectional area of the muscle."—F.J. George, ATC, PT

Adherence to Sports-Injury Rehabilitation Programs
Fisher AC, Domm MA, Wuest DA (Ithaca College, Ithaca, NY; James Caldwell High School, West Caldwell, NJ)
Physician Sportsmed 16:47–51, July 1988   3–40

Adherence to rehabilitation programs is crucial to an injured athlete's ability to return to competition. Why some injured athletes adhere to their rehabilitation program and others do not was investigated in 41 college athletes, 21 men and 20 women, who had sustained sports-related injuries involving either the shoulder, the knee, or the ankle.

Each athlete had started a rehabilitation program of at least 6 weeks. A review of their rehabilitation records and consultation with their trainers revealed that 21 of them had adhered to their program and 20 had not. All 41 study participants completed a 40-item Rehabilitation Adherence Questionnaire that contained 6 scales pertaining to perceived exertion, pain tolerance, self-motivation, support from significant others, scheduling, and environmental conditions. These scales represent personal and situational factors previously shown to discriminate adherents from nonadherents in various contexts.

Statistical analysis of the data showed that support from significant others contributed most to adherence to rehabilitation programs. Adherents perceived that they worked harder at their rehabilitation than did nonadherents, but nonadherents also rated their efforts relatively high. Another deterrent to adherence was inconvenient scheduling. As expected, self-motivation played an important role. Also, adherents tolerated the pain and discomfort of rehabilitation better than did nonadherents. Environmental conditions were the least significant reasons for nonadherence.

▶ The authors make a point that we should all be very much aware of and that is: "The injured athletes who receive support from those around them, including their trainers, are more likely to adhere to their rehabilitation program than the athletes who receive less support." If the athletes know you care about their progress, they will be much more enthusiastic about their rehabilitation program.—F.J. George, ATC, PT

Mental Imagery and Its Potential for Physical Therapy
Warner L, McNeill ME (East Carolina Univ, Greenville, NC)
Phys Ther 68:516–521, April 1988   3–41

Mental imagery refers to the cognitive reproduction or visualization of an object, scene, or sensation as though it were occurring in reality. Mental practice is the symbolic rehearsal of a physical activity in the absence of any gross muscular movements. The sports and motor-learning literature on mental imagery and mental practice was reviewed to assess the feasibility of using these techniques as adjuncts to physical therapy.

Measurable evidence of reactions in the body's musculature during mental imagery has been reported in a number of studies. An early study found that individuals who imagined typing the alphabet showed increased action potentials in their arm muscles. In 1 study significantly greater increases in deltoid muscle activity measured by electromyography were noted in the right arm when the individual imagined lifting the right arm. Later studies on motor learning showed that skillfulness can be enhanced by using mental practice. In 1 study, individuals who mentally practiced basketball free throws or dart throwing demonstrated improved skills similar to those who practiced physically.

Mental imagery has also been used to treat patients with medically incurable cancer and an average life expectancy of 1 year. After participating in a mental imagery treatment regimen, 63 of 159 patients survived twice as long as a matched control population and 22% of them had no evidence of the disease. Biofeedback studies also support the concept that physical functioning can be altered by mental processes.

Mental practice is also used in the area of athletics. Injured or inactive players can continue to practice mentally when they are unable to participate physically in athletic activity. Mental practice is used to practice without making mistakes and to rehearse for desired results. In physical therapy, mental practice allows patients to visualize themselves performing physical movements in real-life situations, to practice with ease, and to envision outcomes beyond what is generally believed to be possible. One author recommends that patients who are recovering from injury or illness start practicing mentally to reduce recovery time. Another application is the use of mental exercises between physical therapy sessions. For instance, patients could visualize themselves using equipment such as pulleys, shoulder wheels, or weights.

A review of the literature supports a mind-body relationship and confirms the benefits of mental imagery. The use of mental imagery has the potential to be a viable tool in physical therapy if patients are motivated and show a willingness to step beyond their limited concepts about what is possible.

▶ I've had patients tell me that they thought about an activity many times after being unable to perform it in the previous treatment session. They were convinced that because of the many times they thought about doing it correctly it helped them to achieve success in the next treatment session.—F.J. George, ATC, PT

4 Epidemiology of Injuries

Epidemiology of Badminton Injuries
Jørgensen U, Winge S (Univ of Copenhagen)
Int J Sports Med 8:379–382, December 1987   4–1

Badminton is an increasingly popular sport that now is played at the professional level. Injuries were registered prospectively in 376 randomly selected elite and recreational badminton players, 81% of whom were followed.

The 257 injuries found resulted in an average of about 3 injuries per player per 1,000 playing hours. Men were injured more often than women were. Three fourths of injuries were related to overuse, and most of the rest were strains and sprains. Nearly 60% of the injuries involved the lower extremities. Only 2 players sustained eye injuries. Overuse injuries were more frequent in elite players than in recreational players. A large majority of the 24 back injuries resulted from overuse. There was only 1 Achilles tendon rupture in the series.

Badminton appears to cause fewer injuries than other popular sports do. Overuse injuries are most prominent. Stretching and better equipment may lower the occurrence of these injuries. Better shock-attenuating ability of equipment would reduce the load produced by the stereotyped movements used in badminton.

▶ This paper represents a rare report dealing with badminton injuries. It is interesting to note the difference in the anatomical distribution of injuries in elite and recreational players. Specifically, in the elite player, injuries are more frequent below the knee, whereas in the recreational player they occurred in the knee, groin, and upper extremities.—J.S. Torg, M.D.

The Mortality Experience of Major-League Baseball Players
Waterbor J, Cole P, Delzell E, Andjelkovich D (Univ of Alabama, Birmingham; Chemical Industry Inst of Toxicology, Research Triangle Park, NC)
N Engl J Med 318:1278–1280, May 12, 1988   4–2

An analysis of the rate and causes of death of American professional baseball players was done to determine whether the conditioning and training of professional athletes influence their length of life or cause of death. The cohort studied comprised all baseball players who played their first games for a professional major league baseball team between

1911 and 1915 and who survived until 1925. The study group included 985 players, all of whom were white.

Follow-up was successful on 958 men; 942 of these were dead. Standardized mortality ratios (SMRs) were calculated. The 10 major causes of death were arteriosclerotic heart disease, cancer, vascular lesions of the central nervous system, respiratory diseases, digestive system diseases, accidents, infective and parasitic diseases, genitourinary system diseases, diabetes mellitus, and suicide. An excess of deaths from cancers of the rectum and pancreas was noted. There was also an excess of deaths from gastric and duodenal ulcers. The total SMRs for length of career showed a weak trend, from 96 in those whose careers lasted for less than 1 to about 4 years to 84 in those with careers lasting 10–14 years. These data suggest that employment as a baseball player had a weak protective effect.

Being a baseball player may confer a minimally protective effect against death. The cohort had only 94% of the deaths expected on the basis of United States death rates for white men. Also, an inverse association of the SMR with length of career was noted. Players who performed best lived longest, and the men known at death as baseball players had the lowest overall mortality.

▶ The observation that baseball confers a "minimally protective effect against death" is interesting but without practical application. Of note, that despite the lower than expected mortality rate among baseball players, the mortality rate for arteriosclerotic heart disease in this group was statistically higher than that of the general population.—J.S. Torg, M.D.

A Study of Urban Bicycling Accidents

Tucci JJ, Barone JE (St Vincent's Hosp and Med Ctr, New York)
Am J Sports Med 16:181–184, March–April 1988   4–3

Because of the large number of bicycle accident victims treated in the emergency room, a study was undertaken to assess the type, frequency, and mechanism of occurrence of bicycle accidents. During a 10-month study period, 182 patients were involved in cycling accidents. Complete documentation was available for 37 female and 135 male patients; the average age was 28.3 years. Of these 172 patients, 153 were cyclists and 19 were pedestrians. Telephone interviews were conducted with 41 cyclists and 10 pedestrians.

The types of injuries sustained included 47 contusions, 34 fractures, 32 lacerations, 30 sprains, 16 abrasions, 9 cerebral concussions, and 4 miscellaneous injuries. There were 72 (42%) upper extremity injuries, 38 (22%) injuries to the head or cervical spine, 39 (23%) lower extremity injuries, 8 (5%) thoracic injuries, 6 (3.5%) lumbar spine injuries, 1 (0.6%) abdominal injury, and 8 (5%) injuries to other anatomical areas.

A review of the accident descriptions by the 51 interviewed patients revealed that 14 (27.5%) were struck by a moving motor vehicle when cycling, 13 (25.5%) had fallen from a bicycle, and 14 (27.5%) were pedestrians who had been struck by a bicycle. Weather and light conditions were not responsible for causing any of the accidents. Thirty-one of the 51 interviewed patients used no form of safety devices, 6 wore a helmet, and 3 wore a reflective vest or gloves. Twenty-nine of the interviewed patients were not at fault in the accident, whereas 11 accidents were caused by the cyclist's carelessness or disregard of traffic regulations.

In addition to an emergency room fee of $65.00, 75% of the patients required radiographic examination at an average cost of $49.00. Patients lost about 7 days of work because of their injury, with fractures accounting for most of the time away from work.

Modification of safety systems may prevent more of the morbidity associated with bicycling accidents and reduce the amount of time lost from work.

▶ This paper underscores the observation of others that bicycle accidents present a significant health problem. Kiburz et al. (1) observed that 500,000 bicycling accidents occur yearly in the United States and comprise the greatest recreational source of emergency room visits. Kruse and McBeath (2) determined that 29% percent of 1,200 randomly selected college students had been involved in an accident during the previous 3 years, with 13% within the immediate year. Interestingly, in the urban environment, 11% of the patients reported by Tucci et al. were pedestrians who were involved in a collision with a bicycle.

More recently, Selbst SM, et al. (3) pointed out that approximately 1,000 deaths resulting from bicycle injuries occur yearly, and that very few studies have been done regarding bicycle accidents and related injuries. Again, reporting on accidents occurring in an urban environment, Selbst reported that between April 1 and October 1, 1983, 10% of all trauma visits to the emergency room at his institution were related to bicycle accidents, with 80% of the patients being between the ages of 5 and 14 years. Clearly, such data establish bicycle-related injuries as a major health problem deserving initiation of appropriate epidemiologic and preventive measures.—J.S. Torg, M.D.

References

1. Kiburz D, et al: *Am J Sports Med* 14:416–419, 1986.
2. Kruse DL, McBeath AA: *Am J Sports Med* 8:342–344, 1980.
3. Selbst SM, et al: *Am J Dis Child* 141:140–144, 1987.

Indoor Cricket Injuries
Forward GR (Royal Perth Hosp, Australia)
Med J Aust 148:560–561, June 6, 1988   4–4

Indoor cricket is played in an enclosed area, surrounded by nylon netting with an all-purpose carpet floor covering that has a high coefficient of friction, with the ball reaching high velocities. All indoor cricket injuries seen at the emergency room at Royal Perth Hospital were evaluated.

Sixty-four patients sustained indoor cricket injuries, including 14 women aged 19–34 years. At the time of injury 72% were fielding and 17% were batting. The upper extremity was most frequently injured, and injury to the finger or thumb was most common. Injuries to the lower limb consisted mostly of grade I–II tears of the ankle and knee ligaments. Five wicket-keepers sustained eye injuries, and 3 others sustained fractured nasal bone. Other injuries were bruised or fractured ribs and shoulders and concussion. More than 50% of injured patients required time off work, with 30% requiring more than 1 week off work.

Injuries sustained while playing indoor cricket occur mostly in the upper extremities, particularly the finger or thumb. These injuries are commonly sustained by fit, young persons who are employed; consequently, time off work as a result of injury becomes significant. Precautions in terms of the technique of playing, wearing protective devices, and optimizing the shoe-surface interface need to be addressed.

▶ The preponderance of hand, eye, and facial injuries is noteworthy. Unfortunately, the data have not been presented in terms of injury rates and do not support the suggested precautionary measures.—J.S. Torg, M.D.

A Historical Perspective of Injuries in Professional Football: Twenty-Six Years of Game-Related Events
Nicholas JA, Rosenthal PP, Gleim GW (Nicholas Inst of Sports Medicine and Athletic Trauma, Lenox Hill Hosp, New York)
JAMA 260:939–944, Aug 19, 1988   4–5

A professional football franchise was studied consecutively from 1960 to 1985 for injuries incurred during regular season games. A "significant" injury caused a player to miss at least 2 consecutive regular season games, whereas a "major" injury caused a player to miss at least 8 games or the equivalent time.

There were 330 significant injuries and 130 major injuries sustained in the 373 regular-season games played. Significant injuries averaged 0.9 per game and major injuries averaged 0.35 per game. Over the entire 26 years there was a significant decline in both the number of significant injuries per game and major injuries per game. However, excluding the high injury rate before 1965, the number of significant injuries was episodic with time, whereas the number of major injuries declined significantly.

Since the team's first games on synthetic surfaces in 1968, the rates of significant or major injuries per game did not differ between those played on grass or artificial turf. The lower extremity, particularly the knee, sustained the most injuries of any site. However, since 1969 there has been a major decline in major knee injuries, whereas the number of significant knee injuries did not change. Major injury rates did not differ among offensive, defensive, and special-team plays, but the rates of major injury on special-team play declined significantly from 1969 to 1985.

Contrary to the high injury rates and more serious injuries perceived by the media, there was a decline in game-related significant and major injuries in this professional football team. Significant injuries showed no trend with time, whereas major injuries, particularly those sustained by the knee, have declined with time.

▶ The conclusion that there has been a decrease in the rate of both significant and major injuries must be questioned. This is in view of the fact that the authors have failed to report these injuries in terms of anatomical parts involved and degrees of tissue disruption. Certainly, when injuries are reported in the manner presented, i.e., on a time loss basis, other factors can affect this parameter, including a less conservative approach on the part of trainers and physicians, improved surgical techniques (ie, arthroscopy vs arthrotomy), and perhaps most important, the obsolescence of the 5–1 knee reconstruction.—J.S. Torg, M.D.

An Epidemiologic and Traumatologic Study of Injuries in Handball
Nielsen AB, Yde J (Aarhus County Hosp; Municipal Hosp, Aarhus, Denmark)
Int J Sports Med 9:341–344, October 1988   4–6

Handball is a popular team sport in Europe, and is reported to be the second most important reason for sports injuries. To understand the risk factors involved in the sport, 221 handball players were followed during a single indoor season in a prospective study. The players included those in both senior and youth divisions. They were surveyed before the season, at the end of play, and at the 6-month follow-up. Injuries that prevented a player from participating in the next game or practice were recorded.

Ninety-one players sustained 105 injuries, 37% of which occurred during practice. Sprains accounted for 61% of all injuries, with sprains of the fingers and ankles being most common. Women and girls were more likely to have ankle injuries, and girls had the highest risk of reinjury. Only men incurred fractures. Contact with another player caused 31% of injuries, and 18% resulted from contact with the ball. Noncontact injuries included some overuse injuries; many occurred during running (29%) or shooting (20%). Offensive movement had a greater association with injury (50%) than did defensive positions (20%).

Absences longer than 1 month were caused by 20% of the injuries, with the knee accounting for the longest removal from play. At the 6-month follow-up, 4 players were found to be unable to return to handball. The overall injury rate, lower than previous estimations, was 4.6 per 1,000 playing hours and 11.4 per 1,000 game hours. This may result from the fact that actual playing time for each team member was not calculated. Many injuries were not treated by a physician. Because rehabilitation was not complete at the time of reentry into play, reinjury was common.

Both prevention and treatment can be improved, and better knowledge of sports injuries, taping procedures, and rehabilitation could decrease the incidence and long-term effects of injuries in handball.

The Risks of Injury in Public Ice Skating
Radford PJ, Williamson DM, London IMR (John Radcliffe Hosp, Oxford, England)
Br J Sports Med 22:78–80, June 1988   4–7

Public ice skating has recently become more popular. A prospective study of the injuries sustained by members of a well-established ice rink in a major city was undertaken to help define plans for health service resources.

Of the 8,361 patients who presented to the Accident Service of the John Radcliffe Hospital, 80 had been injured at the ice rink, for an incidence rate of less than 1%. Minor tissue injuries (e.g., bruises, lacerations, and sprains) commonly affected the upper and lower extremities in 51 patients. Twenty-three patients had 23 definite fractures, 2 had dislocations, and 1 had tendon dislocation; only 2 patients required hospital admission. Serious injuries tended to result from a fall, usually without collision with another skater.

There were 82,193 attendances at the ice rink. The overall risk of injury requiring attention was 0.31%, which was less than the reported 0.38% risk when the ice rink was newly opened to the public. More impressively, the rate of serious injury declined from 0.14% to 0.03% of all attendances. The First-Aid team at the ice rink dealt primarily with minor soft tissue injuries, and less than 1% of the total attendances seen at the Accident Service were patients from the ice rink.

These data show that injuries sustained during public ice skating are relatively minor, and the number of serious injuries is low. Increased safety measures at the rink, as well as the increased experience of the staff, accounted for the reduced rate of serious injuries in public ice skating. The development of properly trained first-aid teams at ice rinks is recommended as this produces definite savings in health service resources.

▶ This is one of the few reports dealing with the occurrence of injury among recreational ice skaters. The authors have based their "incidence rate" on records of the accident service of the John Radcliffe Hospital. They observed a decreased incidence when current figures were compared with a study from the same rink previously performed. They also note that ". . .the increased experience of the staff at the rink has led to greater treatment by first-aiders alone of trivial injuries. . .". Thus the reported decrease in the occurrence of injuries based on hospital records may well be attributable to the activity of the first-aiders rather than a true reduction. In view of the potential for litigation, it is doubtful that public skating rinks in the United States will entertain the notion of becoming involved in the health care business as they appear to have done in Great Britain.—J.S. Torg, M.D.

Incidence, Nature, and Causes of Ice Hockey Injuries: A Three-Year Prospective Study of a Swedish Elite Ice Hockey Team

Lorentzon R, Wedrèn H, Pietilä T (Univ Hosp of Umeå, Sweden)
Am J Sports Med 16:392–396, July–August 1988   4–8

The incidence of injury appears to be high in ice hockey; however because no prospective study with closely controlled clinical examination and continuous registration of injuries has been done, the real incidence of hockey injuries of different severity is unknown. The risk of injuries in a Swedish ice hockey team in relation to exposure was investigated, and the nature and causes of these injuries were assessed in a prospective study, with daily attendance of the same orthopedic surgeon during practice sessions and games. The players were subsidized amateurs on an elite level team. All injuries that occurred during on-ice practice or games during a 3-year period were recorded. The players had a median age of 24 years. An injury was recorded when it caused the player to miss the next practice or game. Minor lacerations or other low-level injuries were not included. Injuries were classified as minor, moderate, or major, and as traumatic or overuse injuries.

Of the 95 injuries recorded, 72 (76%) occurred during games and 23 (24%) during practice. Sixty-nine injuries were judged to be minor; only 8 were major. The game injury rate was 39.2/1,000 player game hours for goalkeepers, 107.8 for defensemen, and 71.8 for forwards. A Swedish elite ice hockey team player can statistically be expected to sustain, 3 minor injuries each year, 1.4 moderate injuries every other year, and 1 major injury every third year. Chances of injury are considerably lower during practice. Overall, 80% of injuries were caused by trauma and 20% by overuse. Contusions, strains, and sprains were the most common types of injuries, and complete tears of the medial collateral ligament of the knee were the most common severe injuries. The 19 overuse injuries were largely adductor and patellar tendinitis. Player contact caused most of the injuries, and foul play was involved in 39% of them.

The individual incidence of injury, 1.4 per 1,000 practice hours, is lower than that associated with soccer, which has an incidence of 7.6 per 1,000 hours. The most common major injuries might be avoided by enforcement of rules against stick violations. Facial injuries can be prevented by wearing a visor during practice as well as games. Although many of these injuries are superficial, serious eye wounds can occur.

Injuries in International Ice Hockey: A Prospective Comparative Study of Injury Incidence and Injury Types in International and Swedish Elite Ice Hockey

Lorentzon R, Wedrèn H, Pietilä T, Gustavsson B (Univ Hosp of Umeå, Sweden)
Am J Sports Med 16:389–391, July–August 1988   4–9

Ice hockey players are at risk for injuries caused by forceful contact with other players, the puck, and sticks. International ice hockey, with its more intense play, was assumed to be more hazardous than national level play. The incidence, nature, and mechanisms of injury in the Swedish national hockey team during 40 international games were studied prospectively. Data on national hockey injuries were compared with international data. The same orthopedic surgeon was present during all games.

During 1984 and 1985 the Swedish national ice hockey team played 40 international games. Injuries that caused the player to miss the next game or practice were recorded. Nineteen injuries occurred during the study period, 7 of which were injuries to the knee (4) or thigh (3). Player contact and intentional tackling caused 14 of the injuries, half a result of foul play.

An individual player had an incidence of injury of 79.2 per 1,000 player-game hours, which was almost identical to the incidence in national games of 78.4 per 1,000 game hours. Although international games are more intense, injuries may not be increased because of the players' higher level of skill, training, and experience. Defensemen were more vulnerable to injury in national play, but in this study forwards had an injury rate 3 times as high as defense players.

Facial lacerations occurred 3.3 times more frequently in Swedish international hockey than in Swedish elite hockey. Stick contact was responsible for 82.3% of facial wounds and elbowing for 11.8%. Although such injuries are mainly superficial, serious eye injuries can occur. The use of visors and strict enforcement of rules can prevent many of these injuries.

▶ The 2 preceding abstracts describe a sound epidemiologic approach to identifying injury problems and present proven preventive methods. Specifically, the data strongly suggest that 47% of the facial injuries could have been prevented by wearing a face shield or visor. However, the authors have failed to deal with the observation of Tator et al. (1) that the advent of the hockey helmet and visor in Canada was associated with a concomitant increase in catastrophic injuries to the cervical spine and cord.—J.S. Torg, M.D.

Reference

1. Tator CH, Edmonds VE: *Can Med Assoc J* 130:875–880, 1984.

Martial Arts Injuries: The Results of a Five-Year National Survey
Birrer RB, Halbrook SP (Geisenger Med Ctr, Danville Pa; Fairfax, Va)
Am J Sports Med 16:408–410, July–August, 1988   4–10

Martial arts are estimated to have at least 1 million participants in the United States, but little research has been reported on the risk of injuries in the sport. A 5-year national survey was conducted using data from the National Electronic Injury Surveillance System that were gathered from a sample of hospitals statistically representative of emergency departments in the United States.

From 1980 through 1984, 1,916 injuries were reported, for an estimated 105, 253 injuries, or 16.9 per 100,000 population. Men sustained 75% of the injuries, although the proportion of men and women participating in the sport is not known. Further, 95% of the injuries were mild to moderate, and most involved the lower extremities (47%), upper extremities (27%), or trunk (18%). Contusions and abrasions and sprains and strains made up approximately two thirds of reported injuries. Of 102 serious injuries 18 required hospitalization and included grade III concussions, retinal hemorrhages, and fractures.

Martial arts is a sport with a low risk for injury. Its estimated rate of 16.9 injuries per 100,000 population compares well, for example, with the rates for football (167), most aquatic activities (46), and basketball (188). Nevertheless, wearing protective gear and having supervision during participation are recommended to avoid potential injury.

▶ Utilizing data from the National Electronic Injury Surveillance System (NEISS), the authors conclude that the martial arts, when compared with other contact activities, are associated with a low risk for injury. However, they also recognize that the estimated risk of injury reported is appreciably less than that observed in other studies. Specifically, McLatchie (1) reported 1 injury for every 4 fights and 1 disabling injury for every 10 fights. Similarly, Birrer and Birrer (2) estimated the risk of serious injury to be 200 per 100,000. It appears to this observer that the reliability of the NEISS data and the manner in which the data were handled must be questioned.—J.S. Torg, M.D.

References

1. McLatchie GR: *Injury* 8:132–134, 1976.
2. Birrer RB, Birrer CD: *Physician Sports Med* 10:103–108, 1982.

Paragliding Injuries: Report of 100 Cases
Reymond MA, de Gottrau Ph, Fournier PE, Arnold T, Jacomet H, Rigo M (Hopital de District, Monthey; Swiss Air Ambulance Service, Zürich)
Chirurg 59:777–781, November 1988   4–11

Because paragliding equipment is inexpensive, lightweight, and easy to transport, the sport is rapidly gaining in popularity in Europe. During the first half of 1987, no less than 1,000 paragliders passed their pilot's test. It is estimated that there are presently about 7,000 paragliders in Switzerland. Concomitantly, the number of paragliding accidents has also increased, with 5 fatalities since 1987. The number of injured paragliders treated in the emergency department of the Monthey hospital increased from 3 in 1985, 11 in 1986, to 25 in 1987, for a total of 39. In 1987 the Swiss Air Ambulance Service transported 61 injured paragliders, 4 of whom had sustained fatal injuries. The records of these 100 injured paragliders, who sustained 138 injuries, were studied retrospectively.

The patients were classified by severity of injury into 4 categories, ranging from grade 1, defined as slight injuries treated on an outpatient basis, to grade 4, denoting fatal injuries. Six patients involved in accidents were not injured. There were 57 (41%) injuries to the lower extremities, 36 (26%) spinal injuries, 8 of which included neurologic trauma, 28 (20%) head injuries, 9 (7%) upper extremity injuries, and 8 (6%) torso injuries. Several patients had calcaneal fractures, usually caused by wearing improper footwear. Most of the serious accidents occurred immediately after takeoff, but the majority of injuries occurred during landing.

Only 8 of the 39 patients were licensed; the other 31 (79%) did not yet have their license. Two paragliders had not had any formal training; the other 37 had had flying lessons. Only 15% of the gliders were wearing safety helmets when the accident occurred. Among the injured patients transported by the Swiss Air Ambulance Service, only 31% had passed their pilot's test, 64% had received training but had not yet passed the test, and 5% had not received any formal training.

These findings demonstrate that paragliders need better training programs, need to be more aware of the risks they are taking, and that takeoff sites should be made safer.

▶ Based on the data presented in this paper, an annual fatality rate of 23/ 100,000 paragliders is estimated. By any standards, this is extraordinarily high. Most accidents in this series were judged to be related to pilot error, and none was caused by failure of the material. Significant observations are that most of the severe injuries occurred immediately after takeoff, whereas the most frequent injuries occurred during landing. Also, there was a correlation between the altitude, wind velocity, and severity of the injuries. This article documents those areas where preventive measures are indicated.—J.S. Torg, M.D.

A Review of Intra-Articular Knee Injuries in Racquet Sports Diagnosed by Arthroscopy
Marans HJ, Kennedy DK, Kavanagh TG, Wright TA (Toronto Western Hosp Sports Medicine Inst)
Can J Surg 31:199–201, May 1988   4–12

Reports on injuries sustained during racquet sports have emphasized facial and upper extremity injuries. Because of the recent increase in knee injuries related to racquet sports, a retrospective study of racquet-sports-related injuries treated over a 5-year period was undertaken.

Of the 404 racquet-sports related injuries, 222 (55%) involved a knee. The mean patient age at presentation was 32.8 years (range, 14–68 years). Two thirds of the patients were male. More than 85% of the patients sustained knee injuries by a twisting mechanism. Almost 50% of the patients consulted a physician within 2 weeks and more than 90% within 3 months of injury.

Arthroscopy, performed in 121 knees, revealed 202 intraarticular lesions in 128 procedures. Meniscal lesions were most common (60%), almost 50% of which were of the oblique or flap type. Medial meniscal tears were frequent and the posterior horn was the most common site of injury. The other lesions were chondromalacia patellae, anterior cruciate ligament injuries, chondral lesions, and pathologic plicae. Arthroscopic surgical procedures included soft tissue resections (37%), articular cartilage shaving (24%), lavage (20%), and trimming (6%). Open operative procedures were required in only 11 knees. During an average follow-up of 27.2 months, 91% of the patients returned to their sport within 3 months of arthroscopy, particularly those with meniscal lesions, chondral lesions, or pathologic plicae, and 80% had regained their preinjury performance level.

These data show that a substantial number of racquet sports injuries occur to the lower extremity, particularly the knee. The use of arthroscopy, rather than the traditional open procedures, plays a major role in the early and successful treatment of these injuries.

▶ Understandably, the authors were not able to present their data in terms of injury rates. Also, their supposition that a recent increase has occurred in knee injuries related to racquet sports is conjectural. If anything, this paper seems to indicate that there has been an increase in the diagnosis of knee injuries in racquet sports with the advent of the arthroscope.—J.S. Torg, M.D.

Injuries in Sailboard Enthusiasts

McCormick DP, Davis AL (Univ of Texas, Galveston)
Br J Sports Med 22:95–97, September 1988   4–13

Sailboarding has increased in popularity as a recreational sport. To determine the rate and types of injuries sustained by boardsailors, 51 men and 22 women admitted for injuries were interviewed.

The mean age of the men was 26 years and that of the women, 28 years. Most described themselves as novice or intermediate sailors. Ten men had gone sailboarding in a 40-knot wind before the arrival of a hurricane.

Minor injuries (e.g., lacerations, sprains, and abrasions) occurred in 73% of the patients. Significant injuries—those requiring treatment by a physician or resulting in the loss of 1 or more days at the sport—were reported by 15%. Women sustained more types of injuries and more significant injuries per 1,000 participant hours: this may have been a result of less experience and conditioning.

The rate of significant injury was 0.22/1,000 participant hours, which places sailboarding in the middle range for injury risk. Those who sail in high winds experience more serious injuries. Many injuries can be prevented by proper training, conditioning, wearing protective gear, using a sunscreen, and using ear drops. As with other water sports, epileptics should be warned of the dangers of a seizure while in or near the water.

▶ This is one of the few reports in the literature dealing with injuries resulting from boardsailing. Of interest is the fact that the authors, members of the faculty of the University of Texas in Galveston, reporting on injuries that occurred in Texas, published the material in the *British Journal of Sports Medicine*. Of note, they have appeared to coin the phrase "hurricane sailors" for those sailboarding in a 40-knot wind of a hurricane. The observation that recreational sailboarding is a relatively safe sport with a low rate of significant injuries is somewhat contradicted by Ullis and Anno (1) and Habal (2), who reported intervertebral disk herniations, significant fractures, cerebral concussions, pneumothorax, cervical spine fractures, cruciate ligament injury, and a drowning death.—J.S. Torg, M.D.

References

1. Ullis KC, Anno K: *Physician Sports Med* 12:86–93, 1984.
2. Habal MB: *J Fla Med Assoc* 73:609–612, 1986.

Skiing Accidents in the Past 15 Years
Matter P, Ziegler WJ, Holzach P (Hosp of Davos, Davos-Platz, Switzerland; Inst for Research Planning, Bettingen, Switzerland)
J Sports Sci 5:319–326, Winter 1987   4–14

Data on alpine skiing accidents in the Davos-Klosters area of Switzerland were reviewed for the past 15 years. Changes in the type of injuries, factors leading to accidents, and ways of lowering the rate of ski-related injuries were analyzed.

About 20 years ago alpine skiing accidents involved mostly below-the-knee fractures. Changes in equipment, especially safety bindings, lowered these figures. But knee injuries, previously rare, now account for half of the lower extremity injuries and about one fourth of injuries overall. Upper extremity injuries are also on the increase, from 17% of all skiing injuries in 1972 to 35% in 1986. A decline was seen, however, in the average injury severity.

A Swiss study on skiing safety revealed that only 32% of bindings had a tolerable frontal release setting. Only 17% of bindings were set to the torsional release values recommended by the Swiss Council for Accident Prevention.

Overall, the number of long-term disabilities resulting from skiing are relatively few. To increase safety, skiers should set safety bindings properly and review skiing techniques. The prevalence of knee injuries suggests that binding release mechanisms need to be improved.

▶ This paper substantiates recent observations that improved equipment, i.e., boots and ski bindings, has resulted in a decrease in tibia and fibular fractures. However, a concomitant increase in knee injuries, as documented by this paper, has been observed. There is a dichotomy in the views expressed by the authors that should be noted. Specifically, they point out that, "According to the statistics of the National Accidents Insurance Company of Switzerland, 28% of the cost of all sporting accidents was due to skiing accidents in the period 1968–1972. This number has decreased to 21% during the observation period 1978–1982." They then go on to conclude, "There is no reason to speak of a high accident risk in Alpine skiing." There appears to be an inconsistency in these 2 statements. Also, they state that ". . .permanent disorders after head injuries are exceptionally rare." Unless they do not consider death a "permanent disorder," this statement is not in keeping with recent experience in the United States.—J.S. Torg, M.D.

Frequency and Aetiology of Injury in Cross-Country Skiing
Steinbrück K (Sportklinik Stuttgart-Bad Cannstatt, West Germany)
J Sports Sci 5:187–196, Winter 1987   4–15

The number of cross-country skiers in West Germany has been growing steadily during recent years. This trend has led to an increased number of injuries associated with the sport. However, the available literature does not contain much information on the frequency, type, and etiology of typical cross-country ski injuries. The records of orthopedic nonhospitalized patients who sustained either downhill or cross-country ski injuries were analyzed.

During a 15-year study period, 13,296 individuals sustained orthopedic sports injuries; 1,263 were downhill skiers and 85 were cross-country skiers. Most of the injuries in downhill skiers involved the lower extremities (77%), whereas most of the injuries in cross-country skiers were to the upper extremities (47.7%). Injuries to the head and trunk were rare. The shoulder was affected in 25% of the patients. The most frequent injuries in cross-country skiing were contusions (31.8%), whereas in downhill skiers 37.8% of the injuries were distortions, torn ligaments (22.8%), or fractures (22.2%). Further, 57% of the downhill skiers were younger than age 30 years and 87% of the cross-country skiers were at least age 30 years. Of the injured cross-country skiers, 5.9% were older than age 70 years. The total number of cross-country skiing injuries was slightly but not significantly higher for women, who also had more ruptures of tendons and more contusions than men.

Lack of skill was a common cause of injury in cross-country skiers, as the sport requires no particular training. Many cross-country skiers were unfit or overweight. Typical causes of injury included falling on steep terrain or icy or badly damaged lanes, or getting a ski stuck in the snow. Cross-country skiing injuries can be prevented with good equipment, a good state of fitness, appropriate choice of cross-country courses, and cross-country skiing lessons to learn proper techniques.

▶ The fact that this report was limited to injuries occurring in "orthopedic nonhospitalized patients" seen over a 15-year period at the Orthopaedic University Hospital in Heidelburg and at the Sports Clinic in Stuttgart-Bad Cannstatt precludes an accurate determination of the frequency and risk of injury in cross-country skiing. The author points out that cross-country skiing is available to almost everyone without any particular training or preparation. Also, it is noted that Kruger and Alt (1) reported only a small number of deaths in middle-aged cross-country skiiers. However, it is doubtful that these deaths, as well as serious injuries and illness, would be forthcoming from data on injuries sustained by "orthopedic nonhospitalized patients."—J.S. Torg, M.D.

Reference

1. Kruger P, Alt M: *Beitraege zur Sportmedizin* 15:283–291, 1981.

Nordic Ski Jumping Fatalities in the United States: A 50-Year Summary
Wright JR Jr (Washington Univ)
J Trauma 28:848–851, June 1988   4–16

Nordic ski jumping competitions have been held in the United States for about 100 years. Six jumping fatalities occurred in the past 50 years, for an estimated fatality rate of about 12 deaths per 100,000 participants per year. The facts that jumping is well organized and jumpers are a tightly knit group make it likely that the list is complete. Takeoff speeds are about 60 mph on a 90-m jumping hill. Most deaths have involved young men who are highly skilled and capable of moving at high rates of speed.

Most downhill skiing and jumping fatalities result from head and neck injuries, but neck injuries probably are more typical of fatal jumping incidents, whereas head injuries predominate in downhill fatalities. Many fatalities associated with alpine skiing result from high-velocity impact with an immovable object such as a tree; jumping deaths are more likely to result from a fall.

▶ The contention of the author, based on deaths occurring in the United States, is that ski jumping fatalities are rare events. This is supported by data from Canada presented by Reed at the Second International Symposium on Catastrophic Neck Injuries Occurring in Sports held this past January at the University of Toronto.—J.S. Torg, M.D.

Injuries Associated With Downhill Sledding
Landsman IS, Knapp JF, Medina F, Sharma V, Wasserman GS, Walsh I (Children's Mercy Hosp, Kansas City, Mo)
Pediatr Emerg Care 3:277–280, December 1987   4–17

Sledding is a popular wintertime activity that is not without risk. During the winter of 1985–1986, 24 boys and 6 girls aged 5–16 years came to the emergency department with injuries related to downhill sledding. All 30 patients were treated during December 1985, which was unseasonably cold, snowy, and icy in Kansas City. There was no significant accumulation of snow for the remainder of the winter season. The records of these 30 patients were reviewed to identify risk factors associated with downhill sledding injuries.

One patient was injured while being pulled by a motorized 3-wheeler; the other 29 patients had been injured while downhill sledding. Six boys required admission because of abdominal trauma or head injuries, 4 of whom were admitted during the 2 weeks when conditions were most icy. One boy who had been inadvertently driven head first into a postal service mailbox died of brain stem herniation. One patient was riding a toboggan, 2 were sliding downhill on a cardboard box, and 27 were using a standard metal runner sled when the accidents occurred. All children were riding alone; 29 were unsupervised by an adult.

Analysis of the type of injuries sustained in association with downhill sledding led to several conclusions. Only sleds that allow for steering should be used. Pulling a sled with a motorized vehicle is extremely dangerous and should be completely avoided. Extreme caution should be observed during icy conditions, as the sled travels faster and is more difficult to control. A helmet would help to absorb impact to the head when riding downhill in the prone position. Heavy-duty gloves and boots would provide protection against serious distal extremity lacerations and abrasions. Observation of certain precautions may minimize injuries related to downhill sledding.

▶ To be noted, the data from this study indicate that older boys and teenage males are at greatest risk for sustaining downhill sledding injuries. The authors note that this is the same at-risk population identified in other unsupervised recreational activities, e.g., swimming, bicycling, and so on. Although the conclusions recommending specific preventive measures have not been subject to clinical evaluation, they are reasonable and appropriate. It appears that the major problem is getting this information out of the medical and into the lay literature.—J.S. Torg, M.D.

Softball Sliding Injuries: A Prospective Study Comparing Standard and Modified Bases

Janda DH, Wojtys EM, Hankin FM, Benedict ME (Univ of Michigan)
JAMA 259:1848–1850, March 25, 1988   4–18

A previous retrospective study revealed that base sliding was responsible for 71% of recreational injuries in softball. Altering base design may be a practical, reliable, cost-effective means of reducing sliding-related injuries. Because most injuries occur after rapid deceleration impact against stationary bases, quick-release bases might modify this mechanism of injury. Quick-release, or breakaway, bases were evaluated.

Breakaway bases are anchored by receiving holes fitting into grommets on a rubber mat that is flush with the infield surface (Fig 4–1). The rubber mat is anchored as a standard stationary base is. Softball teams were assigned to breakaway or standard-base fields on a random and rotating basis. In all, 633 games were played on breakaway-base fields and 627 on the standard stationary-base fields. Base-sliding injuries were recorded and analyzed.

During 2 seasons, 45 sliding injuries occurred on the stationary-base fields, whereas only 2 sliding injuries occurred on the breakaway-base fields. Of the 45 injuries sustained by players sliding into stationary

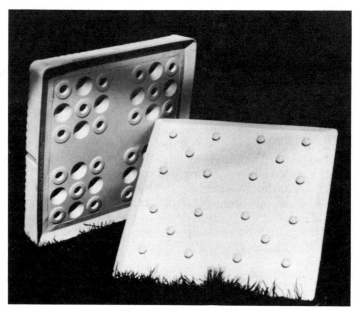

Fig 4–1.—Breakaway base is displayed. Two components fit together by small rubber grommets. (Courtesy of Janda DH, Wojtys EM, Hankin FM, et al: *JAMA* 259:1848–1850, March 25, 1988.)

bases, the lead foot or hand was involved in 43. Of these injuries, 53% involved the ankle. The 2 injuries occurring on breakaway bases were a nondisplaced medial malleolar fracture of the ankle and an ankle sprain; in both instances the bases failed to break away. Field supervisors believed that softball play was not significantly delayed by the use of breakaway bases, although sliding players broke away the bases up to 6 times per game.

Modifying bases can alter the pattern and frequency of sliding injuries in softball. Using breakaway bases could possibly result in a significant, cost-effective reduction of injuries.

▶ This is an excellent prospective study that clearly indicates the efficacy of the breakaway base in decreasing the rate of sliding injuries. Whether the data are presented as 1 injury occurring in every 14 games on stationary bases as opposed to 316 games on breakaway bases, or as a ratio of 23 injuries on stationary bases for every sliding-related injury on a breakaway base, the facts speak for themselves.—J.S. Torg, M.D.

Hand Injury Patterns in Softball Players Using a 16-Inch Ball
Degroot H III, Mass DP (Univ of Chicago)
Am J Sports Med 16:260–265, May–June 1988   4–19

Softball is a popular sport among men and women, but the 16-in. softball can cause a wide range of injuries, some of which may be multiple.

In a retrospective analysis of hand injuries caused by the impact of a 16-in. softball, 119 hand injuries in 108 patients were treated at 1 hand clinic.

Bone was involved in 73% of the injuries. Surgery was needed in 22% of the injuries because of fractures in 23 patients and soft tissue alone in 3. One operative complication occurred, i.e., infection after open reduction and internal fixation, treated successfully with antibiotics.

The finger joints were involved in 86% of all injuries. Thirty-nine percent of the injuries were to the distal interphalangeal (DIP) joint, 40% to the proximal interphalangeal (PIP) joint, and 6% to the metacarpophalangeal joint. Mallet injury was the most common DIP joint injury. This fracture accounted for 27% of all injuries and was the most common single type of injury. Fractures comprised 86% of all mallet injuries. The second most common injury was the volar plate fracture, which was the most common PIP joint injury. Patient's gender, dominance or nondominance of hands, and early or late season play were unassociated with a higher risk of injury. Certain parts of the hand, including the more ulnar digits and the DIP and PIP joints, were at especially high risk.

A significant number of hand injuries occur in softball players playing with 16-in. balls. Injury occurs particularly because of the way the ball must be caught. Use of a 10-in. ball, which permits the wearing of gloves, would help to prevent these injuries.

▶ Despite several inadequacies, this is an excellent and worthwhile epidemiologic contribution. As the authors acknowledge, they were unable to present their data in terms of injury rates. Also, the data do not support the conclusion that the 10-in. softball would necessarily prevent hand injuries. It should be noted that their observations coincide with those of Dawson and Pullos (1), who reported 153 baseball or softball hand injuries that occurred during a single season, 69% of which were caused by the 16-in. softball.—J.S. Torg, M.D.

Reference

1. Dawson WT, Pullos N: *Ann Emerg Med* 10:302–306, 1981.

Illness and Absence Among Wrestlers, Swimmers, and Gymnasts at a Large University
Strauss RH, Lanese RR, Leizman DJ (Ohio State Univ)
Am J Sports Med 16:653–655, November–December 1988   4–20

Less attention has been given to illnesses among athletes than to injuries. The prevalence and consequences of illness were examined in members of university swimming, gymnastics, and wrestling teams. The athletes were studied by questionnaires administered weekly during the season of competition, i.e., January and February. The months chosen are also the peak times for respiratory illnesses.

All except 2 of the 87 athletes reported at least 1 illness, and 86% experienced at least 1 respiratory illness during the 8-week period. Gymnasts had the lowest prevalence of illness. Swimmers reported more gastrointestinal illnesses, an unexplained finding. Wrestlers had more skin problems as a result of abrasions; the difference was not statistically significant, however, when compared with the other groups. In this group of athletes, the higher overall prevalence of illness among swimmers resulted from a period of abnormal water quality in the pool.

Rates of absenteeism from practice or competition were similar for the 3 teams. Furthermore, the athletes were less likely to miss class than to miss practice or competition. When the pool water problem was accounted for, the 3 groups had similar rates of illnesses. Studies including greater numbers of athletes over a longer period of time might reveal recurring patterns. Comparisons have rarely been made between illness differences in athletes and nonathletes.

▶ To this reviewer, the most interesting observation presented by this paper is that during one 8-week study period, 85% of the athletes experienced at least 1 respiratory illness, this in addition to other dermatologic, gastrointestinal, and miscellaneous illnesses. Unfortunately, the authors did not address the question of illness differences between nonathletes and athletes. Certainly, this line of epidemiologic investigation needs to be pursued.—J.S. Torg, M.D.

The Role of a Regional Trauma System in the Management of a Mass Disaster: An Analysis of the Keystone, Colorado, Chairlift Accident
Ammons MA, Moore EE, Pons PT, Moore FA, McCroskey BL, Cleveland HC (Denver Gen Hosp; St Anthony's Hosp, Denver; Univ of Colorado)
J Trauma 28:1468–1471, October 1988   4–21

In a chairlift accident at a ski area in Keystone, Colorado, 60 of 372 skiers were thrown to the ground from heights up to 50 ft. The accident was effectively managed by local medical resources coordinated with a regional trauma system, the Colorado Trauma Institute.

Initial triage and treatment of the victims was carried out by the local ski patrol, the on-duty physician, and volunteer nurses and physicians present at the scene. Victims were rapidly assessed, neck and back injuries were immobilized, oxygen was administered if needed, measures were taken to prevent hypothermia, and obvious fractures were splinted. Injured patients were taken to a clinic at the base of the mountain by snowcat, toboggan, or snowmobile.

At the clinic more seriously injured patients received heart monitoring, intravenous administration of crystalloids, and placement of chest tubes in 6 patients with overt pneumothorax. Thirty-three of 49 patients triaged to the clinic were evacuated to other medical care facilities. Most were evacuated by helicopter to level I and II trauma centers. Eighteen patients were in serious or critical condition. Evacuation was carried out according to an existing disaster plan developed by the Colorado Trauma Institute. Eight patients underwent emergency surgery for a variety of conditions. Fifteen secondary operations were performed on 5 patients during initial hospitalization. The only death occurred in a patient who required 3 delayed procedures and eventually succumbed to persistent sepsis and multiple organ failure.

Communities should formalize a trauma system and practice disaster plans often to prepare for multiple casualty incidents. After the disaster, the involved trauma system should provide leadership for injury prevention and should make their concerns known to legislative policy makers.

▶ This papers describes the effective management of an extraordinary recreational disaster. The role played by the Colorado Trauma Institute was most noteworthy. The paper emphasizes the required components of an effective disaster plan. First is the establishment of an avenue by which the plan can be activated. Second is estimation of the injury severity and number of critically injured persons. The third component involves recruitment of necessary resources to manage multiple casualties, and, lastly, the provision of definitive medical care.—J.S. Torg, M.D.

Helicopter Rescues and Deaths Among Trekkers in Nepal
Shlim DR, Houston R (Himalayan Rescue Assoc; Canadian Internatl Water and Energy Consultants Clinic; US Peace Corps, Katmandu, Nepal)
JAMA 261:1017–1019, Feb 17, 1989   4–22

Trekking in Nepal is a popular vacation activity involving approximately 45,000 persons yearly. To evaluate the risks to tourists who undertake this adventure, the records of all helicopter evacuations and deaths among tourists trekking in Nepal between January 1984 and June 1987 were studied. During that period, 148,000 persons obtained trekking permits.

Twenty-three persons died and 111 were rescued by helicopter. The risk of death while trekking was 15/100,000 permits. Eleven persons died of trauma, 8 died of illness, and 3 died of acute mountain sickness. Deaths occurred equally at higher and lower altitudes, although the number of persons at risk at various altitudes could not be ascertained. The frequency of death among persons older than 50 years was similar to that among younger trekkers, but significantly more older persons were rescued by helicopter.

The overall risk of trekking in Nepal is low. However, the decision to trek should be individualized. Travelers should bear in mind the problems of remoteness, altitude, and illness in the absence of accessible medical facilities.

▶ The authors conclude that their data suggest that trekking in Nepal is a relatively safe activity. However, they do not answer the question as to whether or not helicopter rescues contributed to this observation, i.e., what were the number of deaths per 100,000 trekking permits before the implementation of helicopter evacuation.—J.S. Torg, M.D.

5 Injuries of the Head, Neck, and Spine

Bone Scintigraphy in the Assessment of Spondylolysis in Patients Attending a Sports Injury Clinic
Elliott S, Hutson MA, Wastie ML (Univ Hosp, Nottingham, England; Park Row Orthopaedic and Sports Injury Clinic, Nottingham)
Clin Radiol 39:269–272, May 1988   5–1

Stress fractures of the pars interarticularis can be difficult to evaluate radiographically. There is a "subradiologic" period in which radiographic appearances are normal. In addition, a number of persons have a spondylolysis dating from childhood. Bone scintigraphy, however, can indicate a recent spondylolysis or stress fracture in its subradiologic stage. A comparison was made between the results of radiology and scintigraphy in 33 patients who had clinical diagnoses of stress fracture of the pars interarticularis. Fifteen had normal results on both examinations, 9 had normal scintigraphy but abnormal radiographs, and 9 had abnormal scintigrams.

Boy, 15 years, experienced right low lumbar pain while playing cricket. Clinical examination 9 months later suggested a stress fracture. Radiographs revealed a spondylolysis on the left side. A bone scintigram showed both left and right increased uptake. Rest from athletic activity resolved his symptoms. At 2-year follow-up, the right side was normal on radiographs, indicating healing of the subradiologic stress fracture.

Early diagnosis of acute stress fracture of the pars interarticularis is important so that treatment can be started and development of spondylolysis prevented. A normal scintigram can exclude the diagnosis of stress fracture. When radiology shows spondylolysis but the scintigram is normal, the defect is an old one and recent stress fracture can be ruled out.

▶ The authors' position as to the value of bone scintigraphy in assessment of patients suspected of having spondylolysis is well taken. It has been my experience that in the symptomatic patient with a positive bone scan and negative x-ray appearances, treatment in the form of activity restriction and bracing halts the process. When radiographic spondylolysis becomes established, the defect does not "heal" and, in the active youngster, cyclic episodes of symptoms commonly ensue.—J.S. Torg, M.D.

Injuries of the Spine Sustained During Rugby
Silver JR, Gill S (Stoke Mandebille Hosp, Aylesbury, England)
Sports Med 5:328–334, May 1988   5–2

A previous report described 63 serious cervical spine injuries incurred during rugby games from 1952 to 1982. An additional 19 such injuries can now be included. Most of the recent injuries occurred in forwards and resulted from a blow to the head or from the head being pushed onto the ground. Apart from scrum injuries, several players were injured while tackling or when in a ruck and maul situation, often when trying to pick up the ball. Five of 7 injuries ascribed to foul play involved the head.

Although the current rugby rules seem to be adequate, they are difficult to enforce, especially at a junior level. Additional information gained from video recordings on how injuries actually occur should help in finding ways to lower the risk.

▶ The mechanism of injury alluded to in this article resulting from impact to the head has been vividly described by McCoy et al. (1). Specifically, he described the "vertex restrained against a player or the ground" with continued movement of the trunk, resulting in forced dislocation produced by "extreme flexion of the cervical spine." This is a variation on the theme of what has been described as the mechanism of injury occurring in cervical spine injuries resulting from tackle football.—J.S. Torg, M.D.

Reference

1. McCoy GF, et al: *J Bone Joint Surg [Br]* 66-B:500–503, August 1984.

Maxillofacial and Dental Injuries in Contact Team Sports
Sane J (Univ of Helsinki)
Proc Finn Dent Soc (Suppl 6–7) 84:9–45, 1988   5–3

Contact sports are reputed to be the most hazardous. The incidence and nature of maxillofacial and dental injuries were determined in contact team sports, such as American football, bandy, basketball, handball, ice hockey, and soccer. Also, the effects of facial protection were defined. Data on sports-related accidents to maxillofacial and dental hard tissues and periodontal tissues and to prostheses were obtained from 1,430 patients with maxillofacial fractures seen from 1981 to 1985 and the records of insurance companies were reviewed.

Hospital data showed 80 (5.6%) sports-related maxillofacial fractures during the 5-year period. These fractures were rarely associated with multiple trauma and were less serious than maxillofacial fractures in general. Sixty percent of these injuries occurred in contact team sports. All of the patients injured in contact team sports were male, had more zygomatic and less mandibular fractures, and required surgical treatment most often.

Maxillofacial and dental injuries were highest in ice hockey (11.2%) and bandy (10.6%), in which adequate facial or dental protection was not mandatory for all players; the least number of such injuries were incurred in American football (1.4%), where such protection was mandatory. More than 60% of the injured players were aged 16–30 years. Dentoalveolar injury was the most common type of injury; most dental fractures were crown fractures. There was a preponderance of dental injury in the upper jaw, especially to the maxillary central incisors. Fractures of the lower and middle third of the facial skeleton accounted for the minority of injuries.

Injury was most often caused by a blow from the stick in ice sports, or a blow or kick from another player in all other contact team sports. Falls and blows from the ball or puck caused more extensive injuries to the teeth, and falls and blows or kicks from other players caused more severe injuries to the teeth. Games were much more hazardous than training sessions.

The costs of treatment of maxillofacial and dental injuries were disproportionately high for their number in bandy, basketball, ice hockey, and soccer players. However, in American football where facial protection was adequate, the cost of treatment was well below that in relation to all other accidents. This was further supported by the distinctly lower occurrence of maxillofacial and dental injuries in American football. Further, in ice hockey the occurrence of maxillofacial and dental injuries as well as the cost of treatment were reduced in players aged 18 or younger in whom full cage face mask was mandatory.

Although there are no generalizations that can be made from this study, it appears that the use of good facial and dental protection reduces the occurrence and severity of maxillofacial and dental injuries in contact team sports. Further studies are warranted to define the role of protection in contact team sports more clearly.

▶ This study is basically a retrospective review of hospital records and data collected from insurance companies. It was performed to meet the requirements for an academic dissertation. The bibliography is extensive, and although there is limited statistical analysis of the data, the conclusions indicating that maxillofacial dental injuries resulting in athletic activity can be prevented is sound.—J.S. Torg, M.D.

6 Injuries of the Upper Extremity

Beware the Sprained Wrist: The Incidence and Diagnosis of Scapholunate Instability
Jones WA (Broadgreen Hosp, Liverpool, England)
J Bone Joint Surg [Br] 70-B:293–297, March 1988   6–1

Sprained wrist is a common diagnosis in accident departments. Because variable ligament disruption may result in different degrees of instability, data on 100 consecutive patients with wrist injury, other than those referred with a radial fracture, were reviewed to determine the incidence of acute scapholunate instability. In addition to the routine scaphoid views, a "clenched fist" radiograph also was performed (Fig 6–1). The radiographic signs of scapholunate dissociation include widening of the scapholunate gap (normally 2 mm or less), cortical ring sign, dorsiflexed intercalated segment instability, and increase in the scapholunate angle from a normal value of 40–60 degrees.

Of the 19 patients with an increased scapholunate gap, 5 had significant scapholunate instability, including 2 with associated Colles' fracture.

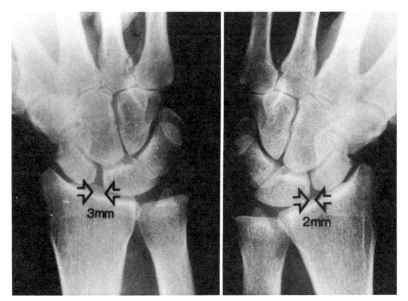

Fig 6–1.—Clenched-fist views of both wrists showing an increase in the scapholunate gap on the left. (Courtesy of Jones WA: *J Bone Joint Surg* [Br] 70-B:293–297, March 1988.)

The difference in mean static scapholunate gap and scapholunate angle was not striking among the 5 patients with significant scapholunate instability and the 14 patients without significant instability, indicating the importance of comparing appearances with the normal wrist.

It appears that significant and potentially serious ligamentous disruption and carpal instability may be as common as fracture of the scaphoid. A dynamic clenched fist view should also be routinely included in the scaphoid series. Patients with a history of falling on the thenar eminence, pain in the anatomical snuffbox or at the scapholunate interval, and static enhanced scapholunate gaps of more than 2 mm should undergo radiographs of the contralateral wrist, and the scapholunate angles should be measured. An angle of 65 degrees or greater strengthens the diagnosis of scapholunate instability, particularly if the unaffected wrist is within normal range.

▶ This paper calls attention to a commonly unrecognized problem. The authors have documented a 19% incidence of "increased scapholunate gap" in a group of patients with wrist injuries. Of note is the fact that they then point out: "The importance of this injury may be doubted; clinics are not full of patients with chronic wrist strains, but many patients do remain symptomatic for prolonged periods after injury, others return with established chronic instability and some may find that minor symptoms are tolerable but may later develop degenerative changes." Increased awareness of these injuries will clarify the natural history. Although the author recommends treatment in a scaphoid cast for 6–8 weeks, then suggests either open reduction of percutaneous pinning for those with persistent diastasis in a cast confirmed by arthrography, he does not document the efficacy of the management guidelines.—J.S. Torg, M.D.

Stress Changes of the Wrist in Adolescent Gymnasts
Carter SR, Aldridge MJ, Fitzgerald R, Davies AM (Coventry and Warwick Hosp, Coventry; New Cross Hosp, Wolverhampton; Royal Orthopaedic Hosp, Birmingham, England)
Br J Radiol 61:109–112, February 1988   6–2

The growth plate in the immature skeleton is particularly vulnerable to chronic trauma such as that occurring with certain types of athletic training. The radiographic appearances of chronic stress to the wrists were reviewed in 8 adolescent boys aged 14–16 years, including 7 competitive gymnasts and 1 champion roller skater. All 8 patients complained of acute or chronic trauma to 1 or both wrists.

Radiographs of the wrists revealed bilateral widening of the distal radial growth plates of 3–5 mm (Fig 6–2). The growth plates had irregular margins, particularly on the metaphyseal side. In the more florid injuries, the margins had a poorly defined cystic appearance and sclerosis. In 6 patients discrete fragmentation was seen within the growth plate. Some degree of flattening of the medial portion of the distal radial epiphysis, predominantly on the palmar aspect, was seen in all 8 patients.

Although the radiographic abnormalities were always bilateral, the de-

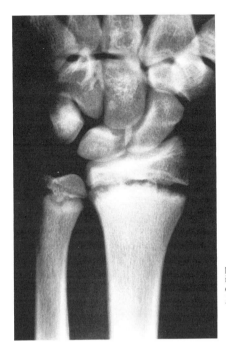

Fig 6–2.—Widening of the radial growth plate with irregularity of the metaphyseal margin in a male gymnast aged 16 years. (Courtesy of Carter SR, Aldridge MJ, Fitzgerald R, et al: *Br J Radiol* 61:109–112, February 1988.)

gree of involvement of each wrist was asymmetric. The distal ulnar growth plate was also bilaterally involved in 5 patients but to a much lesser degree. Two patients had vacuum phenomena in the distal radioulnar joints presumed to be related to the stress. All 8 patients had normal bone density in the affected joints as well as in other joints that had also been radiographed. The only patient who underwent blood tests had no evidence of an underlying metabolic bone disease. However, the radiographic bone age in all 8 patients was retarded by 1–2.5 years.

Healing of the lesions depended on cessation of the sporting activity. One patient who stopped participating in gymnastics experienced significant healing within 3 months, whereas in another patient who continued competitive gymnastics further widening and irregularity of the growth plate occurred until he was forced to take a rest.

The chronic stress of the repetitive motions associated with gymnastics can cause radiographically demonstrable stress changes in the growth plates of the immature skeleton.

Chronic Injury to the Distal Ulnar and Radial Growth Plates in an Adolescent Gymnast: A Case Report
Yong-Hing K, Wedge JH, Bowen CVA (Univ Hosp, Saskatoon, Sask)
J Bone Joint Surg [Am] 70-A:1087–1089, August 1988   6–3

Male gymnasts have been using dowel grips for several years to increase hook-grip strength during bar and rings routines. Injuries sustained by an adolescent national-class gymnast suggest that dowel grips should not be used by younger athletes.

Boy, 13 years, experienced pain over the distal end of the right ulna while training and competing. Wrist movement was not restricted, and pain was not brought about by forced flexion or extension. Radiographs revealed that the wrist had an abnormally wide and irregular distal ulnar growth plate. Almost complete healing ensued after a 4-week period in a palm-to-elbow cast. The distal end of the radius of the same wrist became painful a year later. Clinical signs were similar to those of the previous episode. An abnormally wide distal radial growth plate was visible on radiographs, and the ulnar growth plate appeared to be starting to close. A similar cast treatment brought about healing and resolution of symptoms.

This type of injury has not been described previously. It appears to result from the use of dowel grips, which exert traction on the distal physes of the radius and ulna. Gymnasts should postpone the use of dowel grips until they have reached skeletal maturity.

▶ The lesions described in Abstracts 6–2 and 6–3 involving the distal epiphyseal forearm growth plates appear to be similar, at least from a clinical and radiographic standpoint. Specifically, the problems appear to be caused by repetitive compressive loading, are associated with pain, and are self-limiting and radiographically reversible when activity is curtailed. The conclusion of Yong-Hing et al. (Abstract 6–3) that the dowel grip used by gymnasts in this age group may be ill advised appears to be ill founded. This is based on the observation that the devices were not worn by the 8 individuals described in the article by Carter et al. (Abstract 6–2). Thus these 2 articles caution us regarding definitive recommendations based on a single series. Also, although the lesion does not appear to have been reported in the English literature, it is interesting to note that Auberge et al. (1) demonstrated similar roentgenographic findings in 83% of 105 adolescent gymnasts radiographed at the European Junior Gymnastics Championships in 1980. Also, the lesion appears to be somewhat similar to that reported by Adams (2) occurring in the shoulder and called the "Little League shoulder syndrome," in which there was widening and irregularity at the proximal humeral growth plate in the throwing arm of adolescent baseball pitchers.—J.S. Torg, M.D.

References

1. Auberge T, et al: *J Radiol* 65:555–561, 1984.
2. Adams JE: *California Med* 105:22–25, 1966.

Paralysis of the Ulnar Nerve in Cyclists
Haloua JP, Collin JP, Coudeyre L (Chamalières, France)
Ann Chir Main 6:282–287, 1987   6–4

Only 35 reports of ulnar nerve compression in cyclists have appeared in the literature, but because of the increasing interest in cycling, the incidence of cyclist's palsy is expected to rise. Three additional cyclists with ulnar nerve paralysis were seen.

In cycling, the hands transmit tensile loads to the abdominal and back muscles, which transfer these forces via the seat to the feet, with the seat serving as a pivot. The magnitude of these forces is greater than the cyclist's body weight, particularly during climbing. The ulnar nerve fits tightly in the canal of Guyon. During cycling, the ulnar nerve is stretched taut, because of hyperextension and ulnar deviation of the hand over the unciform articulation as the hand grips the handlebar (Fig 6–3). This type of permanent stress can cause injury to the ulnar nerve, particularly when certain other contributing factors (e.g., poor riding position, unsuitable equipment, faulty grip, or poor road surfaces) also are present.

Symptoms of ulnar palsy may vary depending on where the compression lesion is located in relation to the terminal branches of the ulnar nerve. Of the 35 patients reported, 67% had motor and sensory paralysis, 12.5% pure motor deficit of all intrinsic muscles, and 8% pure sensory paralysis. A number of dissociated impairments unique to cyclist's palsy have also been described. Impairment may be bilateral, but the dominant hand that remains permanently on the handle bar is most often affected. Onset of paralysis may be acute or progressive. Electromyographic examination is used to pinpoint the exact site of the lesion. Treatment consists of total abstinence from cycling. Symptoms usually regress spontaneously, and surgical decompression is rarely indicated. However, motor recovery may be slow, sometimes requiring as long as 3–4 months.

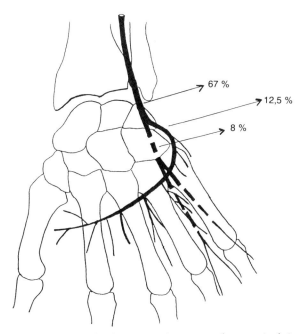

Fig 6–3.—Terminal branches of the ulnar nerve and percentage of compression lesions. (Courtesy of Haloua JP, Collin JP, Coudeyre L: *Ann Chir Main* 6:282–287, 1987.)

In all 3 newly reported patients, the recovery was spontaneous on discontinuing cycling. Precautionary measures (e.g., the use of padded gloves and a properly adjusted bicycle) afford some measure of protection against ulnar nerve paralysis in cyclists.

Distal Sensory Latencies of the Ulnar Nerve in Long Distance Bicyclists: Pilot Study
Wilmarth MA, Nelson SG (Foothill Med Ctr, Sunnyvale, Calif)
J Orthop Sports Phys Ther 9:370–374, May 1988   6–5

Ulnar neuropathy, commonly known as handlebar palsy or cyclist's palsy, is an overuse compression syndrome injury of the ulnar nerve at the wrist associated with bicycling. Because previous studies suggest that severe compression injury to the ulnar nerve results in a change in nerve conduction velocity, it is assumed that bicycling may influence the nerve conduction velocity of the ulnar nerve. Distal sensory latency periods of the ulnar nerve were compared in 15 controls and 10 long distance bicyclists to determine if the latter have altered nerve conduction velocities caused by repeated sustained compression of the ulnar nerve. The controls bicycled a mean 5 miles per week, compared with an average of 169 miles cycled by the long-distance group.

Distal sensory latencies of the ulnar nerve were significantly longer in long-distance bicyclists than in controls. There was no significant correlation between distance bicycled and latency.

These data show a significant difference in the distal sensory latencies between long-distance cyclists and controls, possibly because of adaptive changes in long-distance bicyclists, such as compressive forces that are placed on the hand while cycling. Hand position should be changed at regular intervals; the rider should have the correct bicycle frame size, and foam handlebar pads or well-padded bicycling gloves should be used to avoid undue stress on the hand. Further research is warranted to confirm these findings.

▶ The preceding 2 reports (Abstracts 6–4 and 6–5) help to establish "handlebar palsy" or "cyclist's palsy" as an injury to the ulnar nerve at the wrist associated with bicycling. Unfortunately, the rate at which this injury occurs has not been established. Also, the recommended preventive measures are not supported by data.—J.S. Torg, M.D.

Simple Dislocation of the Elbow in the Adult: Results After Closed Treatment
Mehlhoff TL, Noble PC, Bennett JB, Tullos HS (Baylor College of Medicine, Houston)
J Bone Joint Surg [Am] 70-A:244–249, February 1988   6–6

Simple dislocations of the elbow are thought to have generally favorable prognoses, and there have been few reports of posttraumatic sequelae. The long-term outcome of closed treatment of dislocation of the elbow in 52 adults was reviewed using photographic, goniometric, and radiographic data. All 52 patients had traditional closed reduction, but the period of immobilization varied. Patients were followed for an average of 34 months.

At follow-up, 60% of the patients reported symptoms, usually residual pain (45% of the patients); 35% reported pain on valgus stress. Fifteen percent had a flexion contracture of more than 30 degrees. Prolonged immobilization after trauma was strongly associated with poor results. No excellent results were found when the period of immobilization was more than 2 weeks; after 4 weeks results were always fair or poor. In contrast, when the elbow was immobilized for less than 18 days, there were no fair or poor results.

After simple elbow dislocation, early active mobilization is the key factor in successful rehabilitation.

▶ This is an excellent study and the statistically substantiated observation that "The longer the immobilization had been, the larger the flexion contracture . . . and the more severe the symptoms of pain," indicating that early active motion is a key factor in rehabilitation of the elbow after dislocation, is a major contribution. It should be noted that none of the patients in this series had a redislocation after such treatment. The original paper is recommended reading for those involved in management of elbow dislocations.—J.S. Torg, M.D.

Cineradiographic Studies With Shoulder Instabilities

Maki NJ (Louisiana State Univ)
Am J Sports Med 16:362–364, July–August 1988   6–7

Thirty patients with various shoulder disorders underwent fluoroscopy under general anesthesia. Glenohumeral joint laxity is assessed by applying anterior and posterior directional stress to the proximal arm (Fig 6–4). Posterior translation of up to 50% of the diameter of the humeral head in the glenoid is normal with stress directed posteriorly (Fig 6–5).

Initially, 20 patients with a history of trauma had a diagnosis of unstable shoulder disorder. Cineradiography altered the clinical impression in 3 patients. A patient with impingement syndrome also had an unstable shoulder. One suspected of having anterior subluxation was found to have posterior subluxation instead. In a patient with recurrent posterior dislocations, multidirectional instability was observed on imaging. All of the patients thought initially to have an unstable shoulder had abnormal stress images.

Fluoroscopy under general anesthesia adds little time to surgery. Combined with video recording, it can provide visual documentation at operation. The method may prove helpful in placing staples or screws used in reconstructive surgery, apart from clarifying uncertain diagnoses.

▶ In this the era of computed arthrotomography, magnetic resonance imaging, and ultrasonography, it is gratifying to see a clinician dealing with such mun-

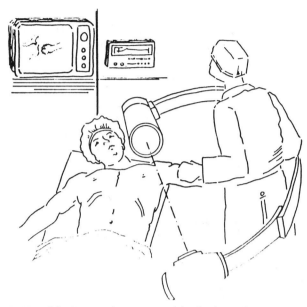

Fig 6–4.—Position of the C arm to obtain imaging of the glenohumeral joint. (Courtesy of Maki NJ: *Am J Sports Med* 16:362–364, July–August 1988.)

dane matters as the basic stress examination of the glenohumeral joint with the benefit of anesthesia. Actually, this is perhaps the most important component of evaluating the patient in whom surgery is being contemplated to rectify instability. The fact of the matter is that this component of the diagnostic workup is little appreciated and performed even less by the nationally reputed

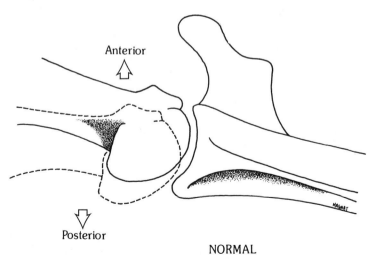

Fig 6–5.—On stress examination there should be no translation beyond 50% of the diameter of the humeral head in the glenoid. (Courtesy of Maki NJ: *Am J Sports Med* 16:362–364, July–August 1988.)

shoulder mavens. One frequently quoted article simply established the subjective experience of "the dead arm" as an indication for performing a Bankart capsulorrhaphy (1). It would be interesting to know how many youngsters with "dead arm syndrome" have stable glenohumeral joints with labrum pathology easily rectified arthroscopically.

Gerber and Ganz (2) published an article concerning clinical assessment of instability of the shoulder with special reference to the anterior and posterior drawer tests. I would also point out that less attention has been given to the diagnosis than to the treatment of chronic shoulder instability.—J.S. Torg, M.D.

References

1. Rowe CR, et al: *J Bone Joint Surg [Am]* 60:1–16, 1978.
2. Gerber C, Ganz R: *J Bone Joint Surg [Br]* 66-B:551–556, 1984.

MR Imaging of Recurrent Anterior Dislocation of the Shoulder: Comparison With CT Arthrography
Kieft GJ, Bloem JL, Rozing PM, Obermann WR (Univ Hosp, Leiden, The Netherlands)
AJR 150:1083–1087, May 1988   6–8

Posttraumatic damage caused by dislocation of the anterior glenohumeral joint may result in recurrent dislocation of the shoulder. Damage to the glenoid labrum and separation of the capsule from the anterior glenoid rim can be visualized by computed tomography (CT) arthrography, which is an invasive diagnostic technique. To determine whether magnetic resonance (MR) imaging can be used to depict posttraumatic changes noninvasively and whether MR can be a possible replacement for CT arthrography, 13 patients with recurrent anterior dislocation of the glenohumeral joint were evaluated by both methods. A diagnosis of

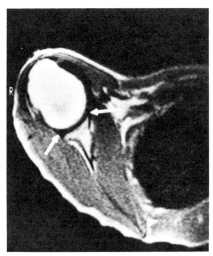

Fig 6–6.—Transverse MR image, 600/30, shows anterior and posterior labrum in cross-section *(arrows)* of normal shoulder anatomy. (Courtesy of Kieft GJ, Bloem JL, Rozing PM, et al: *AJR* 150:1083–1087, May 1988.)

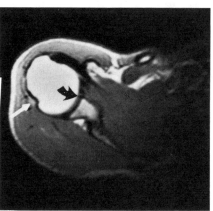

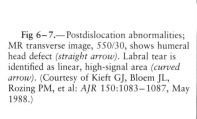

Fig 6–7.—Postdislocation abnormalities; MR transverse image, 550/30, shows humeral head defect *(straight arrow)*. Labral tear is identified as linear, high-signal area *(curved arrow)*. (Courtesy of Kieft GJ, Bloem JL, Rozing PM, et al: *AJR* 150:1083–1087, May 1988.)

damaged glenoid labrum was made if the normal, low-signal-intensity cross-sectional appearance was disrupted, or if abnormal signal intensity was observed (Fig 6–6). Each patient was also assessed by conventional radiography to detect a posterolateral humeral defect or a fracture of the glenoid rim.

Eleven patients had double-contrast arthrography and 10 had CT. Twelve of the 13 patients had arthrotomy, which allowed comparison between surgical findings and the results of MR and CT arthrography. All patients had MR images of adequate technical quality. The patient who had normal findings on all examinations did not undergo operation. The humeral head defects visualized with MR in the other patients were confirmed with CT or plain film radiography (Fig 6–7). Both MR and CT arthrography showed the integrity of the glenoid labrum equally well. All labral changes detected with MR and CT arthrograms were confirmed during operation. However, separation of the capsule from the bony glenoid was seen with MR in only 2 patients, whereas CT arthrography detected capsular stripping in 6 patients. The surgical reports did not provide any information about capsule attachment.

The results indicate that MR is capable of showing osseous damage and important labral pathologic changes related to traumatic anterior dislocation. Although this study was done with a relatively small number of patients, the findings suggest that MR may possibly replace CT arthrography and thus spare the patient invasive presurgical procedures.

▶ This comparative study of MR with CT arthrography is well performed and surgically documented. The authors' concluding sentence, "We believe that MR might possibly replace CT arthrography and thus spare the patient invasive presurgical procedure," however, is extremely premature. First, this assumption is based on findings in 13 patients, all with previous anterior dislocations, and, second, this study was limited to demonstration of glenoid labrum and humeral head defects. The MR and the CT arthrographic examinations are complementary, not competitive, examinations.—J.S. Torg, M.D.

Shoulder Arthroscopy With the Patient in the Beach-Chair Position
Skyhar MJ, Altchek DW, Warren RF, Wickiewicz TL, O'Brien SJ (Hosp for Special Surgery, New York)
Arthroscopy 4:256–259, 1988   6–9

Shoulder arthroscopy is usually performed with the patient in the lateral decubitus position, but this method can cause brachial plexus strain. A simple and successful alternative, the beach-chair position, was developed.

Method.—The patient is placed at an angle of at least 60 degrees on a standard operating table. The patient's shoulder is brought off the side of the table for subacromial decompression and routine shoulder arthroscopy. Arthroscopic shoulder stabilization is performed with the patient's affected side moved off the edge of the table and a sandbag placed under the ipsilateral hip to allow rotation of the upper torso. Because the arm is not placed in traction, it can be easily manipulated and the entire joint visualized.

A review of 50 patients undergoing shoulder arthroscopy in the beach-chair position documented the advantages of this method. Positioning the patient was faster than with the lateral position. No operative or anesthetic complications were recorded, and no postoperative complications (e.g., palsies or paresthesias) occurred. The increased mobility of the arm allows a full view of the entire glenohumeral anatomy. Conversion to an open procedure can be accomplished easily. The only disadvantage of using the beach-chair position for shoulder arthroscopy is that the irrigation solution can run down the arthroscope and cause fogging of the camera lens. A rubber cap placed over the arthroscopic sheath decreases the amount of solution run-down and minimizes this problem.

▶ Shoulder arthroscopy with the patient in the beach-chair position is a technique worthy of consideration. Basically, the authors have challenged the concept that traction is necessary for shoulder arthroscopy. Their observation is that in the beach-chair position, ". . . the capsular anatomy within the glenohumeral joint is not placed in a nonanatomic, stretched-out attitude that occurs with arm traction." Also, they believe that there is more mobility of the arm, and that this technique facilitates a complete view of the entire glenohumeral joint with a minimum of manipulation. Also, to be noted, in the 15 patients who underwent arthroscopic subacromial decompression, 90% were anesthetized with an interscalene brachial plexus block and light sedation.—J.S. Torg, M.D.

Normal and Abnormal Mechanics of the Glenohumeral Joint in the Horizontal Plane
Howell SM, Galinat BJ, Renzi AJ, Marone PJ (Thomas Jefferson Univ, Philadelphia)
J Bone Joint Surg [Am] 70-A:227–232, February 1988   6–10

The glenohumeral joint, which has the widest range of motion of any joint in the body, was studied in a series of axillary roentgenograms. The technique used was designed to determine quantitatively the relationship of the humeral head to the scapula in 4 arm positions within the horizontal plane of motion.

A group of 20 normal persons and 12 patients with anterior instability of the shoulder entered the study. Roentgenograms were obtained with the person lying flat on the x-ray table, positioned at the edge with the thorax on a foam pad (Fig 6–8). Numerous views were obtained in each of the positions before adequate images were acquired. Roentgenograms were taken to show a sharp, sclerotic glenoid margin, the superior lip of the glenoid rim, and a small space between the glenoid and the acromion. Eighteen sets of interpretable roentgenograms were obtained.

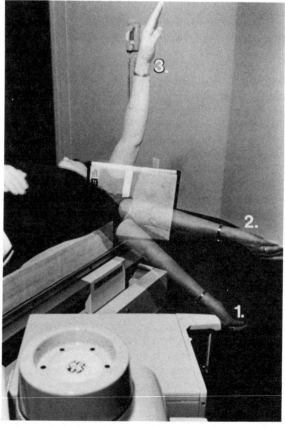

Fig 6–8.—Orientation of the subject for the series of roentgenograms. Position 1: maximum extension and maximum external rotation. Position 1b (not shown): maximum extension and neutral rotation. Position 2: maximum external rotation with the arm held parallel to the floor. Position 3: forward flexion and maximum internal rotation. (Photo is a slight modification of that appearing in the original article). (Courtesy of Howell SM, Galinat BJ, Renzi AJ, et al: *J Bone Joint Surg [Am]* 70-A: 227–232, February 1988.)

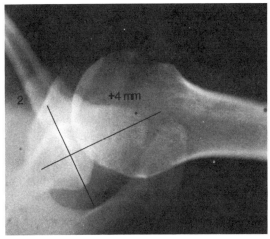

Fig 6–9.—Abnormal anterior translation (4 mm) in a patient who had recurrent anterior instability (position 2). (Courtesy of Howell SM, Galinat BJ, Renzi AJ, et al: *J Bone Joint Surg [Am]* 70-A:227–232, February 1988.)

Precise centering of the humeral head was seen in the control group except when the arm was in maximal extension and external rotation, in which case the humeral head showed posterior translation of about 4 mm in relation to the central axis of the glenoid cavity. In some of the patients with anterior instability, anterior displacement of the humeral head was seen in the first 2 positions (Fig 6–9).

During the acceleration phase of a throwing motion, the humeral head glides anteriorly, resulting in a shearing stress on the articular surface of the glenoid and labrum. In those with anterior instability, the normal rotational motion of the glenohumeral joint is disrupted.

▶ This study is interesting but does have several problems. The authors' observed that precise positioning of the patients was essential so that reproducible and interpretable roentgenograms could be obtained—so much so that 8 of the 20 controls and 6 of the 12 patients with anterior instability did not have interpretable roentgenograms. The authors' attempt to apply static findings, i.e., roentgenographic, to the dynamics of throwing and overhead striking activities must be questioned. Specifically, the statements that "Strengthening exercises therefore would be expected to have no effect on reducing this normal gliding motion. . ." and ". . . flexibility programs that are designed to increase external rotation and extension may aggravate the shearing stress" (in the cocking phase of throwing) are conjectural and not supported by the data.— J.S. Torg, M.D.

Shoulder Instability: Evaluation With MR Imaging
Seeger LL, Gold RH, Bassett LW (Univ of California, Los Angeles)
Radiology 168:695–697, September 1988   6–11

The glenohumeral joint is the most inherently unstable joint in the body and pathologic conditions associated with shoulder instability are common. The accuracy of magnetic resonance (MR) imaging was evaluated in depicting soft tissue abnormalities associated with shoulder instability.

Of 67 shoulders with MR findings indicative of glenohumeral instability, 56 were associated with previous dislocation or subluxation. Surgery was subsequently performed on 27 of these shoulders. All imaging was performed in the axial plane. In 9 shoulders, T1-weighted images were obtained; T2-weighted images were obtained for 4 shoulders, and both T1- and T2-weighted images for the remaining 14.

There were no false positive MR images for labral abnormality in the 27 shoulders for which surgical follow-up was available. On MR imaging the labrum manifested severe attenuation, indistinct borders, diffusely abnormal increased signal intensity, or a discrete band of abnormal increased signal intensity. Labral abnormalities were limited to the anterior labrum in 24 of the 27 shoulders. Of the other 3 shoulders, 1 had a posterior labral abnormality, and 2 had both anterior and posterior labral abnormalities, indicating multidirectional instability. Surgical confirmation of a Bankart lesion in 7 shoulders was supported by MR evidence of either labral detachment or capsular stripping on T2-weighted images, or by abnormal signal intensity within the subchondral bony glenoid on T1-weighted images. Magnetic resonance failed to show capsular Bankart lesions in 5 shoulders for which only T1-weighted images had been obtained. None of the patients had abnormalities of the posterior portion of the rotator cuff on MR images.

Magnetic resonance imaging appears to be a valuable noninvasive diagnostic technique for assessing pathologic conditions associated with glenohumeral instability.

▶ This is an interesting demonstration of the potential usefulness of MR in evaluating shoulder problems. According to the authors, MR evaluation of glenohumeral instability should include 2 pulse sequence scans—a T1-weighted image and a T2-weighted image. The T1-weighted images are used to evaluate the rotator cuff and the T2-weighted images are used to evaluate the glenoid labrum. Unfortunately, of the 56 patients included in the study, only 27 had abnormalities confirmed at surgery and only 1 pulse sequence was available in 13 of these 27 patients. Faster scan speeds, experience, and improved communications between the clinician and the radiologist will improve the diagnostic capabilities of the MR examination.—J.S. Torg, M.D.

The Trillat Procedure for Recurrent Anterior Instability of the Shoulder
Gerber C, Terrier F, Ganz R (Univ of Bern)
J Bone Joint Surg [Br] 70-B:130–134, January 1988   6–12

In the Trillat procedure for recurrent anterior instability of the shoulder, the coracoid process is osteotomized and tilted down to serve as a bone block; a screw is then used to fix it and the Bankart lesion to the anterior scapular neck. The originators of this procedure reported that it was technically simple and gave excellent results with no disabling long-term complications. The long-term results of this procedure were reviewed in 52 unstable shoulders in 48 patients followed up after an average of 69 months (Fig 6–10, p 130).

Results were excellent in 73% of the shoulders, good in 10%, fair in 7%, and poor in 10%. Dislocation recurred in 4%, but a positive apprehension sign was noted in 10 additional shoulders. Some degenerative changes occurred in 62% of the shoulders, a complication known to be associated with bone-block procedures. The most important reason for lateral rotation loss was iatrogenic impingement of the coracoid. This complication could also cause osteoarthritis and posterior subluxation of the humeral head.

This review challenges the conclusions of the originator of the Trillat procedure that the procedure is simple, devoid of disabling complications, and results in more than 80% entirely normal shoulders. In this series, the Trillat technique was found to be exacting, with a potential for serious complications. These complications can result from most bone-block procedures.

▶ This procedure is remarkably similar to the modified Bristow-Helfet-May procedure for recurrent dislocation or subluxation of the shoulder that we have described (1). As in the Trillat procedure, our modification of the Bristow involved positioning of the osteotomized coracoid process with attached conjoin tendon over and not through the subscapularis tendon with screw fixation onto the anterior aspect of the bony glenoid. We believe that utilizing the entire subscapularis tendon and muscle increases its strength as an anterior inferior sling or buttress. Of note is the fact that the redislocation rate in this series was also 4%.—J.S. Torg, M.D.

Reference

1. Torg JS, et al: *J Bone Joint Surg [Am]* 69-A:904–913, 1987.

A Long-Term Retrospective Study of the Modified Bristow Procedure
Ferlic DC, DiGiovine NM (Denver Orthopedic Clinic; Univ of Pittsburgh)
Am J Sports Med 16:469–474, September–October 1988   6–13

A method of treating recurrent dislocation of the shoulder by fixing the coracoid process to the glenoid fossa with a screw was first described in 1954. A modification known as the Bristow procedure has become a popular technique. The modified Bristow procedure was assessed in a long-term study of 51 patients. The mean follow-up was 95 months. There were 37 men and 14 women with an average age of 25 years at surgery. Preoperative radiographs showed Hill-Sachs lesions in 39% of the shoulders and no visible abnormalities in 41%.

Of 25 patients who were examined physically at follow-up, 16 had ex-

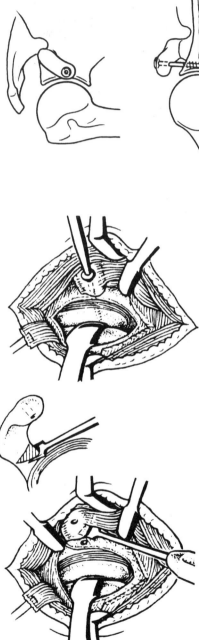

Fig 6–10.—A vertical skin incision is made lateral to the tip of the coracoid, and the deltoid is split. The coracoacromial ligament is divided, and the cranial two thirds of the subscapularis is incised with the arm in full lateral rotation. The capsule is then opened 2 cm lateral to the glenoid rim, and the joint is explored. A 3.2-mm hole is drilled into the coracoid tip to receive a malleolar screw, the base of the coracoid is exposed, and a wedge is resected using a 10-mm chisel. The coracoid is tilted downward, and the screw is introduced to traverse any detachment of the anterior capsule and enter the previously curetted scapular neck, passing above the superior border of the subscapularis. The optimal position of the coracoid and the screw is shown in 2 projections. (Courtesy of Gerber C, Terrier F, Ganz R: *J Bone Joint Surg [Br]* 70-B:130–134, January 1988.)

ternal rotation of more than 80 degrees and 22 had internal rotation of more than 80 degrees. Of the 26 patients interviewed by questionnaire, 17 thought that the procedure had resulted in full range of motion. Overall, 39 patients had no limitations on activity and 37 judged the surgical results to be excellent. Fourteen percent of the patients had complications involving a screw, with 8% requiring screw removal. Another 6% had recurrent anterior subluxation after surgery.

Overall, there was a high level of patient satisfaction with the modified Bristow procedure. Problems seem to occur when athletically inclined patients try to return to a competitive level, especially in sports requiring high impact and throwing. Patients should be given a realistic assessment of the limitations of the modified Bristow procedure.

▶ The results of this series compare favorably with those that we recently reported (1) concerning 212 modified Bristow procedures with recurrent subluxation and dislocation of the shoulder. In our series there was a redislocation rate of 3.8% and a resubluxation rate of 4.7% compared with the postoperative anterior redislocation rate of 6% and recurrent anterior subluxation rate of 4% reported here by Ferlic and DiGiovine. Also, we reported that 92% of our patients said they were happy with the results of the surgery and would have the procedure again. There was an associated 10% complication rate. Ferlic and DiGiovine also report that 92% of their patients assessed the surgical results as excellent or good, and that the associated complication rate was 14%. Of note, both studies identified overhead throwing activities as one area of athletic activity that may be diminished after a modified Bristow procedure. In our series we obtained data with regard to changes in the range of motion and strength in the glenoid-humeral joint indicating that the loss of overhead throwing ability was not caused solely by loss of glenohumeral motion. It appeared also to be a result of the concomitant loss of strength at the extreme of external rotation and initiation of the internal rotation of the humerus in the transition phase between cocking and acceleration in the pitching act.—J.S. Torg, M.D.

Reference

1. Torg JS, et al: *J Bone Joint Surg [Am]* 68-A:904–913, July 1987.

Failed Surgery for Recurrent Anterior Dislocation of the Shoulder: Causes and Management
McAuliffe TB, Pangayatselvan T, Bayley I (Royal Natl Orthopaedic Hosp, Stanmore, Middlesex; North Middlesex Hosp, London)
J Bone Joint Surg [Br] 70-B:798–801, November 1988   6–14

Although the literature on recurrent dislocation of the shoulder is immense, few reports have been made on management after a failed operation. Recurrent anterior dislocation requiring surgery is uncommon, and most clinicians have only limited experience with patients who need it. An average surgeon's experience with failed procedures is even more limited. A series of such patients was reviewed, with special reference to the causes of surgical failure.

The patient group included 10 women and 26 men whose average age was 28 years. Inadequate surgical technique, occurring in 10 patients included failure to use the whole of the subscapularis in a Putti-Platt repair, as shown by intact subscapularis vessels, and a large anterioinferior pouch. Misdiagnosis in 11 patients with habitual dislocation was the third main cause of surgical failure. In patients who had the wrong procedure, the correct procedure was attempted when possible. A Bankart lesion was repaired by suture of the labrum and capsule to the anterior glenoid margin. When there was marked erosion of the anterior glenoid, a bony buttress was fashioned by a coracoid transfer or by free bone graft from the iliac crest. The most frequent finding in habitual dislocation was inappropriate activity of the pectoralis major alone during motions that reproduced symptoms. An important finding in patients who had a simple Putti-Platt reconstruction was that the constant group of vessels at the inferior border of the subscapularis muscle was intact in 12 patients, indicating that only part of the subscapularis muscle had been incorporated into the primary repair. This was the only abnormality in 10 patients and it was judged the cause of failure.

In this series, primary surgical failure could have been avoided in all patients by the correct preoperative diagnosis, selection of appropriate operative procedure, and proper procedure execution. In 14 patients, the wrong operation was done, usually because of failure to recognize a Bankart lesion and to treat it adequately. Most of these patients initially had a simple Putti-Platt procedure, which was inadequate.

▶ Another consideration with regard to failed surgery for recurrent anterior dislocation of the shoulder is the particular procedure used. A review of the literature revealed reports on the rates for redislocation for the Bristow procedure to vary between 2% (1) to 6% (2). Whereas redislocation following the Magnuson-Stack procedure has been reported as being as high as 17% (3) and 13.6% and 19% for the Putti-Platt procedure (2, 4).—J.S. Torg, M.D.

References

1. Lombardo SJ, et al: *J Bone Joint Surg [Am]* 58-A:256–261, 1976.
2. Hovelius KL: *J Bone Joint Surg [Am]* 61-A:566–569, 1979.
3. Miller LS, et al: *Am J Sports Med* 12:133–137, 1984.
4. Morrey BF, Janes JM: *J Bone Joint Surg [Am]* 58-A:252–256, 1976.

Quadrilateral Space Syndrome: A Rare Cause of Shoulder Pain
Cormier PJ, Matalon TAS, Wolin PM (Rush-Presbyterian-St Luke's Med Ctr, Chicago)
Radiology 167:797–798, June 1988   6–15

The quadrilateral space syndrome is a rare disorder caused by occlusion of the posterior humeral circumflex artery (PHCA) in the quadrilateral space. Arteriography reveals occlusion of the PHCA when the arm is abducted and externally rotated. The quadrilateral space syndrome occurred in a baseball pitcher.

Man, 21, complained of progressive shoulder pain over the anterior aspect of the right shoulder while pitching. The pain was exacerbated by abduction and external rotation of the affected arm. During subclavian arteriography the PHCA remained patent when the patient's right arm was at his side (Fig 6–11) and when the Lang maneuver was used, but became occluded when the arm was placed in abduction and external rotation.

Quadrilateral space syndrome usually affects active young persons aged between 22 and 35 years. Symptoms begin as slow, intermittent paresthesias in the upper extremity during forward flexion, abduction, or both, and are exacerbated by external rotation of the humerus. Subclavian arteriography, usually requested to rule out vascular compression syndrome, shows occlusion of the PHCA with the humerus at the side and in abduction with external rotation. Most patients are treated con-

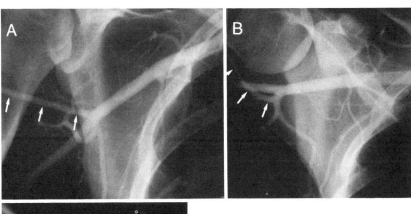

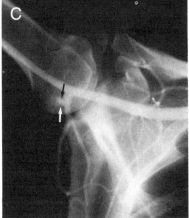

Fig 6–11.—A, subclavian arteriogram obtained with patient's right arm at his side. The PHCA *(arrows)* is patent. **B,** Lang maneuver. The PHCA *(arrows)* remains patent. **C,** in extreme abduction and external rotation, there is complete occlusion of the PHCA *(arrows).* (Courtesy of Cormier PJ, Matalon TAS, Wolin PM: *Radiology* 167:797–798, June 1988.)

servatively whereas others may require surgical decompression of the quadrilateral space and lysis of the abnormal fibrous strands.

▶ The quadrilateral space syndrome was first reported by Cahill and Palmer (1). The pathomechanics involve compression of both the posterior humeral circumflex artery and axillary nerve as they pass through the space bounded by the teres minor superiorly, long head of the triceps medially, the teres major inferiorly, and the surgical neck of humerus laterally. The diagnosis is based on the clinical manifestations of pain associated with abduction and external rotation of the arm and is substantiated at arteriography, usually requested to rule out thoracic outlet syndrome. Depending on the individual situation, treatment may be either conservative or surgical. Surgical treatment is directed toward decompressing the quadrilateral space by lysis of abnormal fibrous bands. Cahill and Palmer reported that in a series of 18 patients who underwent surgery, 8 had dramatic and complete relief of symptoms, 8 were improved, and 2 had no improvement.—J.S. Torg, M.D.

Reference

1. Cahill BR, Palmer RE: *J Hand Surg* 8:65–69, 1983.

Rotator Cuff Injuries in Baseball: Prevention and Rehabilitation
Jobe FW, Bradley JP (Kerlan Jobe Orthopedic Clinic, Inglewood Calif; Centinela Hosp Med Ctr, Inglewood)
Sports Med 6:378–387, December 1988   6–16

Chronic stress caused by repeated high-velocity overhand throwing disposes the shoulder to rotator cuff pathology and impingement syndrome. Pitchers are especially at risk. Chronic overuse can cause healing to lag as a result of repeated microtrauma. After years of throwing, increased external rotation is present along with attenuation of the anterior capsule and subluxation. In addition, muscle/joint imbalance can alter the throwing mechanics of the shoulder. The basic pathophysiology involves stretching or breakdown of the static ligament stabilizers, producing silent subluxation and secondary impingement. Eventually, anterior subluxation impinges the rotator cuff against the acromion and coracoacromial ligament.

Pain often is present at rest and at night in those with a rotator cuff tear. In rotator cuff tendinitis, pain occurs with progressive shoulder activity. Initially, rest is prescribed, but use of a sling should be avoided as it may lead to further rotator cuff contracture. Kinesiologic repair is most helpful when used preventively or as early treatment. A highly specific exercise program is designed and nonsteroidal anti-inflammatory drugs are administered. Stretching exercises generally are contraindicated in this phase. If kinesiologic repair fails, capsulolabral reconstruction is indicated. Early reconstruction is preferable if pure instability is present.

Muscle attachments should be respected at reconstruction. The capsule must not be unduly shortened, and the anterior labrum must be built up. A full range of motion is regained through abduction splinting and specific rehabilitative measures. When full range of motion returns, muscle reeducation is undertaken with isokinetic devices.

▶ This is an excellent primer on the subject of rotator cuff injuries in baseball players written by recognized authorities. The interested reader is referred to the original article.—J.S. Torg, M.D.

Comprehensive Functional Analysis of Shoulders Following Complete Acromioclavicular Separation
MacDonald PB, Alexander MJ, Frejuk J, Johnson GE (Univ of Manitoba, Winnipeg)
Am J Sports Med 16:475–480, September–October 1988   6–17

There is much controversy in the literature concerning the best approach to treatment of acromioclavicular injuries. Some authors are proponents of conservative treatment, whereas others favor surgical treatment of complete acromioclavicular separation. Recovery of shoulder strength and function after treatment for a complete acromioclavicular separation was evaluated in 10 patients aged 19–50 years with grade III acromioclavicular separations treated nonsurgically by taping or an acromioclavicular immobilizing sling, 10 patients aged 18–44 years with grade III separations treated surgically with Bosworth screw or Steinmann pin fixation, and 10 normal controls aged 20–32 years. All participants were tested for shoulder strength, using the Kin-Com isokinetic dynamometer, shoulder flexibility using a Leighton flexometer, and grip strength, using a standard grip dynamometer. Each participant also completed a questionnaire to evaluate subjectively the results of treatment.

There was no significant difference between surgically and nonsurgically treated patients for most of the strength and flexiblity test scores. However, results in the nonsurgically treated patients were statistically slightly superior to those in surgically treated patients with regard to test scores for eccentric abduction, concentric external rotation, eccentric external rotation, eccentric abduction, and flexibility in external rotation. The nonsurgically treated patients also recovered faster than the surgically treated ones, probably because rehabilitation could be initiated earlier; also, the nonoperated-on patients had less pain during recovery.

A nonsurgical approach is favored in the treatment of complete acromioclavicular separation.

▶ The conclusions stated in this paper are in keeping with those of Taft et al. (1) and Dias et al. (2) as well as myself, i.e., anatomical reduction of an acromioclavicular joint separation is not necessary to obtain a good result. In addition to the end results being equal to those of similar injuries treated surgically, conservative management is cost effective and, importantly, associated with a much lower complication rate. One of the problems with this paper is that the current trend to divide complete separations into 3 subgrades is not dealt with.—J.S. Torg, M.D.

136 / Sports Medicine

References

    1. Taft TN, et al: *J Bone Joint Surg [Am]* 69-A:1045–1051, 1987.
    2. Dias JJ, et al: *J Bone Joint Surg [Br]* 69-B:719–722, 1987.

The Mumford Procedure in Athletes: An Objective Analysis of Function
Cook FF, Tibone JE (Palm Beach Gardens, Fla; Inglewood, Calif)
Am J Sports Med 16:97–100, March–April 1988   6–18

The Mumford procedure, used to treat degenerative changes after a grade I or II dislocation, was first described in 1941. Some reports have claimed that muscle weakness and fatigue can occur after the procedure. The first objective muscle testing after distal clavicle resection was carried out in 23 athletes (mean age, 33 years) an average of 3.7 years after the Mumford procedure. Seventeen performed the rigorous Cybex II muscle testing, and all 23 completed a questionnaire and underwent physical examinations and radiography.

Results of the Mumford procedure were judged satisfactory by all but 1 of the athletes. Most were able to return to sports at preinjury levels within 3 months, and these sports usually involved overhead movements. Full shoulder motion was not impaired in any of the individuals. Radiographs showed 8 joints to have some degree of ossification between the remaining clavicle and acromion.

The unaffected limb was significantly stronger during extension and flexion at 60 degrees per second than the involved limb, but the 2 limbs performed similarly at 240 degrees per second. In the abduction-adduction plane both limbs performed equally at 60 or 240 degrees per second. Cybex data showed that loss of acromioclavicular joint ligaments affected muscular stability, but this loss was apparent only in maximum bench press motions.

The Mumford procedure gave excellent results overall, and the few deficits may be overcome by strengthening exercises. The procedure is not recommended for acute injuries in nondislocated acromioclavicular joints.

▶ The observations and conclusions regarding the efficacy of the Mumford procedure for managing posttraumatic degenerative changes after grade I or grade II acromioclavicular dislocations agree with our own clinical experience. Also to be mentioned is the role that this procedure plays in the management of osteolysis of the distal clavicle not associated with acute trauma, as described by Cahill (1). Phenomena seen in weight-lifters are the degenerative changes in the acromioclavicular joint, probably caused by subchondral stress fractures resulting from repetitive microtrauma.—J.S. Torg, M.D.

Reference

    1. Cahill BR: *J Bone Joint Surg [Am]* 64-A:1053–1058, 1982.

7 Injuries of the Lower Extremity

The Natural History and Treatment of Delayed Union Stress Fractures of the Anterior Cortex of the Tibia
Rettig AC, Shelbourne KD, McCarroll JR, Bisesi M, Watts J (Methodist Hosp, Indianapolis)
Am J Sports Med 16:250–255, May–June 1988   7–1

Stress fractures of the tibia in athletes have been discussed often in medical literature, but those involving the anterolateral cortex of the midshaft of the tibia are less frequently noted. Eight basketball players with this type of stress fracture were followed through treatment and recovery. The athletes, 7 males and 1 female, ranged in age from 14 to 23 years. They had experienced pain and tenderness for an average of 4.4 months before seeking treatment.

Male, 19 years, had a "sawtooth" type of stress fracture at the anterior cortex of the tibia (Fig 7–1). The patient was treated for 2 months with pulsing electromagnetic field therapy, which resulted in incomplete healing. After 3 months of limited activity the patient reported little pain, and healing was found to have progressed. Final radiographs approximately 1 year after the start of treatment showed solid union of the fracture.

Stress fractures of the anterior tibial cortex are relatively difficult to treat and slow to heal. Delayed union and complete fracture are possible complications. In this study, pulsing electromagnetic field therapy and rest brought about recovery and allowed return to competitive sports without surgery. Any athlete with pain and tenderness at the anterior tibial cortex should be examined for stress fracture.

▶ What the authors describe as a "sawtooth" type of stress fracture at the anterior cortex of the tibia has been more aptly termed the "dreaded black line" by Bergfeld (personal communication). This report should be viewed in terms of that of Green et al. (1) who reported 6 similar nonunion stress fractures of the tibia, 5 that went on to complete fractures. These authors noted that they had not encountered a stress fracture of the mid-tibia that healed without bone grafting. Certainly, the suggestion that rest and pulsating electromagnetic field therapy may result in healing in some patients appears more optimistic. However, in view of the impracticality of using a randomized, double-blind study, with or without implementation of a pulsating electromagnetic field, no conclusion can be made regarding its effect. It should also be pointed out that Brigh-

137

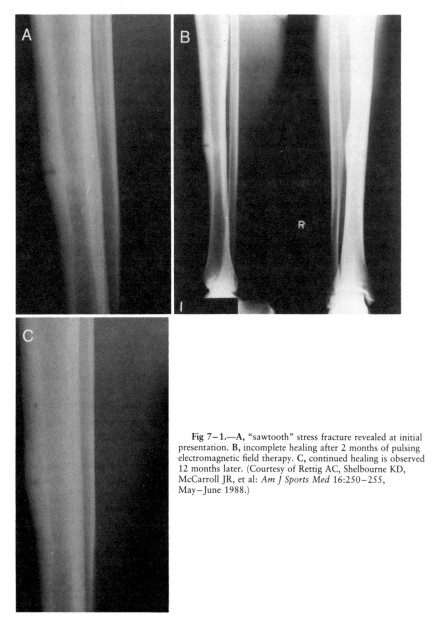

Fig 7–1.—A, "sawtooth" stress fracture revealed at initial presentation. B, incomplete healing after 2 months of pulsing electromagnetic field therapy. C, continued healing is observed 12 months later. (Courtesy of Rettig AC, Shelbourne KD, McCarroll JR, et al: *Am J Sports Med* 16:250–255, May–June 1988.)

ton's success in treatment of nonunion of the tibia with a capacitively coupled electrical field (2) did not deal with this type of fracture. The recommendation of the authors that ". . . initial treatment of this type of stress fracture (should) consist of rest and electrical stimulation for 3 to 6 months before considering surgical intervention" will only tend to prolong the agony.—J.S. Torg, M.D.

References

1. Green NE, et al: *Am J Sports Med* 13:171–176, 1985.
2. Brighton CT: *J Trauma* 23:153–155, 1984.

Diagnosis of Exercise-Induced Pain in the Anterior Aspect of the Lower Leg
Styf J (East Hosp, Göteborg, Sweden)
Am J Sports Med 16:165–169, March–April 1988   7–2

The diagnosis of recurrent exercise-induced pain in the lower leg is difficult because there are many possible causes and few specific signs. Ninety-eight patients (average age, 27 years) experiencing pain in this region, specifically the anterior compartment with the anterior ridge of the tibia and the anterior intermuscular septum, were examined. Of these, 53 had pain in both legs. The anterior aspect of the lower leg was the only location of pain in 47 patients, whereas 51 had pain in other leg areas. The patients were studied by physical examination, intramuscular pressure recording, electromyography, determination of nerve conduction velocity, radiography, and questionnaire.

Although all 98 patients had been given a preliminary diagnosis of chronic compartment syndrome, only 26 fulfilled the criteria. Thirteen were found to have compression of the superficial peroneal nerve. The largest group of patients (41) had periostitis—not a definite diagnosis but a symptom not caused by muscle strain, stress fracture, myositis, or tendinitis. Those with periostitis had soreness dominating over the anterior ridge of the tibia.

Chronic compartment syndrome is not a common cause of recurrent pain in the lower leg. Pressure recordings should be obtained at rest and during and after exercise to avoid false positive diagnoses. Thorough testing using the methods described can aid in the difficult diagnosis of chronic pain in the anterior compartment of the lower leg.

Study of Pressure of the Normal Anterior Tibial Compartment in Different Age Groups Using the Slit-Catheter Method
Nkele C, Aindow J, Grant L (Weymouth and District Hosp, Weymouth; Dorset County Hosp, Dorchester; Royal United Hosp, Bath, England)
J Bone Joint Surg [Am] 70-A:98–101, January 1988   7–3

Compartment syndromes of the leg can be diagnosed by measuring pressure in the anterior tibial compartment. The slit-catheter method was used to determine normal resting pressure in 30 volunteers aged 17–85 who were divided into 3 groups: those under age 35 (group I), those between ages 35 and 54 (group II), and those aged 55 or older (group III). After catheter insertion, measurements were taken at rest, after a weight

140 / Sports Medicine

was applied to the foot, when the foot was placed horizontally, and when the trunk was raised to 60 degrees.

The average resting pressure in the anterior tibial compartment was +5.1 mm Hg. During dorsiflexion of the foot, peak pressure rose to an average of 25.4 mm Hg. When the trunk was raised the average change in resting pressure was +1.7. A wide variation was found among participants, although in more than 95%, resting pressure was less than 12 mm Hg. Changes or variations in pressure were not age related.

Chronic compartment syndrome should be diagnosed according to these criteria: resting pressure in the compartment of more than 12 mm Hg, pain in the area during exercise, and failure of pressure to return to preexercise levels within 5 minutes.

Chronic Exercise-Induced Compartment Pressure Elevation Measured With a Miniaturized Fluid Pressure Monitor: A Laboratory and Clinical Study
Awbrey BJ, Sienkiewicz PS, Mankin HJ (Massachusetts Gen Hosp, Boston; Harvard Med School)
Am J Sports Med 16:610–615, November–December 1988   7–4

Acute compartment syndrome, if left untreated, can result in muscle fibrosis and contracture. Chronic or recurring pain at exercise occurs in the arm or leg when tissue pressure within a closed fascial space exceeds the critical closing pressure of the local microcirculation. Diagnosing the condition requires intracompartmental pressure measurements during exercise. A new measuring device, a miniaturized fluid pressure monitor, was compared with the widely used needle manometer.

The digital monitor was faster and more accurate than the needle manometer. In the clinical setting, it was twice as precise in obtaining reproducible pressure measurements. The device can provide either intermittent or continuous monitoring, enabling the clinician promptly to differentiate chronic compartment syndrome from conditions with similar symptoms.

The small size of the fluid pressure monitor (5 × 3 × 1 in.) allows it to be held in one hand or attached to a patient's limb. The device offers a significant advance in the diagnosis of suspected chronic exercise-induced compartment syndrome.

The Compartment Syndrome: An Experimental and Clinical Study of Muscular Energy Metabolism Using Phosphorus Nuclear Magnetic Resonance Spectroscopy
Heppenstall RB, Sapega AA, Scott R, Shenton D, Park YS, Maris J, Chance B (Philadelphia VA Med Ctr; Univ of Pennsylvania)
Clin Orthop 226:138–155, January 1988   7–5

Compartment syndrome is caused by elevated pressure within a closed osteofascial compartment that, if high enough, can reduce muscle perfusion below the level required for cellular viability. Because none of the available invasive techniques to monitor compartment pressure in animal models of compartment syndrome can determine the presence of ischemia directly, many critical compartment pressure thresholds at which muscle ischemia supposedly sets in have been proposed as a guide to determine when fasciotomy should be performed.

Nuclear magnetic resonance scanning was used in an experimental dog model of compartment syndrome to determine the pressure threshold at which resting skeletal muscle begins to use anaerobic energy sources because of insufficient cellular oxygen delivery. Muscle biopsy and electron microscopy were used concomitantly to study the severity of cell injury produced by various degrees of compartment pressurization. In addition, 9 patients with clinical signs of compartment syndrome in either the anterior tibia or the volar forearm compartments were prospectively studied to provide clinical correlation to the data from the dog studies.

The difference between mean arterial blood pressure (MABP) and compartment pressure was a more accurate indication of tissue ischemia than the absolute compartment pressure by itself. Correlation between animal and clinical data showed that the lowest difference between the MABP and the compartment pressures at which a normal cellular metabolic state can be maintained is approximately 30 mm Hg in normal muscle and 40 mm Hg in moderately traumatized muscle. Thus no single absolute tissue pressure automatically denotes tissue compromise.

In clinical practice, absolute tissue pressure measurements should be considered together with the degree of soft tissue trauma sustained and with the patient's MABP in determining when to perform a fasciotomy.

The Role of Tissue Pressure Measurement in Diagnosing Chronic Anterior Compartment Syndrome
Rorabeck CH, Bourne RB, Fowler PJ, Finlay JB, Nott L (Univ Hosp, London, Ont)
Am J Sports Med 16:143–146, March–April 1988   7–6

An attempt was made to determine whether chronic anterior compartment syndrome can be diagnosed successfully by tissue pressure measurement. The syndrome, in which exercise-related pain interferes with athletic performance by impairing neuromuscular function, can be treated by surgical fasciotomy.

Of 55 individuals who entered the study, 31 (group I) were healthy recreational athletes who served as controls. The other 24 (group II) had been given tentative diagnoses of chronic anterior compartment syndrome. The 2 groups had a similar male/female ratio, but those in group

I had an average age (22.5 years) that was 9 years younger than in group II. The slit-catheter system was used to obtain intramuscular pressure measurements after treadmill exercise.

A resting pressure above 15 mm Hg at 15 minutes after exercise was the parameter used to diagnose the condition. Pressure in the control group averaged 10.9 mm Hg. Seven of the patients in group II had normal pressure. The 17 patients in whom the condition was diagnosed had an average resting pressure of 18.1 mm Hg. These patients successfully underwent fasciotomy.

Dynamic pressure studies, however, did not reveal significant differences among the 3 groups, and there was potential overlap at the 15 mm Hg resting pressure. The increased pressures at rest and after exercise can be helpful, nevertheless, in diagnosing chronic anterior compartment syndrome and in distinguishing those patients who could benefit from fasciotomy.

▶ The 5 articles reviewed in Abstracts 7–2 through 7–6 present the current thinking, with high-tech embellishments, concerning the diagnosis of both acute and chronic compartment syndrome. Styf (Abstract 7–2) points out that the diagnosis is difficult and that chronic compartment syndrome ". . . seems to be a rather uncommon reason for recurrent pain in the lower leg." Using the slit-catheter method, Nkele et al. (Abstract 7–3) and Rorabeck et al. (Abstract 7–6) both establish criteria for a clinical diagnosis of chronic anterior compartment syndrome. Awbrey et al. (Abstract 7–4) demonstrate the practicality of a prototype electronic digital monitor consisting of a pressure transducer, solid-state miniaturized electronic circuitry, 9-volt battery with electric calibration, and a digital LCD readout. We currently use such a device in our clinic and can attest to its practicality. However, it should be mentioned that its utilization requires experienced personnel and that the device itself costs approximately $2000. Lastly and most important are the criteria established by Hepenstall et al. (Abstract 7–5) for surgical intervention in acute compartment syndrome. This selection of articles on compartment syndromes is excellent and the originals are recommended to the interested reader.—J.S. Torg, M.D.

Proximal Tibial Osteotomy in Patients Who Are Fifty Years Old or Less: A Long-Term Follow-Up Study
Holden DL, James SL, Larson RL, Slocum DB (McBride Clinic, Oklahoma City; Orthopaedic and Fracture Clinic, Eugene, Ore)
J Bone Joint Surg [Am] 70-A:977–982, August 1988   7–7

Whereas it is widely accepted that proximal tibial osteotomy is an effective treatment for unicompartmental osteoarthritis of the knee, regardless of the patient's age, it has been suggested that this procedure should be reserved for younger patients who have an active life-style. The results of proximal tibial valgus osteotomy were evaluated in 45 patients younger than 50 years (average age, 41 years; range, 23–50 years) with unicompartmental osteoarthritis of the knee. The average length of follow-up was 10 years (range, 5–13 years).

Using the knee rating of the Hospital for Special Surgery, results were rated as good or excellent in 36 of 51 knees (70%) and fair or poor in 15 (30%). The degree of osteoarthritis at the time of osteotomy, age of the patient at osteotomy, or length of follow-up did not significantly affect the quality of the result. An increased angle of correction after osteotomy was associated with better results, but the values were not statistically significant. The most accurate determinant of the success of proximal tibial osteotomy over time was the severity of disease preoperatively as reflected by the knee score. Of the 18 knees that had a preoperative score of 70–84 points, there were 11 excellent and 4 good results, for a total of 83%. Deficiency of the anterior cruciate ligament at the time of osteotomy did not prevent a good result.

Proximal tibial osteotomy for unicompartmental arthritis of the knee provides the best long-term result when performed early in the course of the disease, and the opportunity to do this occurs most often in the young patient. Proximal tibial valgus osteotomy can thus be an effective procedure for patients younger than 50 years who are living an active life-style.

▶ On the basis of a very limited personal experience, I would agree with the conclusion of the authors that ". . . proximal tibial osteotomy for unicompartmental arthritis of the knee is a good and effective procedure for patients who are less than fifty years old and have an active life-style, and that lasting results can be achieved if the procedure is done early in the course of the disease." Several additional points should be made, however. As is noted in the article, it is unreasonable to expect patients to return to sports that require a great strain on the knee, such as occurs in jumping and cutting, after a successful osteotomy. Also, because of the basic problem, deterioration following successful results should be expected in that it reflects the inevitable progression of the disease process and does not necessarily reflect failure of the procedure.—J.S. Torg, M.D.

Femoral Neck Stress Fractures
Fullerton LR, Snowdy HA (Martin Army Community Hosp, Fort Benning, Ga; Med College of Georgia, Augusta)
Am J Sports Med 16:365–377, July–August 1988   7–8

The current emphasis on increased physical activity has prompted many reports concerning stress fracture in the femoral neck. A prospective study was made of 54 of these fractures to clarify the natural history of the injury. Because previous classification methods were found to be inadequate, a classification system was developed combining the biomechanical and degree of displacement elements from previous classification systems. Femoral neck stress fractures were divided into 3 categories:

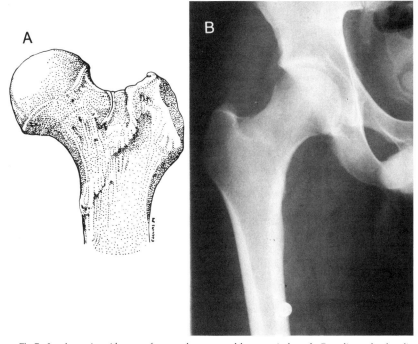

Fig 7–2.—**A**, tension-side stress fracture demonstrated by a cortical crack. **B**, radiograph of undisplaced crack in the tension side of a femoral neck. (Courtesy of Fullerton LR, Snowdy HA: *Am J Sports Med* 16:365–377, July–August 1988.)

tension-side fractures (Fig 7–2), compression-side fractures (Fig 7–3), and displaced fractures. Of 9 fractures treated operatively, 3 were displacement fractures.

Factors that should alert the physician to a diagnosis of femoral neck fracture are hip or groin pain in a patient subjected to repetitive loading of the femoral neck in an exercise situation in which exertion to the point of muscle fatigue is common. In this study, neither tension fractures nor compression fractures progressed to displacement during treatment.

The findings differ from earlier studies in that apparently greater racial diversity exists among patients than has been heretofore noted. Nonprogression of tension-side fractures and return-to-function data also differed.

Displaced Stress Fractures of the Femoral Neck in Young Male Adults: A Report of Twelve Operative Cases
Visuri T, Vara A, Meurman KOM (Central Military Hosp, Helsinki)
J Trauma 28:1562–1569, November 1988   7–9

Stress fractures are a common form of injury among runners and military trainees. Fractures of the femoral neck comprise only a small per-

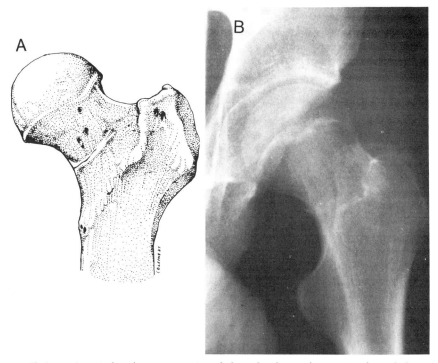

Fig 7—3.—**A,** cortical crack in a compression-side femoral neck stress fracture. **B,** radiograph showing a compression-side stress fracture with an undisplaced cortical crack. (Courtesy of Fullerton LR, Snowdy HA: *Am J Sports Med* 16:365—377, July—August 1988.)

centage of these injuries, but they are the most serious and most likely to cause permanent handicap. Twelve patients were seen with displaced stress fractures of the femoral neck. All 12 were military conscripts (mean age, 19.8 years). They were treated operatively at a mean of 4.9 days after sustaining the injury. In 10 hips a sliding hip compression screw was used. A Jewett nail was used in 1 patient, and a 130-degree AO-nail in another.

Man, 20, underwent closed reduction and compression screw fixation. At 6 months the screw was removed because of perforation of the femoral neck. Two months later delayed union required osteotomy fixed by a sliding compression screw. Avascular necrosis was visible 3 years after surgery (Fig 7—4).

Primary osteosynthesis achieved acceptable results in only 6 patients. Other studies also have reported poor results in young patients treated operatively for femoral neck fractures. Three months of total non-weight-bearing seems to improve the outcome. Patients complaining of hip pain after running or training should be examined by scintigraphy, which can show stress fractures before they are visible on x-ray examination.

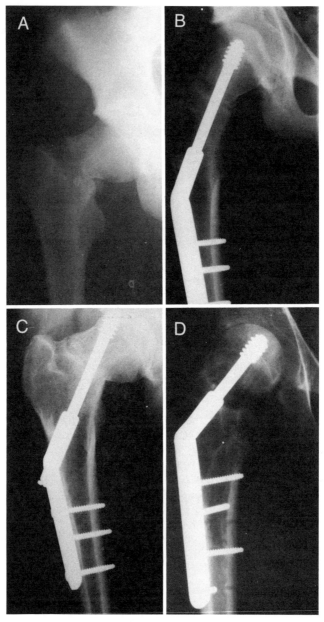

Fig 7–4.—**A,** displaced stress fracture with typical posteromedial cortical fragmentation. **B,** good alignment of the fracture and good position of the nail after closed reduction and compression screw fixation. **C,** perforation of the femoral head by the nail and delayed union 6 months after surgery. **D,** result after varus osteotomy and refixation with compression screw. **E,** final result 3 years after surgery. Total aseptic necrosis of the femoral head is visible. (Courtesy of Visuri T, Vara A, Meurman KOM: *J Trauma* 28:1562–1569, 1988.)

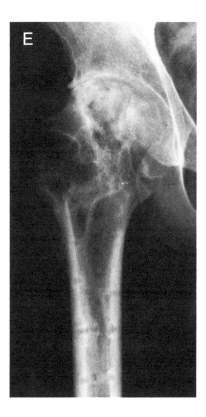

Fig 7–4. (cont.).

▶ Ill-defined hip pain in the physically active individual arouses suspicion of a stress fracture of the femoral neck. Appropriate diagnostic studies include a bone scan as well as roentgenographic examination. The classification by Fullerton and Snowdy (Abstract 7–8) of femoral neck stress fractures into tension, compression, or displaced is not necessarily complete. We prefer the following: (1) preradiographic: positive history, positive bone scan, and negative x-ray appearance; (2) radiographic: tension fracture nondisplaced and compression fracture nondisplaced; (3) tension fracture partially displaced and compression fracture partially displaced; (4) displaced fracture.

Early diagnosis and firm conservative non-weight-bearing management of grades I and II fractures necessitate a more comprehensive classification. Early diagnosis and treatment should prevent the problem from entering the third and fourth stages where, as indicated by Visuri et al.'s paper (Abstract 7–9), surgical management leaves a lot to be desired. Specifically, of the 12 displaced stress fractures surgically treated by Visuri et al., aseptic necrosis of the femoral head developed in 5 and 3 went on to nonunion. Only 6 patients had what they considered acceptable results. The fact that Fullerton and Snowdy do not state their operative results certainly arouses one's curiosity.—J.S. Torg, M.D.

Torn Acetabular Labrum in Young Patients: Arthroscopic Diagnosis and Management

Ikeda T, Awaya G, Suzuki S, Okada Y, Tada H (Koga Hosp, Shiga-ken, Japan; Kokura Mem Hosp, Kitakyushu, Japan)
J Bone Joint Surg [Br] 70-B:13–16, January 1988   7–10

Reports of a torn acetabular labrum without major trauma have been infrequent. This lesion was found in 7 young patients in 3 of whom the pain began suddenly and in 4 occurred gradually. Hip arthroscopy enabled the diagnosis of tears of the labrum. Arthrography revealed the lesion in only 1 case; plain radiographs offered no positive findings. A period of non weight-bearing on crutches brought relief from pain in 6 patients. The seventh patient required partial resection of the anterior part of the labrum with freeing of the psoas tendon before she was able to resume normal activities.

The posterosuperior part of the labrum appears to be subject to inquiry from a sudden twist or repeated stress. A tear in the labrum does not seem to heal naturally, and without treatment, osteoarthritis or locking may develop. Arthroscopy is recommended for the diagnosis of a torn acetabular labrum. Arthroscopic treatment by resection or repair is likely to be a future development.

▶ The authors clearly establish the feasibility of the diagnostic and therapeutic potential of hip arthroscopy. Having made the diagnosis of tears of the anterior superior attachment of the acetabular labrum, they note that all cases were managed conservatively with a period of non-weight-bearing, with all but 1 responding well to this regimen. They then note that, "A labral tear does not seem to heal naturally," without attempting to explain this apparent inconsistency.—J.S. Torg, M.D.

Longstanding Groin Pain in Athletes: A Multidisciplinary Approach

Ekberg O, Persson NH, Abrahamsson P-A, Westlin NE, Lilja B (Univ of Lund, Malmö, Sweden)
Sports Med 6:56–61, July 1988   7–11

In athletes with chronic groin pain of insidious onset, signs of musculoskeletal injury usually are vague or absent. The pain can impede sports activities and training. Data on 21 men aged 20–40 years with groin pain for longer than 3 months were reviewed. Most of them were soccer players. Nuclear diagnostic studies were done using ^{99m}Tc-methylene diphosphate.

Herniography showed pathology in the symptomatic groin in 11 patients, 7 of whom had indirect (lateral) herniation. None of these patients had a palpable hernia, but 1 had a widened external canal ring. Two others had clinical signs of incipient hernia. Fifteen patients had evidence of symphysitis, some without positive scan findings; 11 of 14 with positive scans had clinical findings of symphysitis. All 10 patients with prostatitis had signs of other illness as well.

Chronic groin pain in athletes often has a complex pathogenesis. For this reason, those with pain of obscure origin are best managed on a multidisciplinary basis.

► This paper presents an interesting and what in all probability is a practical approach to a not uncommon, and in most instances, difficult problem. The interested reader is referred to the original article.—J.S. Torg, M.D.

8 Injuries of the Knee

Knee Injuries in Sports
Zarins B, Adams M (Harvard Med School)
N Engl J Med 318:950–960, Apr 14, 1988   8–1

The knee is the most commonly injured joint in many sports, and knee injuries are the leading cause of long-term athletic disability. Improvements in football shoes and in rules have lowered the rate of knee injury. However, knee injuries from skiing have increased, particularly anterior cruciate ligament injuries.

In the Lachman test for anterior cruciate ligament function, the tibia is pulled forward at 25 degrees of knee flexion. The pivot shift test reproduces the event that occurs when the knee gives way because of loss of the anterior cruciate ligament. Operative arthroscopy has shown that an anterior cruciate tear is present in more than two thirds of knees with acute hemarthrosis. A small avulsion fracture of the lateral tibial condyle just below the joint line also signifies anterior cruciate injury. Magnetic resonance imaging is a sensitive means of diagnosing soft tissue injuries about the knee but remains too expensive for routine use.

Most intra-articular conditions now can be treated by arthroscopic surgery. However, primary surgical repair of the torn anterior cruciate ligament without added augmentation has a very low rate of success. Autogenous tissue, therefore, should be used in the repair. Most young patients who are active in sports should have reconstruction. A complete tear of the medial collateral ligament can be treated with a cast brace or hinged brace. The injured meniscus should be saved if possible, and partial removal is preferable to complete meniscectomy. Satisfactory surgical treatment remains to be developed for posterior cruciate ligament injury. In patellar injuries, débridement can lessen symptoms, but removal of the damaged cartilage probably does not improve the long-term outcome to a marked degree.

▶ This article is an excellent primer on the current state of the art on the diagnosis and management of knee injuries in sports. It is based on an extensive bibliography of 119 articles; however, it is concise and well written. The interested reader is referred to the original article.—J.S. Torg, M.D.

Magnetic Resonance Imaging of the Knee
Jackson DW, Jennings LD, Maywood RM, Berger PE (Southern California Ctr for Sports Medicine, Long Beach, Calif; Univ of California, San Francisco; Mem Magnetic Resonance Ctr, Long Beach; Del Amo Diagnostic Ctr, Torrance, Calif)
Am J Sports Med 16:29–38, January–February 1988   8–2

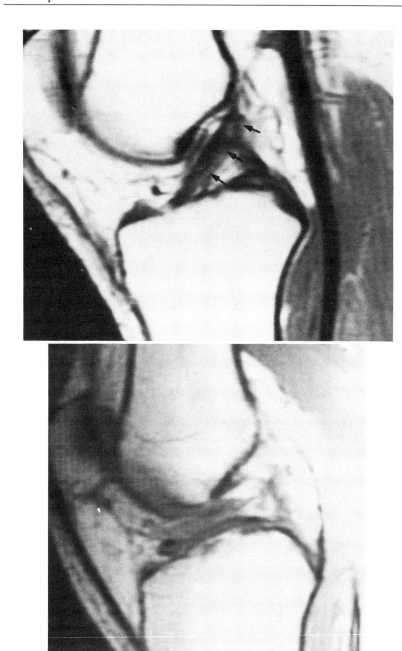

Fig 8–1 (top).—Normal *(arrows)*.
Fig 8–2 (bottom).—Torn anterior cruciate ligament is absent on this and adjacent images.
(Courtesy of Jackson DW, Jennings LD, Maywood RM, et al: *Am J Sports Med* 16:29–38, January–February 1988.)

Magnetic resonance (MR) imaging is a noninvasive method of evaluating soft tissue pathologic changes. When used to examine the knee for suspected tears of the menisci, MR imaging could have advantages over arthrography, now the standard diagnostic tool. Arthrography causes discomfort, is invasive, and uses ionizing radiation; whereas MR imaging has none of these disadvantages and affords improved soft tissue contrast.

The findings at MR imaging and arthrography were compared to assess the accuracy of diagnosis in meniscal and cruciate ligament disorders. Of 155 patients on whom MR images were obtained, 86 subsequently underwent arthroscopic surgery; the results of the 2 procedures in these patients were evaluated.

At MR imaging the anterior cruciate ligament was considered to be present when most of the ligament was identifiable (Fig 8–1). When the anterior cruciate ligament could not be identified, it was classified as torn (Fig 8–2). Treatment was planned according to MR findings, past history, and clinical evaluation.

Forty-one patients were found at arthroscopy to have tears of the medial meniscus. The MR images depicted 40 of these tears and gave 5 false positive results. On the whole, MR imaging and arthroscopic observations corresponded closely. The findings show that MR imaging can be highly accurate in the diagnosis of tears of the menisci and cruciate ligaments, and its accuracy should increase as physicians become more familiar with the method. Because arthroscopy is a procedure that is at once therapeutic and diagnostic, it may still be preferable when the clinical diagnosis is straightforward.

▶ This is an excellently controlled study and confirms that MR imaging has the potential to be an accurate noninvasive method to diagnose internal derangement of the knee provided the examination is performed and interpreted by experienced practitioners.—J.S. Torg, M.D.

Pitfalls in MR Imaging of the Knee
Herman LJ, Beltran J (Ohio State Univ)
Radiology 167:775–781, June 1988   8–3

Magnetic resonance (MR) imaging is a sensitive procedure for diagnosing meniscal tears in the knee, but false positive findings range from 10% to 40% as verified by arthroscopy. Fifty-two knee examinations were reviewed retrospectively to determine the areas of discrepancy between the findings on MR imaging and arthroscopy.

Some of the pitfalls were noted on normal structures with inherently low signal intensity. The transverse ligament and the lateral inferior geniculate artery mimicked a meniscal tear in the anterior horns of the medial and lateral menisci, respectively. The popliteus tendon mimicked a tear in the posterior horn of the lateral meniscus. Pitfalls were also caused by volume averaging at the outer margin of the meniscus. The attachment of the joint capsule produces a concavity at the outer margin of the meniscus that is filled with periarticular fat and neurovascular structures. Sagittal images through this periphery demonstrated a high-signal-intensity linear artifact within the normally dark meniscus. This was caused by volume averaging of the high-signal-intensity fat in the concavity of the meniscus with the low-signal-intensity fibrocartilage of the meniscus.

Of the 10 patients who underwent MR imaging only in the axial and sagittal planes, 1 bucket-handle tear of the medial meniscus was not identified. In retrospect, this tear on the posterior horn of the meniscus was abnormally small to be seen. One bucket-handle tear was seen on the coronal image but not on the sagittal image. No tears were missed on the 48 knees imaged in both the sagittal and coronal planes, but a peripheral detachment beginning at the popliteus tendon and another suspected tear of a suspensory ligament were noted only in the coronal image.

Errors in interpreting anatomical structures with inherently low-signal intensity, such as the transverse ligament, lateral inferior geniculate artery, and popliteal tendon, can be avoided by tracing these structures on adjacent sagittal images and by comparing sagittal images with the corresponding coronal images. The use of a 5-mm, instead of a 3-mm, section thickness is also helpful. Pitfalls caused by volume averaging at the outer margin of the meniscus can be avoided by using a 5-mm section thickness and additional images in the coronal plane. Familiarity with the appearance of these pitfalls can prevent misinterpretation of MR images. In addition to the sagittal images, imaging in the coronal plane improves the accuracy of the MR imaging.

▶ Inexperience and unfamiliarity with normal structures are not pitfalls. Magnetic resonance imaging is in its infancy and, as with arthrography and arthroscopy, more experience is necessary to improve its accuracy and prevent both false positive and false negative diagnoses.—J.S. Torg, M.D.

The Accuracy of Selective Magnetic Resonance Imaging Compared With the Findings of Arthroscopy of the Knee
Polly DW Jr, Callaghan JJ, Sikes RA, McCabe JM, McMahon K, Savory CG (Walter Reed Army Med Ctr, Washington, DC; Riverside Hosp, Newport News, Va; US Army Hosp, Würzburg, West Germany)
J Bone Joint Surg [Am] 70-A:192–198, February 1988   8–4

Arthroscopy and arthrography improve the accuracy of diagnosis when there is injury to the soft tissues of the knee, but these invasive procedures often cause complications. Selective magnetic resonance (MR) imaging is noninvasive and without ionizing radiation. The accuracy of selective MR imaging was compared with findings from arthroscopy in 50 patients. The protocol for imaging produced T1 sagittal images interleaved at 4 mm with the patient's foot in 20 degrees of external rotation.

Selective MR imaging produced excellent visualization of the posterior cruciate ligament, medial meniscus, and lateral meniscus in all patients; the anterior cruciate ligament was well visualized in 76% of the patients. The sensitivity, specificity, and accuracy of MR imaging, when compared with arthroscopy, were 96%, 100%, and 98%, respectively, for tears of the medial meniscus. For tears of the lateral meniscus, rates were 67%, 95%, and 90%. For tears of the posterior cruciate ligament, they were undefined as to sensitivity and 100% for both specificity and accuracy. When the anterior cruciate ligament was well visualized, sensitivity was 100%, specificity, 97%, and accuracy, 97%.

Selective MR imaging is a safe, noninvasive, and valuable adjunct to clinical evaluation of the knee. The procedure can be performed in 15 minutes at a cost comparable to arthrographic procedures.

▶ The authors state, "The reported accuracy of arthrography has ranged widely, from 60 to 97 per cent . . .". They also state, "Diagnostic arthroscopy is an important advance, improving diagnostic accuracy to 64 to 94 per cent." I question how this is an improvement. The authors add that their technique of MR imaging can show tears that are difficult to detect arthroscopically. However, despite the reported accuracy and the failure to find meniscal tears, arthroscopy is used as the gold standard for this study.

The statement that ". . . the interpretations of experienced radiologists are reproducible" is not fact and should be supported by ROC curves (1).

The authors conclude that their technique ". . . adequately demonstrated the status of the cruciate ligaments and menisci, with some limitations." In their study 50% of degenerative tears were not identified, 24% of anterior cruciate ligaments could not be visualized, extremely lateral and medial findings were missed, cartilaginous loose bodies and articular cartilage defects were not well delineated, and isolated patella femoral problems were not identified. It would seem that "some" limitations are "major."—J.S. Torg, M.D.

Reference

1. Metz CE: ROC methodology in radiologic imaging. *Invest Radiol* 21:720–733, 1986.

Anterior Cruciate Ligament Tears: MR Imaging Compared With Arthroscopy and Clinical Tests
Lee JK, Yao L, Phelps CT, Wirth CR, Czajka J, Lozman J (Albany Med College and Albany Med Ctr Hosp, NY)
Radiology 166:861–864, March 1988   8–5

Timely evaluation of the extent of ligamentous damage is essential for appropriate management of significant knee injury. A study was conducted to determine the effectiveness of magnetic resonance (MR) imaging as a noninvasive method of diagnosing tears of the anterior cruciate ligament (ACL).

Seventy-nine MR studies of the knee were reviewed, and the findings were compared with the findings of 2 commonly applied clinical tests of

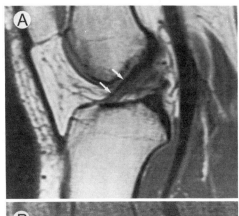

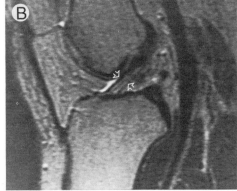

Fig 8–3.— Normal knee. **A,** sagittal image through the intercondylar notch (2,000/20) shows the ACL as an oblique, low-signal-intensity band *(arrows)*. **B,** delayed-echo image (2,000/80) of the same sagittal section demonstrates the "arthrographic" effect of high-signal-intensity joint fluid outlining a smooth, straight synovial reflection along the anterior margin of the ACL *(arrows)*. **C,** sagittal image (2,000/20) 1 cm medial to those in **A** and **B** shows the normal curvature of the posterior cruciate ligament. (Courtesy of Lee JK, Yao L, Phelps CT, et al: *Radiology* 166:861–864, March 1988.)

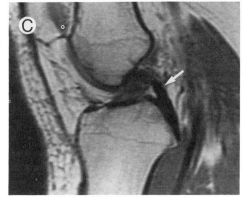

ACL instability, the Lachman test and the anterior drawer test. The sensitivity of MR imaging was 94%, compared with 78% for the anterior drawer test and 89% for the Lachman test. The specificity of all 3 was 100%. A diagnosis of ACL tear was based on the presence of any of 3 findings: an irregular, wavy contour to the anterior margin of the ACL; high signal intensity in the substance of the ACL on T2-weighted images;

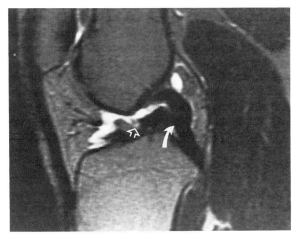

Fig 8–4.—Sagittal image (2,000/80) of knee in a man aged 34 years shows disruption of the midportion of the ACL *(open arrrow)* and associated anterior bowing of the posterior cruciate ligament *(curved arrow)* related to anterior subluxation of the tibia. Joint effusion is also noted. (Courtesy of Lee JK, Yao L, Phelps CT, et al: *Radiology* 166:861–864, March 1988.)

and discontinuity of the substance of the ACL on sagittal images. A fourth finding, anterior bowing of the posterior crucial ligament (Fig 8–3), was often seen as a supportive sign of ACL tear when 1 of the other major findings was present; however, this finding depended in part on patient positioning and the degree of ligament laxity. The sagittal T2-weighted image was particularly helpful, producing an arthrographic effect in which the anterior margin of the ACL was outlined by high-signal intensity joint fluid (Fig 8–4).

These findings support the efficacy of MR imaging in demonstrating tears of the ACL, as predicted by earlier studies. By demonstrating ACL and other extrameniscal lesions, MR imaging may help to clarify the mechanisms of injuries to the knee.

▶ The difference between MR imaging of the anterior cruciate ligament and a properly performed Lachman test is about $900.00—J.S. Torg, M.D.

Tears of the Meniscus as Revealed by Magnetic Resonance Imaging
Silva I Jr, Silver DM (Orthopaedic Hosp, Los Angeles; Beverly Hills Med Ctr, Los Angeles)
J Bone Joint Surg [Am] 70-A: 199–202, February 1988   8–6

Magnetic resonance (MR) imaging was evaluated for its accuracy in detecting tears of the meniscus. Forty-four patients were examined with both MR imaging and arthroscopy. Group I (28 patients) had no previous knee surgery. Group II (16 patients) had previously undergone surgery for meniscal injury.

A grading system was adopted for evaluating the severity of each tear. Grade 0 indicated that there was no tear. Grade I meant that there was a

95% chance that no tear was present. The patterns seen in grade II suggested an 80% chance that no tear would be found. A grade III pattern indicated an 80% probability that a tear would be found. Grade IV patterns increased the chance that a tear would be found to 98%.

In group I the findings at MR imaging were false positive in 10 cases and false negative in 12; thus the rate of accuracy was only 45%. In group II the results were no better; MR imaging allowed a correct diagnosis in 48% of the cases. With false negative scans eliminated, the accuracy rate for the 2 groups would be 65% and 56%, respectively.

The findings suggest that arthroscopy may facilitate detection of as many as 92% of tears of the posterior horn of the meniscus. Because the accuracy of MR imaging is considerably lower, surgeons and radiologists should not rely on data obtained with this modality.

▶ The authors conclude that, ". . . the surgeon and radiologist should exercise caution in interpreting the data that are derived from magnetic resonance imaging." Certainly, this is a correct statement and is true for data received from any modality, be it imaging, the history and physical, the clinical examination, or arthroscopy. It is the expertise of the individual performing and interpreting these examinations that determines the accuracy of the study.—J.S. Torg, M.D.

An Electron Microscopic Study of Early Pathology in Chondromalacia of the Patella

Ohno O, Naito J, Iguchi T, Ishikawa H, Hirohata K, Cooke TDV (Kobe Univ, Japan; Kanebo Hosp, Kobe; Queen's Univ, Kingston, Ont)
J Bone Joint Surg [Am] 70-A:883–899, July 1988   8–7

Biopsy specimens from 12 young patients obtained during knee surgery were examined. The changes found in the articular cartilage were characteristic of chondromalacia. To distinguish chondromalacia patellae from other lesions, ultrastructural changes in a variety of specimens were studied. The patients were evaluated clinically and their biopsy samples submitted for analysis by light microscopy and electron microscopy.

Girl, 14 years, experienced instability of the patella for a year. Jumping brought on sudden pain followed by swelling. An axial patellar radiograph revealed the patella to be tilted and laterally displaced. Surgeons noted a chondral defect (2 × 1.2 cm) with fraying and splitting of the surface. Photomicrographs showed the early stage of chondromalacia patellae, with chondrocytes sparsely distributed in the superficial layer. Eighteen months after surgery the girl had no major symptoms in the knee.

Cartilage specimens with closed chondromalacia (stage 1) were soft and swollen and had a dull appearance. The surfaces were relatively intact. Compared with normal articular cartilage, those with closed chondromalacia have fewer chondrocytes, and these appeared in scattered clusters. In open chondromalacia (stage 2), surface fissures were noted and matrix streaks seldom observed. These ultrastructural changes are likely to be load and stress related.

▶ Several important points are derived from this paper. First, the authors' ultrastructural observations on the specimens from patients who had clinical chondromalacia are compatible with the pathogenesis resulting from mechanical overload. Second, the assumption is made that there is progression from stage I closed to stage II open chondromalacia during the course of the disease, indicated by the location of the 2 stages in adjacent areas of cartilage in the same patient. Also, a "limited repair reaction" was observed in some specimens, an observation having potentially significant clinical import. Lastly, an attempt was made to answer the question of whether the pathogenic events proposed for chondromalacia patella also apply to osteoarthritis. This view is not supported by the observation that the initial changes of osteoarthritis seem to occur at the surface of the cartilage, whereas the changes of chondromalacia patella appear to begin initially in the matrix beneath the surface.— J.S. Torg, M.D.

Contact Pressures in Chondromalacia Patellae and the Effects of Capsular Reconstructive Procedures
Huberti HH, Hayes WC (Harvard Med School)
J Orthop Res 6:499–508, July 1988   8–8

Patellofemoral contact areas and pressures were measured using pressure-sensitive film in 10 human cadaver knees with degenerative lesions in the patellar cartilage. The specimens were obtained from adults of both sexes aged 61–84 years. Contact pressures were measured on flexion from 20 to 90 degrees and after various capsular reconstructive procedures. Medial and lateral capsular plication and lateral and bilateral capsular release procedures were carried out.

When the capsule was intact, a 50% reduction in pressure was achieved in localized grades I–II lesions. In more severe lesions a loss of contact pressure exceeding 90% was observed. The reduction in pressure was associated with loss of stiffness in low-grade lesions and with loss of cartilage thickness in grades III–IV lesions. Highly localized peak pressures were found for normal cartilage bordering the lesions. No form of capsular reconstruction consistently lowered pressures or created a more uniform distribution of pressure.

Substantial reductions in contact pressure are found overlying chondromalacic lesions. The increased peak pressure found on the bordering normal cartilage is a possible means of lesion extension. Release procedures do not predictably lower pressures in the cadaver knee.

Subluxation of the Patella: Computed Tomography Analysis of Patellofemoral Congruence

Inoue M, Shino K, Hirose H, Horibe S, Ono K (Osaka Univ, Japan)
J Bone Joint Surg [Am] 70-A:1331–1337, October 1988   8–9

Adolescents often experience instability of the patellofemoral joint. Axial radiographs are commonly used to assess subluxation of the patella. It has been recommended that the articulation of the knee be examined with the knee at nearly full extension. Computed tomography (CT) has made this possible. The effectiveness of CT was compared with that of axial radiographs with the knee in various angles of flexion in diagnosing patellar subluxation.

The study was done with 50 patients aged 15–25 years who had a provisional clinical diagnosis of patellar subluxation and 30 normal controls aged 16–40 years. The patellofemoral joint of each participant was examined by CT with the knee in full extension and by axial radiography with the knee in 30 and 45 degrees of flexion. The CT examination was done at the midpatellar level, with the patient supine on the table; the radiographs were taken with the patient seated. The amount of lateral patellar tilt was assessed quantitatively using the lateral patellofemoral angle and the congruence angle.

The lateral angle changed significantly when the knee was flexed from full extension to 30 degrees in both the controls and the patients. The difference between the groups was statistically significant at each angle of knee flexion. Both normal and subluxating patellae usually tilted laterally when the knee approached full extension. However, most patients with patellar subluxation had more lateral tilt of the patella when the knee was fully extended than when it was flexed 30 degrees. Therefore, an increase in lateral patellar tilt as the knee is extended should be considered diagnostic of subluxation.

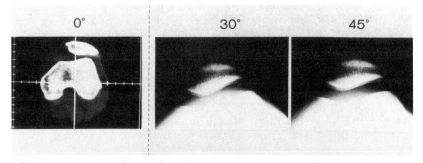

Fig 8–5.—A patient in whom patellar subluxation was demonstrated on CT but not on axial roentgenograms. This patient was playing rugby when he felt acute pain on the medial side of the knee. He had a positive apprehension sign on lateral thrust to the patella. Examination under general anesthesia did not reveal ligamentous instability. Arthroscopy demonstrated no abnormal intra-articular findings. The findings on CT were abnormal; the lateral patellofemoral angle was −8 degrees. Axial roentgenograms showed a shallow femoral groove, but the patella was not seen to be subluxated when the knee was flexed 30 degrees. (Courtesy of Inoue M, Shino K, Hirose H, et al: *J Bone Joint Surg [Am]* 70-A:1331–1337, October 1988.)

The sensitivity of the congruence angle for diagnosing patellar subluxation was low when axial radiography was used. However, the difference in amount of tilt between the controls and the patients doubled when CT was used. In patients with less severe patellar subluxation, CT demonstrated subluxation even at slight flexion of the knee. Four patients in whom an abnormal amount of lateral patellar tilt was observed on CT did not have findings of subluxation on axial radiographs at 30 degrees of flexion (Fig 8–5). The condition would have been overlooked with axial radiography alone.

Patellar subluxation can be detected more accurately by CT with the knee in full extension, particularly in patients with less severe subluxation.

▶ This is an extremely well-planned and executed study with significant clinical usefulness.—J.S. Torg, M.D.

Habitual Dislocation of the Patella in Flexion
Bergman NR, Williams PF (Royal Children's Hosp, Melbourne)
J Bone Joint Surg [Br] 70-B:415–419, May 1988   8–10

Habitual dislocation of the patella in flexion refers to dislocation that occurs each time the knee is flexed. In contrast to recurrent dislocation that occurs as isolated episodes, often in response to trauma, habitual dislocation is painless. Although recurrent dislocation usually involves surgical procedures distal to the patella, habitual dislocation of the patella always requires releases proximal to the patella. The condition is caused by contracture of one or more elements of the quadriceps muscle, but the vastus medialis is rarely affected.

Habitual dislocation of the patella in flexion was treated in 18 boys and 17 girls aged 3–15 years with 43 affected knees; 8 patients had bilateral involvement. All had undergone a quadricepsplasty and were followed for 3 months to 19 years 10 months after operation. Fifteen dislocations were detected when the mother reported an odd-looking knee, 7 were detected at routine examination, and 7 were detected during examination for unrelated trauma to the knee. Only 4 patients had pain. Lateral dislocation of the patella each time the knee is flexed is the most important physical sign of this condition (Fig 8–6).

During operation well-defined bands or muscular contractures within the quadriceps could be detected. Contractures were found in the rectus femoris in 18 knees and in the vastus intermedius in 7. The vastus medialis was felt to be tight in only 1 knee. Operation consisted of release of the tight lateral bands from the patella. The incision was continued proximally, lateral to the rectus femoris tendon to release the vastus lateralis (Fig 8–7). Lengthening the rectus femoris was done in 16 knees, medial plication in 7, and advancement of the vastus medialis in 19. Six patients required transfer of the patellar tendon to achieve stability. In 4 knees significant complications developed during the early postoperative period.

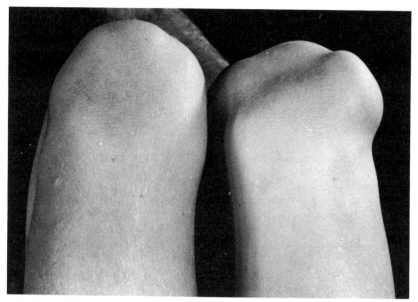

Fig 8–6.—Dislocation occurs each time knee is flexed. (Courtesy of Bergman NR, Williams PF: *J Bone Joint Surg [Br]* 70-B:415–419, May 1988.)

Twelve knees had patellar redislocation and 10 of them were treated with a repeat quadricepsplasty. All 10 reoperations were successful. The other 2 redislocations occurred in children with Down's syndrome; further operations were not deemed justifiable. At follow-up after an average of 6 years 9 months, 34 knees had normal function and 6 occasionally gave way. Three patients complained of pain in the patellofemoral compartment. Nine knees had an ugly scar.

Habitual dislocation of the patella in flexion always requires quadri-

Fig 8–7—Quadriceps lengthening is performed sequentially. First, lateral structures are released; medial structures are then released; the rectus femoris is lengthened at the musculotendinous junction. (Courtesy of Bergman NR, Williams PF: *J Bone Joint Surg [Br]* 70-B:415–419, May 1988.)

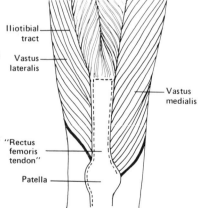

cepsplasty, but good results in terms of patellofemoral pain and function can be expected.

Lateral Retinacular Release of the Patella
Schonholtz GJ, Zahn MG, Magee CM (George Washington Univ)
J Arthroscopic Related Surg 3:269–272, 1987   8–11

In more than 2,300 arthroscopic procedures done on the knee between 1977 and 1984, 35 lateral retinacular releases were accomplished through minimal lateral incisions. Twenty-two patients were available for follow-up. Indications included repeated patellar dislocation, multiple subluxations without dislocation, and anterior knee pain without evident patellar instability. Follow-up averaged 4 years.

Satisfactory results were obtained in 11 of the 22 operated-on knees. Six of 8 patients with a history of dislocation and 4 of 7 with subluxation had a satisfactory outcome. However, just 1 of 7 patients with pain only did well. Complications included 4 hemarthroses. The x-ray findings did not help to predict the results of lateral retinacular release.

Two thirds of the patients in this series operated on for recurrent subluxation or dislocation did well after lateral retinacular release of the patella. This is a reasonable first operative step in patients with symptomatic patellar instability refractory to conservative measures.

▶ I would agree with the authors' observation that success of lateral retinacular release in the surgical treatment of patients with subluxation and or dislocation of the patella is not nearly as high as previously reported (1). However, the numbers presented here are small and were not subjected to tests of statistical significance. Also, classifying the results as "normal," "improved," "unimproved," or "worse" appears less than desirable. I would disagree with the conclusion that knees with symptoms of pain without instability to not benefit from this procedure. Our own experience has been to the contrary (2).—J.S. Torg, M.D.

References

1. Chen SC, et al: *J Bone Joint Surg* 66-B:344–348, 1984.
2. Torg JS, et al.: *Clin Orthop*. In press.

Treatment of Acute Patellar Dislocation
Cash JD, Hughston JC (Hughston Orthopaedic Clinic, Columbus, Ga; Tulane Univ)
Am J Sports Med 16:244–249, May–June, 1988   8–12

Several studies have advocated closed reduction and immobilization in the treatment of acute patellar dislocations, but others recommend acute surgical repair. To help formulate a rationale for determining future treatment, the results were reviewed of nonoperative and operative treatment of initial acute patellar dislocation in 100 patients seen during a 30-year period. Treatment included 1 of 3 methods: immobilization and exercises, arthroscopic surgery, or surgical repair such as arthrotomy and ligament repair. The average age at time of injury was 21.7 years (range, 9–72 years). The most common mechanisms of injury were twisting, valgus stress, or a direct blow to the knee. The average duration of follow-up was 8.1 years (range, 2–26 years).

Retrospectively, the patients were divided into 2 groups. Group I included 69 knees in 66 patients with evidence of congenital abnormality of the extensor mechanism in the unaffected knee, indicating a predisposition to dislocate with less significant trauma. Group II included 34 knees in 34 patients who had no perceptible congenital predisposition to dislocation in the unaffected knee.

In the nonoperatively treated knees, excellent or good results were obtained in 52% of group I and 75% of group II knees. The patient's age at initial dislocation was inversely related to the incidence of redislocation; recurrence was less frequent when the initial dislocation occurred at later than age 14 years, and no patient older than 28 years at initial injury ever had redislocation. Arthroscopic surgery on the knees of 13 patients did not demonstrate significant improved results over those treated conservatively. No redislocations occurred in the 16 patients whose knees were treated with acute open repair, and excellent or good results were obtained in 91% of group I and 80% of group II patients. Of the 29 knees with osteochondral fractures observed on x-ray examination, 20 had undergone acute open repair and only 1 had poor result; the remaining 9 knees were treated conservatively and 5 of them had poor results.

Primary acute patellar dislocations can be treated nonoperatively with good or excellent results. The initial evaluation of all patients with acute patellar dislocations should include a thorough examination of the uninvolved knee, and, if a palpable defect in the vastus medialis obliquus or a large osteochondral fragment is noted, early surgical repair should be considered.

▶ The authors' position that in the absence of significant osteochondral fractures or vastus medialis obliquus (VMO) disruption, initial nonoperative management in the face of primary acute patella dislocation in both the congenitally predisposed and non-predisposed patient is sound. Not dealt with in this study is the potential of arthroscopic lateral retinacular release in group II patients. Two interesting observations were that acute dislocation of the patella occurred more frequently in males, and that recurrence was less frequent when the initial dislocation occurred in those older than 14 years. Although on one occasion they referred to "no statistically significant relationship," they fail to identify the test of statistical significance used or the level of significance obtained.—J.S. Torg, M.D.

Arthroscopic Treatment of Acute Patellar Dislocations
Dainer RD, Barrack RL, Buckley SL, Alexander AH (Naval Hosp, Oakland, Calif)
Arthroscopy 4:267–271, 1988   8–13

Surgery has been recommended for treatment of acute patellar dislocation because of a high incidence of recurrent dislocation and subluxation.
Findings and clinical outcome were surveyed in 29 patients undergoing
arthroscopic treatment for dislocation of the knee; most had sustained a
noncontact twisting injury with the kneecap "going out." None had previous knee symptoms. The average age was 21 years and the average
length of follow-up, 25 months. Fifteen patients had percutaneous lateral
release performed at arthroscopy.

Twenty-four patients had excellent or good results and 1 had a fair result. The 4 poor results were in those who had lateral release. Three of
these had been treated with early motion. No patient without lateral release had recurrence. Osteochondral defects not visible in radiographs
were found in 40% of the patients. In addition, 2 meniscal tears and 1
anterior cruciate tear were noted.

Results in this patient group were better than those reported earlier in
the nonoperative treatment of acute patellar dislocations. Among patients
such as these, with no previous symptoms or predisposition to dislocation or subluxation, reconstructive surgical treatment does not seem necessary.

▶ The position that arthroscopic treatment is indicated in the face of a suspected acute patella dislocation is sound. This approach is not only important
from the standpoint of establishing an accurate diagnosis but will also facilitate
management of osteochondral fractures. I would disagree with the position
that the lateral retinacular release predisposes to a poor result. The problem
with this study was that there were no prospective criteria for performing the
procedure, i.e., hypermobile vs. tight patella. Also, the nature and location of
chondral lesions in the 4 poor results were not noted. Our experience has been
that an arthroscopic lateral retinacular release performed in individuals with
tight lateral structures is quite effective in relieving patella pain as well as in
reducing subluxation and dislocation (1).—J.S. Torg, M.D.

Reference

1. Torg JS, et al.: *Clin Orthop*. In press.

Lateral Release and Proximal Realignment for Patellar Subluxation and Dislocation: A Long-Term Follow-Up
Scuderi G, Cuomo F, Scott WN (Lenox Hill Hosp, New York)
J Bone Joint Surg [Am] 70-A:856–861, July 1988   8–14

A group of patients with patellar subluxation or dislocation underwent a
surgical procedure consisting of lateral release and proximal realignment of
the patella. The results in a long-term follow-up were evaluated and vari-

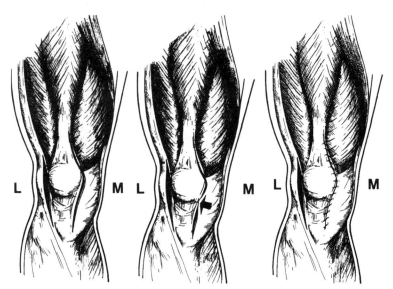

Fig 8–8.—**A,** the lateral release includes intrasynovial dissection that extends from the intrapatellar fat pad, parallels the patellar ligament, and continues proximally into the vastus lateralis. **B,** the patella is centralized in the intercondylar sulcus of the femur. Several trial sutures *(arrow)* are used to ensure that medialization has been accomplished. **C,** before closure of the incision and with all medial capsular sutures in position, the tourniquet is deflated and tracking of the patella is assessed. *M,* medial; *L,* lateral. (Courtesy of Scuderi G, Cuomo F, Scott WN: *J Bone Joint Surg [Am]* 70-A:856–861, July 1988.)

ous factors that might be related to a successful outcome were examined.

Symptoms of patellar subluxation or dislocation include persistent pain, effusions, disability, or recurrent dislocation. Of the 52 patients who entered the study, 21 (group I) had a history of patellar dislocation; 31 patients (group II) had anterior, anterolateral, anteromedial, or occasional popliteal pain. Some patients in both groups had undergone previous surgery.

Technique.—The surgeon makes a medial parapatellar capsular incision that extends from the upper edge of the vastus medialis to the tibial tubercle (Fig 8–8). The medial flap is pulled laterally and distally for at least 1 cm after realignment and then held with provisional sutures. The patella is considered to be centralized if it tracks entirely within the intercondylar sulcus. The medial capsular incision is then closed and the tourniquet deflated. Tracking of the patella is then assessed. After surgery the patient is given a knee immobilizer. Rehabilitation consists of quadriceps-setting exercises followed in a month with range-of-motion exercises.

Of the 52 patients, 42 had good or excellent results. The degree of chondromalacia found did not affect outcome, nor did the fact that the patella had been dislocated. Men and younger patients fared better than women and older patients. In those patients followed for as long as 9 years, those with excellent and good results had no deterioration or recurrence.

► The question that this paper raises is what would have been the effect of a lateral retinacular release alone. Of course, this would have required a randomized study. It has been our experience that in individuals with patellofemoral pain secondary to malalignment with tight retinacular structures, a lateral retinacular release affords comparable results (1).—J.S. Torg, M.D.

Reference

1. Torg JS, et al.: *Clin Orthop.* In press.

Evaluation of the Results of Extensor Mechanism Reconstruction
Cerullo G, Puddu G, Conteduca F, Ferretti A, Mariani PP (Univ of Rome)
Am J Sports Med 16:93–96, March–April 1988   8–15

The many surgical techniques available for treating the malaligned knee can be divided into proximal, distal, or proximal and distal reconstructions. Even with valid techniques properly executed, relatively high incidences of fair to poor results were reported. The long-term outcome was assessed in a series of patients who underwent extensor mechanism reconstructions to determine which factors, if any, influenced the quality of the results.

During an 8-year period, 116 patients underwent operation because of extensor mechanism malalignment associated with dislocating, subluxating, or painful kneecaps. Twenty-two patients were lost to follow-up; the remaining 94 returned for objective and subjective evaluation 3–11 years after operation. Of the 116 patients 80 underwent proximal and distal reconstruction and 36 had only proximal reconstruction. Patients were immobilized postoperatively for 30 days with a plaster cast in extension. All were encouraged to actively exercise the foot and ankle, beginning on the first postoperative day. Exercises for regaining knee flexion were started immediately after cast removal.

Objective evaluation of knee function at follow-up showed that 85% of the patients had excellent or good results and 15% had fair or poor results. Subjectively, 74% of the patients had excellent or good results and 26% had fair or poor results. The excellent and good results were achieved mainly in patients who were treated for a dislocating or subluxating patella. Patients with either fair or poor results had a stable or only mildly unstable patella before operation. Proximal reconstruction was the more effective method for treatment of a stable or mildly unstable patella; proximal and distal reconstruction yielded a very poor outcome in these patients.

Patients with anterior knee pain who have a stable or only mildly unstable patella are better treated by conservative methods as they do not benefit from operation. If operation is unavoidable, only proximal reconstruction should be considered.

► The authors state that in the 116 patients subjected to extensor mechanism reconstruction the indication for surgery was "extensor mechanism malalignment" associated with a dislocating, subluxing, or painful kneecap. However, they fail to establish their criteria for "extensor mechanism malalignment." It is interesting that they express surprise over the fact that in patients with what they describe as a stable or mildly unstable patella, proximal and distal reconstruction had a very poor outcome, i.e., 75% fair or poor subjectively and 50% fair or poor objectively. It appears that the failure of the authors to recognize the role that the lateral retinacular release plays in the surgical management of the "stable" patella associated with patella pain syndrome may account for their quandary. Specifically, they do not describe a lateral retinacular release being performed concomitantly with the proximal and distal realignment. In patients with patella pain syndrome and tight lateral structures associated with the so-called stable patella, a realignment procedure without a concomitant lateral retinacular release only intensifies the patella femoral contact pressures, not only not relieving the problem but perhaps even making it worse. Also, it has been our experience (1) that patella pain associated with the stable patella is managed effectively with an arthroscopic or open lateral retinacular release without associated realignment procedures.—J.S. Torg, M.D.

Reference

1. Torg JS, et al.: *Clin Orthop.* In press.

Osteochondritis Dissecans in the Lateral Patellofemoral Groove
Kurzweil PR, Zambetti GJ Jr, Hamilton WG (St Luke's-Roosevelt Hosp Ctr, New York)
Am J Sports Med 16:308–310, May–June 1988   8–16

Osteochondritis dissecans was encountered in the superior portion of the lateral patellofemoral groove in 2 patients; the defect has never before been reported in this location. The exact size and position of the defects were determined on computed tomographic (CT) scans. Arthroscopic surgery yielded excellent results in both cases.

Case 1.—Boy, 17 years, injured his left knee playing football. After mild pain persisted for 2 weeks, a physical examination was performed, and the sensation of a loose body was detected in the intercondylar notch. A CT scan revealed an area of osteochondritis dissecans along the anterolateral aspect of the patellofemoral groove (Fig 8–9). Two fragments were removed during arthroscopy, and the patient recovered normal movement after rehabilitative exercises.

Case 2.—Man, 47, a marathon runner, had experienced pain in the patellofemoral area for 2 years. A fragment 2 × 1 cm in size was removed, the base of the lesion was curetted to the bone, and a lateral patellar retinacular release was performed. Straight-leg exercises for 3 months returned the patient to a level of vigorous activity.

In both patients, anteroposterior radiographs did not depict the defects, but CT scans defined the problems, and arthroscopic surgery was successful. In patients with patellofemoral symptoms, a diagnosis of os-

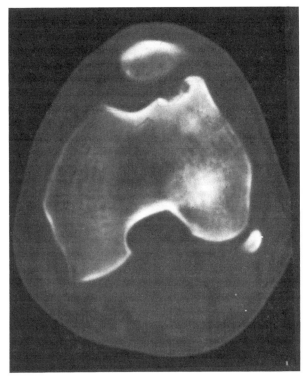

Fig 8–9.—Defect in anterolateral patellofemoral groove is depicted on CT scan. (Courtesy of Kurzweil PR, Zambetti GJ Jr, Hamilton WG: *Am J Sports Med* 16:308–310, May–June 1988.)

teochondritis dissecans of the patellofemoral groove should be considered.

▶ Although certainly no meaningful conclusion can be drawn from a series of 2 cases, there is an interesting comparison between the apparent satisfactory results in osteochondritis dissecans of the lateral patellofemoral groove as compared to the lesions reported by Schwarz et al. involving the patella (see Abstract 8–17).—J.S. Torg, M.D.

The Results of Operative Treatment of Osteochondritis Dissecans of the Patella
Schwarz C, Blazina ME, Sisto DJ, Hirsh LC (The Blazina Orthopedic Clinic, Sherman Oaks, Calif)
Am J Sports Med 16:522–528, September–October 1988   8–17

Osteochondritis dissecans (OCD) of the patella is a rare condition characterized by localized excavation of the patella in which a fragment of articular cartilage and underlying bone have become separated. This fragment should include a true bony layer to be considered as true OCD.

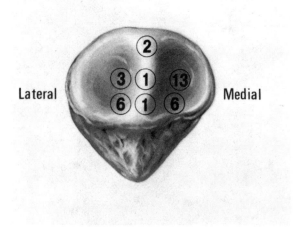

Lateral   Medial

Fig 8–10.—Diagram of undersurface of left patella showing distribution of 32 reported patients with osteochondritis dissecans of the patella. (Modified from Edwards DH, Bentley G: *J Bone Joint Surg [Br]* 59-B: 58–63, 1977). (Courtesy of Schwarz C, Blazina ME, Sisto DJ, et al: *Am J Sports Med* 16:522–528, September–October 1988.)

A review of the literature revealed that the medial facet of the patella is the most commonly involved site (Fig 8–10).

The case reports of 25 patients with OCD in 31 knees who underwent 44 operations were reviewed retrospectively. Preoperative data were extracted from a nationwide Surgical Knee Registry, representing 0.15% of all knee operations listed in the Registry. Follow-up data were obtained by personal interview and physical examination in 20 of the 31 patients and by a telephone interview with 1. Outcome was evaluated with a newly designed patellofemoral rating scale. The average follow-up period in these 21 patients was 73 months.

The average age of the patients at onset of OCD was 18 years. Most (90%) of the patients were men. The most common presenting complaints were pain (87%) and swelling (61%). A loose body was detected by 38% of the patients; locking of the knee was reported by 32%. Patellofemoral crepitus was the most common preoperative finding (74%), followed by generalized effusion (45%) and subpatellar pain with compression (41%). A history of trauma associated with the lesion was reported by 38% of the patients.

The diagnosis of OCD may easily be missed. In a 12-year-old girl who had injured her knee while ice skating, OCD was not discovered during an arthroscopic subcutaneous lateral release for a patellar subchondral cyst. The correct diagnosis was made 2½ years later when she underwent a second operation (Fig 8–11).

Surgical treatment most commonly consisted of curettage of the patella, removal of the loose body, and patellar realignment. Nearly one third of the patients required multiple operations. The outcome, as determined by the new patellofemoral rating scale, was excellent in 5 patients,

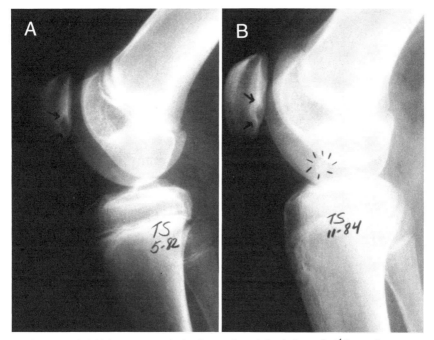

Fig 8–11.—**A,** initial roentgenograph showing patellar subchondral cyst. **B,** $2^{1/2}$ years later, roentgenograph shows defect in patella with presence of loose body. (Courtesy of Schwarz C, Blazina ME, Sisto DJ, et al: *Am J Sports Med* 16:522–528, September–October 1988.)

good in 3, fair in 3, and poor in 10. Only 6 patients experienced no residual pain after operation.

Although OCD of the patella is rare, it should be considered in patients who have patellofemoral symptoms. The prognosis for full recovery of knee function after operation for OCD is considered guarded.

▶ There are several noteworthy aspects of this paper. Although OCD apparently is a rare lesion, the fact that a comparatively large series has been collected by the authors speaks well for the approach through a nationwide surgical knee registry. The means by which the diagnosis of OCD was determined is not stated. Perhaps some or all of the lesions were osteochondral fractures. The fact that a number of the patients also had malalignment problems with various concomitant surgical procedures performed also tends to obscure the issue. With 48% of the group having poor results, it appears that a more innovative surgical approach (e.g., fresh osteochondral allografts) may well be in order.—J.S. Torg, M.D.

Problems Associated With Acute Medial Ligament Ruptures of the Knee: Analysis of Sports Trauma Cases From 1981 to 1987
Paar O (Technischen Univ of München, West Germany)
Chirurg 59:749–754, November 1988   8–18

Acute rupture of the medial collateral ligament of the knee is a common sports injury. The rupture may occur either alone or in combination with an anterior cruciate ligament (ACL) or medial meniscus injury. Incomplete healing of a ruptured medial collateral ligament (MCL) results in permanent abnormal knee function. The MCL may rupture in different places, with no preference for a specific site. The rupture may occur at the tibial or femoral insertion; it may be diffuse, extending over the entire length of the ligament; or it may be isolated deep within the layers of the ligament. Whether there is any association between the site of rupture and the severity of knee injury was examined.

Between 1981 and 1987, 637 knee ligament operations were performed, 311 of which were repairs for acute injuries. Complete data were available for 126 operations. There were 41 proximal, 16 distal, 29 diffuse, and 40 deep intraligament ruptures. More than half of the patients sustained their knee injuries in ski accidents. All ski injuries were combined ligament ruptures, also involving the ACL and/or the posterior portion of the medial meniscus. Soccer was the second most frequent cause of injury; most of these injuries were isolated ruptures. The isolated ruptures were about evenly divided between proximal ruptures at the femoral insertion and single, deep intraligament ruptures, whereas all distal ruptures were combined with rupture of the ACL and the medial meniscus. One patient had complete disinsertion of the medial capsule band apparatus.

Various techniques were used to repair the ruptured ligament, including the use of sutures, small surgical screws, fibrin glue, ligament transfer, PDS strips, or Gore-Tex patches. All 126 ruptured medial collateral ligaments were repaired successfully.

▶ The author has attempted to segregate medial collateral ligament injury into various types as well as establish an association with ACL disruption. The contention that "incomplete healing of a ruptured medial collateral ligament will result in permanent abnormal knee function" is not substantiated by the data or correlated with treatment type, i.e., surgical vs. nonsurgical management. As indicated above, most MCL tears can be managed nonoperatively (see Abstract 8–19).—J.S. Torg, M.D.

The Non Operative Treatment of Isolated Complete Tears of the Medial Collateral Ligament of the Knee: A Prospective Study

Ballmer PM, Jakob RP (Univ of Berne, Switzerland)
Arch Orthop Trauma Surg 107:273–276, 1988   8–19

Good results have been reported after nonoperative treatment in patients who sustain isolated medial collateral ligament (MCL) sprains. A prospective study was conducted to compare the results of 2 different methods of nonoperative treatment of complete grade III MCL injuries in 20 patients. The injury was defined as complete disruption of the ligament with resulting instability.

Selection criteria included valgus instability of 2+ with the knee in 30 degrees of flexion. None of the patients had sustained previous trauma to either the involved or the contralateral knee. Sixteen patients had been injured in sporting activities. All patients underwent arthroscopic evaluation under anesthesia 0–14 days after the injury. One patient refused arthroscopic examination.

Ten patients were treated with an elastic wrap for 8 weeks, allowing immediate mobilization, and early physical therapy. The other 10 were treated with immobilization in a plaster cast for 4 weeks, followed by an elastic wrap and rehabilitation for the next 4 weeks. Patients were evaluated at a follow-up examination 8–30 months after injury.

Eight patients in the early mobilization group and 7 in the rigid mobilization group had excellent ratings at evaluation. Results in the other 5 patients were rated good. None of the patients had any medial laxity with the knee in extension, and 15 had slight laxity with the knee in flexion. The maximal medial opening in 30 degrees of flexion was 1+, both clinically and radiographically. All knees had a normal range of motion compared with the normal knee. All patients were able to return to their previous level of activity or sports without limitation. No subsequent injuries occurred. However, patients in the immediate mobilization group were able to return to work 30% sooner than those in the rigid mobilization group.

The findings of this prospective study confirm that isolated grade III MCL injuries of the knee can be treated successfully by immediate mobilization. Arthroscopic evaluation is indicated in all patients with a medial instability of 2+ to exclude the presence of additional intra-articular injuries that may require surgical intervention.

▶ This prospective study confirms the observations of Ellsasser (1) and Indelicato (2) that injuries involving the MCL with associated laxity can successfully be managed nonoperatively. This study carries the nonoperative concept a step further, i.e., lesions with medial openings up to 10 ml are best treated by early mobilization. However, in interpreting these data, attention must be paid to the classification used. Specifically, grade I and grade II MCL sprains do not demonstrate valgus instability. What they describe as a third-degree sprain is further graded depending on the degree of opening demonstrated on stress test: 1+(3- to 5-mm opening), 2+(6- to 10-mm opening) and 3+(more than 10 mm of opening). Furthermore, they have failed to define anatomically what they consider a complete tear of the MCL. In that the medial supporting structures are really 4 in number (deep layer medial capsular ligament, anterior capsular ligament, posterior oblique ligament, and tibial collateral ligament), a clear definition of the anatomical pathology is lacking. Also, they fail to mention the implications of an anterior cruciate ligament disruption associated with a grade III lesion. I agree with their conclusions based on the data presented; however, I have great reservations about the implication that "complete tears of the medial collateral ligament" is an accurate description of the pathology involved.— J.S. Torg, M.D.

References

1. Ellsasser JC, et al: *J Bone Joint Surg* 56:1185–1190, 1974.
2. Indelicato PA: *J Bone Joint Surg* 65:323–329, 1983.

Acute Tears of the Anterior Cruciate Ligament: Surgical Versus Conservative Treatment
Clancy WG Jr, Ray JM, Zoltan DJ (Univ of Wisconsin, Madison; Univ of Kentucky, Lexington)
J Bone Joint Surg [Am] 70-A:1483–1488, December 1988   8–20

Reports comparing nonoperative and surgical treatment of tears of the anterior cruciate ligament have yielded conflicting results. A prospective study was developed to evaluate the outcomes of the 2 methods through long-term follow-up. Treatment was determined on the basis of the pivot-shift test. Those patients with absent or mild pivot shift were treated conservatively (group I); those with a moderate or severe pivot shift had surgery (group II). Patients in group I underwent arthroscopy followed by a rehabilitation program. The index procedure was performed in group II patients.

Technique.—After arthroscopy, the torn anterior cruciate ligament was identified. Tunnels were drilled in the bone and a whip suture placed on both sides of the largest portion of a proximal or distal tear, or on both ends of a midsubstance tear. A 10-mm wide free graft was harvested from the midportion of the patellar tendon. Sutures of the repaired ligament were drawn through appropriate tunnels; the graft was then drawn into the tunnels and positioned anteriorly on the repaired ligament.

There were 23 patients in group I and 76 in group II. All patients in group I had arthroscopy and 10 also had a meniscectomy. The patients in group II had the index surgical procedure, and 52 had meniscal tears. At an average follow-up of 4 years, 8 patients in group I had excellent results, 10 had good or fair results, and 4 results were judged failures. Good or excellent results were obtained in these 4 patients when the index operation was done at least 2 years after conservative treatment. Of 70 evaluable patients in group II, all except 2 had excellent or good results. No failures were reported in this group.

Even in those patients with absent or mild pivot shaft, nonoperative treatment gave an unsatisfactory outcome in half of them. Primary repair of the anterior cruciate ligament together with augmentation of the patellar tendon yields the best results and is more successful than primary repair alone.

▶ It appears that the authors' conclusion that primary repair and augmentation with the patellar tendon is the treatment of choice for a patient who has an acute tear of the anterior cruciate ligament is all too inclusive and not necessarily supported by their data. To be noted, although prospective, the study was not randomized. The fact that half of the patients in group I, those with negative to mild pivot shift, did well without surgery raises a question as to this group's characteristics; i.e., age, sex, activities, associated meniscal derangement, associated collateral ligament laxity, and so on should have been evaluated. Perhaps in addition to a mild or negative pivot shift there are other characteristics that can differentiate between those patients in group I who will do well conservatively and those who should have ligament reconstruction.—J.S. Torg, M.D.

Lateral Substitution for Chronic Isolated Anterior Cruciate Ligament Deficiency
Frank C, Jackson RW (Orthopaedic and Arthritic Hosp, Toronto)
J Bone Joint Surg [Br] 70-B:407–411, May 1988   8–21

Patients with anterior cruciate ligament (ACL) deficiency syndrome experience episodes of giving way of the knee. One reconstructive surgical technique, the pivot-shift operation (MacIntosh procedure), has been recommended for this condition. The value of this procedure was assessed in 35 patients with gross lateral pivot-shift and arthroscopic evidence of isolated ACL insufficiency.

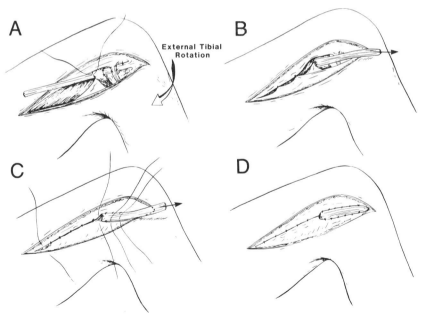

Fig 8–12.—**A,** the strip is sutured under tension to the lateral collateral ligament and the tunnel with the tibia laterally (externally) rotated and flexed to 90 degrees. **B,** the strip is then folded distally and used as a patch for the distal iliotibial band defect (**C**). **D,** strong interrupted sutures complete the lateral closure. (Courtesy of Frank C. Jackson RW: *J Bone Joint Surg [Br]* 70-B: 407–411, May 1988.)

Technique.—A 1.5-cm-wide strip of iliotibial band is passed under the proximal part of the lateral collateral ligament (LCL) and through an oblique tunnel in the tendinous lateral head of the gastrocnemius. The iliotibial graft is sutured to both the proximal LCL and the gastrocnemius tunnel (Fig 8−12). The proximal iliotibial defect is closed with heavy interrupted sutures.

Twenty-seven patients considered that their knee was "definitely better" after the operation. Six reported slight improvement, whereas 2 had no improvement. Six patients experienced arthritic pain, and half of the group felt some degree of pain in the knee. Overall, approximately 75% of the results were judged satisfactory and 25% unsatisfactory.

Because 83% of the patients in this series continued to have symptoms after the pivot-shift operation, the procedure cannot be considered a cure. Other ACL reconstructive methods have resulted in more permanent joint stiffness, however. The pivot-shift procedure can offer low-risk and long-lasting improvement for many patients.

▶ This report puts lateral extra-articular surgical procedures for ACL deficiency in proper perspective. Despite the initial enthusiastic acceptance of such procedures as described by Ellison (1), Losee et al., (2) and MacIntosh and Darby (3), current standards require an intra-articular approach to this problem.—J.S. Torg, M.D.

References

1. Ellison AE: *J Bone Joint Surg [Am]* 61-A:330−337, 1979.
2. Losee RE, et al: *J Bone Joint Surg [Am]* 60-A:1015−1030, 1978.
3. MacIntosh DL, Darby TA: *J Bone Joint Surg [Br]* 58-B:142, 1976.

Reconstruction of the Anterior Cruciate Ligament Using a Torn Meniscus
Ferkel RD, Fox JM, Del Pizzo W, Friedman MJ, Snyder SJ, Dorey F, Kasimian D (Southern Calif Orthopedic and Sports Med Group, Van Nuys; Univ of California, Los Angeles; Valley Presbyterian Hosp, Van Nuys)
J Bone Joint Surg [Am] 70-A:715−723, June 1988   8−22

Patients with a torn anterior cruciate ligament experience giving-way of the knee during normal activities. Reconstructive surgery, which attempts to restore stability to the knee, can be accomplished by a variety of procedures. A torn meniscus was used to repair the anterior cruciate ligament in 100 patients aged 16−57 years. The average follow-up time was 52 months. Forty-four patients had undergone previous surgery for the condition. The success of the procedure was evaluated by means of a questionnaire, clinical testing apparatus, and radiographs.

The meniscus is suitable for repair because it is easily accessible, autogenous, and of sufficient length. In all of these cases the meniscus was already torn and would have to be excised; a normal meniscus should not be used.

Of the results, 80% were judged satisfactory. Most patients returned to work about 5 months after surgery and could engage in sports at an average of 8.5 months after operation. Those who were injured at work tended to have a higher percentage of unsatisfactory results. Of those under age 30, 90% reported satisfactory results, whereas only 65% of older patients had a satisfactory outcome.

Although results were good, this procedure should be used rarely and only under the conditions described. Improvements in arthroscopic technology now enable surgeons to use partial meniscectomy or repair of all but severe meniscal tears: thus, in most cases, a torn meniscus need not be fully excised.

▶ This interesting approach to the age-old problem of managing the anterior-cruciate-deficient knee was reported previously by Collins et al. (1). The well-documented preference for meniscal repair would appear to preclude this approach.—J.S. Torg, M.D.

Reference

1. Collins MR, et al: *Am J Sports Med* 2:11–21, 1974.

Maturation of Allograft Tendons Transplanted Into the Knee: An Arthroscopic and Histological Study
Shino K, Inoue M, Horibe S, Nagano J, Ono K (Osaka Univ, Japan)
J Bone Joint Surg [Br] 70-B:556–560, August 1988   8–23

The remodeling and maturation of an implanted allogeneic tendon in vivo for anterior cruciate ligament repair was investigated in 69 patients. The serial alterations in appearance of the allografts were observed arthroscopically, and biopsy specimens from the midzone of the grafts were studied histologically. The allografts consisted of part of the calcaneal tendon, anterior tibialis tendon, posterior tibialis tendon, or a few bundled flexor tendons.

Arthroscopic examinations from 6 weeks to 55 months postoperatively showed that the grafts were viable. At 6 weeks the graft was covered with a thick hypervascular synovial sheath. At 3–6 months the synovial sheath had thinned out and longitudinally oriented thick fibers were noted. The hypervascularity subsided with time. At 11–12 months the grafts closely resembled the normal anterior cruciate ligament and did not change thereafter. Overall, the functional grafts appeared thick and taut. Histologic studies were performed from 3 to 55 months.

At 3–6 months after operation the surface was covered with a thick synovial sheath infiltrated with many fibroblasts and longitudinally aligned collagen bundles. At 12 months the surface was covered with a thin synovial sheath, and the hypercellularity and hypervascularity decreased with time. At 18 months the substance of the graft showed well-arranged collagen bundles and normal cellularity and remained unchanged thereafter. There was no evidence of immunologic rejection. In contrast, arthroscopy in a patient with a mildly positive Lachman sign at

36 months showed a hypervascular graft, although it seemed relatively taut. The histology showed immaturity consisting of amorphous hyper-cellular and hypervascular scar tissue.

Allograft tendon transplanted into the human knee as an anterior cruciate ligament is infiltrated with vascular buds from the host tissues within 6 weeks. The graft then gradually remodels with time, as hypervascularity and hypercellularity in its substance subside; it reaches maturity by 18 months and survives as a viable anterior cruciate ligament thereafter.

Arthroscopic Reconstruction of the Anterior Cruciate Ligament Using Allograft Tendon

Wainer RA, Clarke TJ, Poehling GG (Wake Forest Univ)
Arthroscopy: J Arthroscopic Related Surg 4:199–205, 1988   8–24

The technique and exact material for reconstruction of the anterior cruciate ligament (ACL) after injury remains controversial. The results of a prospective study of 23 patients who underwent arthroscopic ACL reconstruction using freeze-dried allograft tendons were evaluated. Criteria for reconstruction were failed rehabilitation program and functional instability. The most commonly used tendons were the flexor hallucis tendon, posterior tibialis, and toe extensors. Follow-up ranged from 12 to 24 months (mean, 15 months).

All other intra-articular lesions were treated first; procedures included 6 partial meniscectomies, 2 meniscal repairs, 1 abrasion chondroplasty, and 1 lateral collateral ligament repair. All meniscal repairs were performed arthroscopically. A standard arthroscopic approach combined with a 3-cm incision on the medial tibial flare was used. Two allograft tendons doubled over a ligamentous repair staple were inserted through the tibial hole into the femoral hole. With the knee in 30 degrees of flexion, the tension on the graft was adjusted and its tibial insertion secured with a Stryker ligament staple.

Knee rating values, as assessed with a Lysholm knee rating scale, Lachman test with KT-1,000 arthrometric quantitation, pivot shift, Biodex test, and radiographs, improved in all knees, except for 1 with significant deterioration in the KT-1000 reading. Radiographs showed no change in position of staples and no evidence of advancement of degenerative changes. There were no deep infections and no signs of graft rejection.

All patients with at least 20 months of follow-up had resumed their preinjury activity level. Four patients had subsequent arthroscopy, and a loose tendon, loose staple, loose particle, and medial compartment adhesions were noted. In the patient with a loose tendon, necrotic tissue was found on biopsy. In contrast, the patient with medial compartment adhesions had a taut, revascularized tendon, and histologic examination showed stress-oriented viable fibrocytes with small areas of resorbing necrotic tissue.

This simple arthroscopic procedure using allograft tendon for ACL reconstruction is accurate and causes less morbidity than conventional open procedures. In addition, it allows treatment of other intra-articular disease at the time of grafting. The long-term efficacy of this technique needs to be defined.

▶ The preceding 2 abstracts (8–23 and 8–24) concerning the use of allograft tendons to replace the ACL are certainly encouraging. However, it must be mentioned that the question of the potential transmission of the acquired immunodeficiency (AIDS) virus remains unanswered. And although there has been only 1 reported case of transmission of human immunodeficiency virus from a transplanted organ (1), it is my opinion that, at this point in time, autogenous tissue is preferable to a potential AIDS implant.—J.S. Torg, M.D.

Reference

1. *MMWR* 36:306–308, 1987.

The Gore-Tex Anterior Cruciate Prosthetic Ligament: New Questions and Opportunities in Anterior Cruciate Management
Carstens J (Washington State Univ, Pullman)
Athletic Training 23:253–258, Fall 1988   8–25

The Gore-Tex Anterior Cruciate Prosthetic Ligament (ACPL) is a new option in the management of anterior cruciate ligament (ACL) instability. The Food and Drug Administration approved its use for salvage procedures, but it is also available for primary application. Although it has certain advantages over previous methods, there is uncertainty as to its functional use.

The Gore-Tex ACPL is made of 1 continuous looped, braided strand of polytetrafluoroethylene, 1 of the most inert polymers and biocompatible materials known. It is indicated for use as a permanent replacement for the ACL in patients with at least 1 failed autogenous intraarticular ACL reconstruction and is contraindicated in patients with an incomplete epiphyseal plate and infection. Its use in a primary procedure remains controversial. The Gore-Tex ACPL is similar to the human ACL in tensile strength, design, and longevity; however, unlike the human ACL, its strength is not positionally dependent. It can withstand tensile forces of an average 4,830 ± 28 newtons throughout the full range of motion and absorb up to 4,300 newtons of tensile strain, with only 8% to 10% elongation at failure. Graft longevity was estimated at 20 years in an 84-million-cycle bending fatigue test.

The device is placed using open or arthroscopic procedures, similar to the technique of autogenous reconstruction. The reconditioning process begins immediately after surgery, as the graft strength is maximal at implantation. The athlete can work at his or her reconditioning program using as much effort as the knee can tolerate. During a 2-year trial, 186 patients were given the Gore-Tex ACPL. At 26.2 months the postoperative knee status was rated as improved in 92% of 158 patients, worse in 4%, and unchanged in 4%. During a 3-year follow-up certain complications (e.g., device failure, instability, infection, effusion, screw revision, and other associated problems) occurred in 20.9% of 187 grafts.

The Gore-Tex ACPL is advantageous in terms of surgical implantation, reconditioning time, and graft strength. However, it is not the ultimate answer to improving tibiofemoral joint instability. Questions regarding the anticipated return and degree of disability, possible sacrifice of full extension, and misconception of prosthesis capabilities in ACL instability management remain unanswered.

The goal of managing ACL injuries with any graft, artificial or natural, is to return the athlete to competition and maintain knee stability. The physician and athletic trainer should present sound medical information to the athlete; it is up to the athlete to decide on what is to be done with his unstable knee.

Gore-Tex Prosthetic Ligament in Anterior Cruciate Deficient Knees
Glousman R, Shields C Jr, Kerlan R, Jobe F, Lombardo S, Yocum L, Tibone J, Gambardella R (Kerlan-Jobe Orthopedic Clinic, Inglewood, Calif)
Am J Sports Med 16:321–326, July–August 1988   8–26

Surgeons have reported varying success with reconstruction for symptomatic anterior cruciate ligament (ACL) deficient knees. A potentially promising alternative is the prosthetic cruciate replacement using the Gore-Tex polytetrafluoroethylene ligament as a permanent replacement.

Eighty-two patients with documented symptomatic ACL deficiency underwent reconstruction with the Gore-Tex ligament. Patients were followed for an average of 18 months. Subjective evaluation included pain, giving way, negotiating stairs, locking, and swelling. Objective evaluation included range of motion, thigh circumference, instability tests, and Cybex and KT-1000 Arthrometer evaluation.

Patient scores improved in all subjective evaluations. Patients returned to daily activities at 3 weeks and to athletic activities at 8 months. At 12 months patients lacked 0 degrees of extension and 4 degrees of flexion in range-of-motion evaluation. At final follow-up, all objective data had improved, although an early nonprogressive shift toward loosening was observed. There were 14 reoperations, 15 complications, and 7 permanent complications.

The Gore-Tex ligament may provide an alternative for ACL reconstruction in selected patients. Older, less-active patients and those in whom previous reconstructions have failed may be good candidates. Long-term follow-up studies are necessary before expanded indications for use can be recommended.

Early Experience With the Gore-Tex Polytetrafluoroethylene Anterior Cruciate Ligament Prosthesis
Indelicato PA, Pascale MS, Huegel MO (Univ of Florida)
Am J Sports Med 17:55–62, January–February 1989   8–27

With the current emphasis on fitness and exercise, patients who sustain injuries to the anterior cruciate ligament (ACL) often elect to undergo reconstruction of the knee. The desire for a synthetic ligament prosthesis with biomechanical properties sufficient to withstand the forces applied to the ACL led to the development of the Gore-Tex poltetrafluoroethylene (PTFE) ACL prosthesis (Fig 8–13).

Thirty-nine patients with ACL deficiency who underwent reconstruction with the Gore-Tex PTFE ACL prosthesis were studied by questionnaire, clinical examination, and instrumented ligamentous laxity tests. Reconstruction was performed to repair 8 acute injuries and 31 chronic insufficiencies.

Thirty-four patients returned to full activity with negligible symptoms. Four patients had complete rupture of the prosthesis; the other failure resulted from residual symptomatic posterior cruciate ligament insufficiency. Nine patients had 23 episodes of sterile effusion. These episodes were atraumatic in origin and were associated with swelling and pain. Arthroscopy in 5 patients with recurrent effusions showed partial tears of less than a third of the prosthesis; in synovial biopsy specimens obtained from 3 patients, particles of PTFE were found. Patients responded well to treatment. One patient who had immediate postoperative infection has retained the prosthesis and currently has a stable knee.

The Gore-Tex PTFE ACL prosthesis is a satisfactory method for recon-

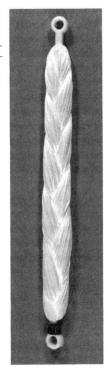

Fig 8–13.—The CORE-TEX PTFE ACL prosthesis. (Courtesy of Indelicato PA, Pascale MS, Huegel MO: *Am J Sports Med* 17:55–62, January–February 1989.)

struction of the ACL in most patients. The device appears to be technique sensitive. Appropriate placement of the graft, anterior and posterior notchplasty, and removal of sharp edges from bony tunnels can help avert failure.

▶ It should be noted that the Gore-Tex anterior cruciate ligament prosthesis was used initially under protocol as an experimental device. In 1986 the Food and Drug Administration gave approval for use of the ligament only in failed intra-articular reconstructions for ACL deficiency. All of the initial clinical studies have been somewhat encouraging; however, in view of the propensity of the device to wear as well as any except for an "early nonprogressive shift toward loosening," its current role in the management of ACL deficiency appears to be limited.—J.S. Torg, M.D.

Pathomechanics of Posterior Sag of the Tibia in Posterior Cruciate Deficient Knees: An Experimental Study
Ogata K, McCarthy JA, Dunlap J, Manske PR (Kyushu Univ, Fukuoka, Japan; Washington Univ)
Am J Sports Med 16:630–636, November–December 1988   8–28

Injuries of the posterior cruciate ligament (PCL) are often diagnosed with the posterior drawer test at 90 degrees of flexion, or by clinical assessment of posterior sagging. However, these methods do not classify the severity of the injury or the rotational changes that occur. In a study using fresh cadaver knees, posterior sag of the tibia was investigated with roentgenographic methods to determine factors associated with sagging. Nine cadaver knees with intact menisci and cruciate ligaments were obtained. To simulate postoperative conditions, 30 newtons of posterior stress were applied to the knees. The actual strain of the PCL and the collateral ligaments was measured with strain gauges.

Posterior sagging of more than 15 mm in a resting, flexed knee did not occur with an isolated PCL and posterior capsular injury. This degree of posterior sagging was seen only after an associated medial collateral ligament (MCL) or lateral collateral ligament (LCL) injury. An increase in tibial rotation at full extension of the knee is also seen with these associated injuries.

The posterior capsule contributes little to the stability of an isolated PCL-deficient knee. An isolated PCL injury requires full extension of the knee after surgical reconstruction, and an intact MCL and LCL are needed to prevent posterior sagging with full extension. Posterior sag at full extension, suggesting an associated collateral ligament injury, can be assessed partially by rotation of the tibia. Roentgenographic evaluation is required to assess the severity of PCL injury and the possibility of associated injuries.

▶ This study makes a significant contribution to the understanding of the clinical behavior of the PCL-deficient knee. Thus an isolated injury to the PCL results in straight posterior laxity, limited to 15 mm extension, whereas greater laxity is associated with involvement of the collateral ligaments. We have reported (1) a series of 47 PCL-deficient knees in which the torn ligament was not repaired or reconstructed. In this group, those with isolated or straight posterior instability did well. On the other hand, those with combined or multidirectional instability did poorly. It appears that the poorer results observed in the knees with combined laxity are explained in part by the findings of Ogata et al.—J.S. Torg, M.D.

Reference

1. Barton TM, et al: *Clin Orthop* 245:95–103, April 1989.

Use of the Quadriceps Active Test to Diagnose Posterior Cruciate-Ligament Disruption and Measure Posterior Laxity of the Knee

Daniel DM, Stone ML, Barnett P, Sachs R (Kaiser Permanente Med Ctr, San Diego; Univ of California, San Diego)
J Bone Joint Surg [Am] 70-A:386–391, March 1988   8–29

Rupture of the posterior cruciate ligament is a condition that has been difficult to assess. The quadriceps active test was developed to diagnose such ruptures and locate the neutral position of the knee in the anterior-posterior plane.

In a series of 92 patients, 25 had no history of a knee injury, 24 had chronic rupture of the posterior cruciate ligament, 18 had an acute pos-

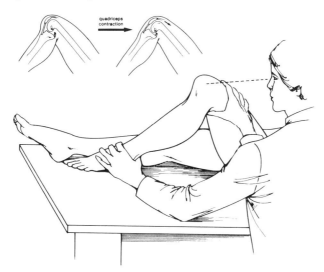

Fig 8–14.—The 90-degree quadriceps active test. Keeping the eyes at the level of the individual's flexed knee, the examiner rests the elbow on the table and uses the ipsilateral hand to support the individual's thigh and confirm that the thigh muscles are relaxed. The foot is stabilized by the examiner's other hand and the individual is asked to slide the foot gently down the table. Tibial displacement resulting from the quadriceps concraction is noted. (Courtesy of Daniel DM, Stone ML, Barnett P, et al: *J Bone Joint Surg [Am]* 70-A:386–391, March 1988.)

terior cruciate ligament rupture, and 25 had chronic rupture of the anterior cruciate ligament. During the test the patient lies on a table with the injured knee flexed. The examiner stablizes the foot and asks the patient to slide the foot down the table. The examiner observes the knee and notes tibial displacement resulting from the quadriceps contraction (Fig 18–14).

The quadriceps neutral angle occurs between 60 and 90 degrees. In a normal knee this is the angle of flexion at which there is no shear component and the tibia does not shift anteriorly or posteriorly when the quadriceps is actively contracted. The individual's normal knee can be compared with the injured knee, allowing anterior and posterior tibial displacement to be measured.

The test correctly diagnosed 41 of 42 knees that had documented posterior cruciate ligament disruption. Anterior translation of the tibia did not occur in any of the normal knees or in those with known unilateral anterior cruciate ligament disruption. The quadriceps active test is not useful, however, if the orientation of the patellar ligament has been changed because of surgery or previous injury.

▶ In this the era of double-contrast arthrography, magnetic resonance imaging, and arthroscopic examinations, it is gratifying to see that some clinicians are able to develop and use diagnostic techniques that rely on physical findings. This paper is in keeping with such a modus operandi. I would, however, challenge the assertion that active anterior translation of the tibia does not occur in the anterior cruciate ligament deficient knee. Gurtler graded the Lachman test on the basis of anterior tibial excursion, the first 3 grades resulting from passive subluxation of the tibia and grade IV caused by active contraction of what in all likelihood is the popliteus muscle (1).

Another interesting observation is that when passive laxity tests are performed with the knee resting in 90° of flexion, knees with the posterior cruciate ligament rupture demonstrate more anterior laxity than do the knees in which the anterior cruciate ligament is ruptured.—J.S. Torg, M.D.

Reference

    1. Gurtler R: *Clin Orthop* 13:13–26, 1984.

The Natural History of Rupture of the Posterior Cruciate Ligament
Dejour H, Walch G, Peyrot J, Eberhard Ph (Ctr Hosp Lyon-Sud, Pierre Bénite, France)
Fr J Orthop Surg 2:112–120, March 1988   8–30

The posterior cruciate ligament (PCL) is the strongest ligament in the knee. Although its rupture often causes only mild functional disability, its ability to become osteoarthritic in time indicates its importance in the biomechanics of the knee. Forty-seven patients with unrepaired, old rupture of the PCL with an intact anterior cruciate ligament were studied to define the natural course of rupture of this ligament. Eleven patients replied to questionnaires only. The mean follow-up was 15 years (range, 5–44 years).

Of the 36 patients who were reexamined radiographically, 21 had isolated posterior laxity, 8 had posterolateral laxity, and 7 had posteromedial laxity. Rupture of the PCL did not significantly disturb the resumption of sports activities. In patients with a follow-up of more than 15 years the outcome worsened over time with regard to stability and pain as well as onset or progression of cartilaginous lesions, compared with patients followed for less than 15 years. Overall, osteoarthritis appeared to develop early and continued to progress for 25 years. True patellofemoral osteoarthritis was noted in 33% of the patients, tibiofemoral osteoarthritis in about 69%, arthrotic remodeling in 41.6%, early tibiofemoral osteoarthritis in 11.1%, and established osteoarthritis in 16.1%, including generalized osteoarthritis in 3 patients.

The natural course of rupture of the PCL can be defined in 3 phases. The first phase is a period of functional adaptation lasting for 3–18 months after injury. Most patients have marked functional derangement with pain and a sensation of instability, especially in full flexion and when using stairs. Reeducation of the quadriceps significantly helps in this adaptation. The second phase is that of functional tolerance, allowing return to sports. This phase lasts about 15 years; however, disturbance to the kinematics of the knees results in early, but slowly progressive deterioration of the patellofemoral and tibiofemoral articular surfaces.

Development of osteoarthritis, mainly tibiofemoral, characterizes the third phase. It appears that 15–20 years may elapse between the presence of cartilaginous lesions and the development of true osteoarthritis. Two forms of osteoarthritis may develop: medial tibiofemoral with progressive tilting into varus or bicompartmental with balance in the frontal plane. Because the disturbance of the kinematics of the knee leads, after an average of 25 years, to osteoarthritis, surgical repair of recent lesions is justified in young persons. However, great care must be exercised in repair of chronic laxities during the first year of adaptation.

▶ The main point of this paper was the authors' observation that their ". . . study of the natural history of isolated posterior cruciate rupture shows that it is not considerations of the functional outcome, even with regard to sports, which should encourage us to repair this ligament. Against this, the incidence of osteoarthritis is not negligible even if it arises late, and this seems to justify surgical treatment to repair it in recent injuries in young subjects. This indication, which is not absolute when there is an isolated rupture of the posterior cruciate ligament, becomes much more necessary when there are combined lesions."

We have recently reported on what we described as the natural history of the PCL-deficient knee (1). A retrospective study of 43 patients with PCL disruption treated nonsurgically established that the functional outcome could be predicted on the basis of instability type. Specifically, those knees with PCL disruption without associated ligamentous laxity will probably remain symptom free. However, with PCL disruption associated with combined instabilities a less than desirable functional result will probably occur. Application of logistics modeling to the data demonstrated that the functional result was not attributable to the type of instability per se, but rather to associated factors, i.e., chondromalacia of the patella, meniscal derangements, quadriceps atrophy, or degenerative changes. A direct correlation was established between combined multidirectional instability and the occurrence of the secondary problems, resulting in patients' complaints of functional disability.

We believe that these data support the thesis that individuals with unidirectional instability caused by PCL deficiency do not require repair or reconstruction. However, in view of the much less favorable prognosis for PCL-deficient knees with multidirectional instability, consideration may be given to surgical stabilization.—J.S. Torg, M.D.

Reference

1. Barton TM, et al: *Clin Orthop* 245:95–103, 1989.

Functional Analysis of Untreated and Reconstructed Posterior Cruciate Ligament Injuries
Tibone JE, Antich TJ, Perry J, Moynes D (Centinela Hosp Med Ctr; Kerlan-Jobe Orthopaedic Clinic, Inglewood, Calif)
Am J Sports Med 16:217–223, May–June 1988   8–31

The posterior cruciate ligament (PCL) has been called the primary stabilizer of the knee, but documentation of functional deficits caused by an absent PCL is limited. Surgical reconstruction of an absent PCL was done using the semitendinosus, iliotibial band, popliteal tendon, lateral meniscus, patellar tendon, and medial head of the gastrocnemius. Although each procedure has proponents, only a few reports of each have been cited as evidence. A functional analysis was made of data concerning 20 patients with untreated PCL tears and with a PCL reconstruction using the medial head of the gastrocnemius.

Ten injuries were untreated and 10 underwent reconstruction. Gait was analyzed using high-speed photography, footswitches, electromyography, and force plate. Patients were studied during walking, running, and stair climbing. A Cybex muscle strength evaluation also was done. All patients had moderate to severe posterior instability clinically. Five also had posterolateral instability. Quadriceps deficits were seen in both reconstruction and untreated groups. Deficits on hamstring Cybex testing were also found in the reconstruction group. Gait velocity of walking was 91% of normal velocity with a normal cadence. There was a tendency for increased knee flexion during the midstance phase of the gait cycle. Knee flexion angles during midstance were comparable in patients with posterior instability when compared with patients with additional posterolateral instability. A decreased foot-floor reaction was seen in the untreated group during terminal stance while walking. Similar findings were seen in the reconstruction group during running. Early activation of the gastrocnemius-soleus complex during the stance phase of the gait cycle was observed.

No conclusions were drawn concerning the advantages or disadvantages of a reconstructed PCL. Clinically, both treated and untreated groups had similar results. Patients who underwent reconstruction had greater subjective and functional disability preoperatively than the untreated group, which prompted surgery.

▶ With regard to the conclusions expressed by the authors that ". . . this paper makes no statement on the advantages or disadvantages of a reconstructed PCL. Clinically, both the untreated and the reconstructed patients have similar results. . .", the data and conclusions can only pertain to this specific procedure, i.e., using the medial head of gastrocnemius to reconstruct the ligament. The way the conclusion is worded is misleading, inferring that their observations are all conclusive regarding reconstruction of the ligament. Although this may well be true, it is not supported by the data presented.—J.S. Torg, M.D.

Postsurgical Knee Rehabilitation: A Five Year Study of Four Methods and 5,381 Patients
Timm KE (St Luke's Hosp, Saginaw, Mich)
Am J Sports Med 16:463–468, September–October 1988   8–32

What is the effect of rehabilitation on the long-term outcome of knee surgery? Various rehabilitative approaches were correlated with outcome in more than 5,000 patients operated on in 1981 and followed through 1986. Success was defined as the resumption of necessary activities without symptoms recurring for 5 years after operation. Whereas 2% of patients did not exercise, 25% performed exercises at home, 42% used isotonic exercise, and 31% performed isokinetic exercise. The mean age was 33 years.

The mean time to rehabilitation was 12 weeks with isotonic exercise, 10 weeks with home exercise, and 9 weeks with isokinetic exercise. Isokinetic exercises correlated with a successful outcome at a level of 0.92. Only 1% of patients in this program had recurrent symptoms in the first year of follow-up. Rates of success differed significantly between the isokinetic program and all other approaches.

Isokinetic exercise was the most effective rehabilitative approach in this series of patients having knee surgery. However, the findings do not necessarily apply to certain problems, e.g., anterior cruciate ligament disorders.

▶ The author's position is that, although the literature is replete with many long-term follow-up studies of knee surgery patients, few if any deal with the effect of the rehabilitation process as a factor in the postsurgical results. On this basis alone, this paper is a significant contribution in that it clearly demonstrates the effect of different rehabilitative modalities on the subjective responses of postsurgical patients. Specifically, there was an absence of a statistically significant difference between no exercise and home exercise programs, a statistically significant difference between these 2 programs and the isotonic exercise program, and a significant difference between the isokinetic program and each of the other 3 rehabilitation methods. With such large numbers, it appears that each of the 4 groups should have been broken down further into subgroups based on lesion types, e.g., meniscal tear, degenerative changes, and so on, and cross-correlated with similar lesion types in each grouping. With this approach the question is whether intensive rehabilitation is indicated in the postsurgical knee that evidences significant degenerative arthritis.—J.S. Torg, M.D.

Rehabilitation of the Anterior Cruciate Ligament in the Athlete
Silfverskiold JP, Steadman JR, Higgins RW, Hagerman T, Atkins JA (US Ski Team, Wheat Ridge, Colo; Tahoe Fracture and Orthopedic Med Clinic, South Lake Tahoe, Calif; Mississippi Sports Medicine Clinic and Orthopedic Ctr, Jackson)
Sports Med 6:308–319, November 1988   8–33

Because of the disastrous effects of the anterior cruciate deficient knee in the athletically active person, a more aggressive approach is taken today that involves reconstruction and rehabilitation. The question of the best surgical approach remains open, but the importance of proper rehabilitation after reconstruction or repair cannot be overemphasized.

Healing tissues must be appropriately stressed but never overloaded. The value of ultrasound and electrical stimulation remains unproved. Goals should be set preoperatively. A full unrestricted range of motion should be achieved at surgery. It seems preferable in general to avoid variable-resistance and isokinetic exercises in the first 6–8 months. The long brace may be replaced by a smaller one, allowing full range of motion within 8–12 weeks after surgery. Slow running forward and backward in water is added in the intermediate phase. At about 16 weeks formal testing is done to determine whether more advanced training is feasible.

The rehabiiltative program must be individualized. The process is a highly dynamic one, and both staff and patient can help to improve and refine the program, because rehabilitation should be enjoyable. Although perfection may be sought, the ultimate goal is the patient's safe return to work and to athletic activity.

▶ The authors clearly indicate that their goal in anterior cruciate ligament (ACL) reconstruction is to use a rehabilitation program that avoids such problems as periarticular contractures, disuse atrophy, degenerative cartilage changes, and cardiopulmonary deconditioning. Presented is an organized, although somewhat regimented, pre-, peri-, and postoperative ACL rehabilitation program. Although not specifically stated, presumably this particular program is for reconstruction using patella bone-tendon-bone with interference fit screw fixation technique. The authors state that "It is imperative to understand that any reha-

bilitation should not be used as a 'cookbook recipe.' " Implied are modified programs for different surgical approaches to ACL reconstruction.—J.S. Torg,
M.D.

**Effects of Electrical Muscle Stimulation Combined With Voluntary Con-
tractions After Knee Ligament Surgery**
Wigerstad-Lossing I, Grimby G, Jonsson T, Morelli B, Peterson L, Renström P
(Univ of Göteborg, Sweden)
Med Sci Sports Exerc 20:93–98, February 1988   8–34

The results of studies on the effects of electrical muscle stimulation in
postoperative muscle weakness and wasting are varied. The effect of electrical muscle stimulation combined with voluntary muscle contractions
was compared with that of a program of voluntary muscle contractions
only during immobilization in casts after anterior cruciate ligament
(ACL) surgery in 23 patients. All patients were immobilized for 3 weeks
in a full leg cast with the knee flexed at an angle of 20–30 degrees, and
then in a knee cast for another 3 weeks. All patients followed a standard
program with quadriceps muscle contractions. In addition, 13 patients
received simultaneous electrical stimulation of the quadriceps muscle 4 ×
10 minutes, 3 times a week at a frequency of 30 Hz (experimental
group); the other 10 did not have electrical stimulation (control group).

Six weeks postoperatively the experimental group exhibited significantly less reduction in isometric muscle strength for knee extension than
the control group. This difference remained significant when only data
for male patients were compared. The cross-sectional area of the quadriceps muscle, as measured with computed tomography, was significantly
less reduced during the immobilization period in the experimental group.
The relative fiber area of type I fibers was significantly reduced in the
control group, whereas the experimental group exhibited a significantly
increased ratio between type II and type I fibers, indicating more intense
muscle contractions in the experimental group. The activity of citrate
synthetase and triphosphate dehydrogenase was significantly reduced in
the control group, whereas no changes were noted in the experimental
group.

These data indicate that electrical muscle stimulation in combination
with voluntary muscle contractions can limit muscle weakness, muscle
wasting, and the reduction in oxidative and glycolytic muscle enzyme activity during immobilization after knee surgery. Electrical muscle stimulation should be part of the treatment during immobilization in casts after
knee surgery.

**Measurement of Stability of the Knee and Ligament Force After Implanta-
tion of a Synthetic Anterior Cruciate Ligament: In Vitro Measurement**
More RC, Markolf KL (Univ of California, Los Angeles)
J Bone Joint Surg [Am] 70-A:1020–1031, August 1988   8–35

Reconstruction of the anterior cruciate deficient knee has been accomplished with either autogenous tissues or a prosthetic ligament. For those requiring a prosthetic device, the Gore-Tex ligament, which functions as a permanent load-carrying implant, has been developed. The Gore-Tex ligament was used in 13 cadaver knees to determine the most advantageous operative and postoperative procedures.

Technique.—After excision of the anterior cruciate ligament (ACL), the prosthetic ligament was inserted with an over-the-top femoral placement. The ligament passes through the tibial hole, into the knee, and out through a small incision in the posterior part of the capsule. Tension is applied to the ligament, and the strain-gauge post is locked on a tibial slider track to record forces in the ligament. A preconditioning procedure is applied to the knee, and the final position of the strain-gauge post on the track is adjusted. The anterior-posterior laxity of the knee was matched within 0.1 mm to that of the preoperative knee.

Tests were undertaken to study the relationship between tension of the ligament and flexion of the knee. The anterior-posterior laxity of the knee decreased 1.0 mm for each mm that the tibial eyelet was moved distally.

It is important to precondition the Gore-Tex ligament after its positioning in the knee and before fixation of the tibial eyelet to prevent excessive stretch-out of the ligament. This also allows soft tissues between the ligament and bone to compress and stabilize. When the knee is at full extension, 200 newtons (45 lb) of pressure result in overtightening, which compensates for a degree of in vivo relaxation. Full extension of the knee should be avoided postoperatively so that initial fixation of the ligament is preserved.

▶ The clinical relevance of this study pertains to the prevention of progressive increases in anterior-posterior laxity with the use of the Gore-Tex device in vivo. Specifically, on the basis of these cadaver studies ". . . the ligament must be preconditioned in the knee at operation, before fixation of the tibial eyelet, to allow proper orientation of the strands of fibers and to allow the soft tissues that are entrapped between the ligament and the bone to compress and stabilize." The authors further describe a clinical procedure for manual preconditioning: "In this procedure, the femoral eyelet is first secured into bone with a screw. An assistant then places an appropriately sized Steinmann pin through the eyelet, grasps the pin transversely with the fingers, and pulls on the eyelet with approximately 200 newtons (forty-five pounds) of tension as the surgeon takes the knee through a series of cycles of flexion and extension."—J.S. Torg, M.D.

Long-Term Evaluation of Knee Stability and Function Following Surgical Reconstruction for Anterior Cruciate Ligament Insufficiency

Harter RA, Osternig LR, Singer KM, James SL, Larson RL, Jones DC (San Jose

State Univ, Calif; Univ of Oregon, Eugene; Orthopaedic and Fracture Clinic of Eugene, Ore)
Am J Sports Med 16:434–442, September–October 1988   8–36

Results of surgical reconstruction for anterior cruciate ligament insufficiency are often paradoxical. The outcome may be successful from the surgeon's point of view, but the patient reports limited functional abilities. Or the patient may be well satisfied even with poor knee stability. A number of subjective evaluation and clinical assessment tests were used to clarify the relationship between function and stability and identify the variables most predictive of outcome.

Fifty-one patients (mean age, 24 years) were evaluated an average of 48 months after surgery. Thirty-three patients had experienced episodic giving way of the knee for an average of 22 months at the time of surgery. The remaining 18 underwent acute reconstruction within 2 weeks of injury. Six parameters were evaluated: subjective assessment of knee function in a 100-point questionnaire; joint position sense; activity level on a 180-point scale; orthopedic clinical examination with a 100-point rating scale; isokinetic strength and work capacity; and instrumented measurement of knee laxity.

The patients' subjective rating was the factor most reflective of knee status after surgery, but this rating did not significantly correlate with other variables. Although there were many statistically significant relationships among the tests, no intercorrelations were found that could be used to predict results of other clinical tests.

Because no one measure of function or stability was able to define another, it seems inappropriate to apply the results of static ligament tests to dynamic situations. Knee function is complex, and more specific dynamic tests are required to develop stronger relationships between test results and patients'evaluations.

▶ This interesting and well-done study clearly documents a surprising lack of correlation between the patients' subjective perception of their knee function after anterior cruciate ligament reconstruction and the standard functional, clinical, and objective tests commonly performed for postoperative evaluation. It is suggested that more specific dynamic tests may be necessary before stronger relationships between clinical tests results and the patients' perception of their knee status can be realized. The other side of the coin may well be that the methods used to evaluate patients' perception of results may be faulty and perhaps changes in this area are needed.—J.S. Torg, M.D.

Long-Term Followup of Anterior Cruciate Ligament Reconstruction Using the Quadriceps Tendon Substitution for Chronic Anterior Cruciate Ligament Insufficiency

Kornblatt I, Warren RF, Wickiewicz TL (Hosp for Special Surgery, New York)
Am J Sports Med 16:444–448, September–October 1988   8–37

Surgical treatment for knee instability resulting from chronic anterior cruciate ligament (ACL) insufficiency is controversial. Some surgeons favor an intra-articular procedure, and others advocate extraarticular repair. Results of quadriceps tendon substitution, an intra-articular procedure, were evaluated in 38 patients, 37 of whom incurred their initial injury while engaged in sports activities. Follow-up averaged 5.5 years, and the patients' average age at reexamination was 29 years. Seventeen patients had undergone previous surgery. In 37 patients episodes of giving way of the knee was the main complaint.

Torn medial menisci were found in 27 knees; 9 had torn lateral menisci, and 5 had both medial and lateral tears. All had evidence at surgery of proliferative osteophyte formation. In 22 of the ACL reconstructions the graft was brought over the top of the lateral femoral condyle. Surgeons brought the graft through a bony tunnel in the remaining 16 patients. A period of rehabilitation followed surgery, and full resumption of sports was delayed for a year.

Results were assessed on a 50-point scale. Average scores rose from 27 preoperatively to 40.6 after surgery. All patients thought that their knees were improved, but none were engaging in competitive sports at long-term follow-up. Most patients experienced local numbness. In 3 patients giving way persisted. Another 5 patients had "loose" knees but were able to feel a "slip" and prevent actual giving way.

Intra-articular reconstruction of the ACL using quadriceps tendon substitution resulted in a 21% failure rate in this series. The rate can be lowered with addition of a lateral fascial sling and by using a stiffer infrapatellar ligament graft to eliminate stretch during the first year after surgery.

▶ This is an important and significant paper with regard to the historical perspective of the development of reconstructive knee surgery in the United States. The series represents patients operated on by Marshall to rectify knee instability, which the surgeon perceived as being caused by ACL deficiency. During this period, 1973–1980, all other knee surgeons in the United States approached the problem with the Slocum, Ellison, or Nicholas 5–1 procedure, or used posterior oblique ligament reefing. Needless to say, these procedures have not withstood the test of time and have since been discarded. However, Marshall's concept of intra-articular ACL reconstruction using autogenous tissue is firmly established. Although the quardriceps tendon substitution technique, as described by Marshall, has been improved upon, the basic principle remains.

Clearly, John Marshall remains a pioneer who overcame adversity, as well as unwarranted and misguided criticism by his peers, and is firmly established as the "Father" of modern ACL reconstructive surgery.—J.S. Torg, M.D.

Patterns of Meniscal Injury With Acute Anterior Cruciate Ligament Tears
Cerabona F, Sherman MF, Bonamo JR, Sklar J (Staten Island Hosp, NY; St Vincent's Med Ctr, New York)
Am J Sports Med 16:603–609, November–December 1988   8–38

Meniscal injury should be evaluated carefully in patients with acute tears of the anterior cruciate ligament (ACL). To design a successful treatment plan, it is necessary to be familiar with the types of meniscal tears that can occur. A group of 102 patients underwent arthrotomy to repair an acute ACL tear. Preoperative examination had revealed a positive Lachman sign, which provided the diagnosis. The mean age was 23 years, and 72% of the patients were male. Only 4 had a history of knee injury.

Patients in group 1 (67) had an acute isolated ACL tear with no associated collateral ligament injury. The 35 patients in group 2 had concomitant collateral tears. An arthroscopic nerve hook probe was used to examine both menisci. Attempts were made to repair peripheral tears— longitudinal tears in the outer 30% of the body of the meniscus. A partial menisectomy was performed if the tear was judged not repairable. A multiple suture technique was used to repair the ACL.

Moderate to severe pivot shifts were noted in 66 patients, 48 in group 1 and 18 in group 2. A total of 47 patients had 50 meniscal injuries. The most common tear in group 1 was a peripheral posterior longitudinal tear of the medial meniscus. Peripheral posteromedial longitudinal tears were most often noted in group 2. Lateral meniscal tears in group 1 tended to be not repairable, whereas medial meniscal tears were easily sutured in group 2.

Meniscal injuries often occur in patients with ACL tears. These complex injuries are probably the result of a combination of mechanisms. A thorough preoperative and intraoperative evaluation must be carefully undertaken to avoid overlooking the presence of medial or lateral meniscal injuries. Arthroscopy clearly reveals the meniscal injury, but it is not necessary in most instances when the Lachman sign is positive.

▶ This paper more precisely documents the observations of many others of the frequent association of injury of the ACL and meniscal tears.—J.S. Torg, M.D.

Arthroscopic Partial Meniscectomy in the Anterior Cruciate Deficient Knee
Aglietti P, Buzzi R, Bassi PB (Univ of Florence, Italy)
Am J Sports Med 16:597–602, November–December 1988   8–39

Controversy remains concerning treatment of the anterior cruciate ligament (ACL) deficient knee. Arthroscopic partial meniscectomy has been variously reported to have a success rate of 52% to 84%. A series of 86 men and 14 women underwent arthroscopic partial meniscectomy for 100 ACL-deficient knees. Most had been injured in sports activities. Patients were followed for an average of 3.5 years.

Excellent results were obtained in 28 knees, good in 24, fair in 34, and poor in 14. Reconstruction of the ACL was required subsequently in 10 knees. The average knee score increased from 63 to 81. Eighty-three patients had little or no pain on performance of strenuous activities. Swelling, instability, and activity level scores also improved, but only 41 patients could participate in high-risk sports without experiencing symptoms. Eleven of 31 patients who were competitive soccer players returned to their prevous level of competition; however, 7 dropped to a recreational level, 9 had to switch to another sport, and 9 were unable to participate in any sport.

Analysis of predictive factors for knee score and instability score showed that age was not a factor, but female sex, generalized laxity, and contralateral recurvatum of more than 10 degrees significantly decreased both scores. The best results were achieved in knees with isolated ACL insufficiency. Complete rather than partial ACL lesions, grade III tibiofemoral or patellar chondromalacia, associated peripheral ligamentous laxity, pivot shift of grade II or greater, and anterior tibial displacement of more than 5 mm also were negative predictors.

Arthroscopic partial meniscectomy is a useful procedure for the ACL-deficient knee, but it should be used selectively.

▶ This paper emphasizes several important points with regard to partial arthroscopic meniscectomy in the ACL-deficient knee. First, only 41% of the patients were able to participate in strenuous activities. The type of meniscal lesion was found to be irrelevant. Also, a strong correlation was found between pivot shift grades and a negative functional result. Specifically, when the pivot shift was absent or minimal, 95% of the patients obtained a stable knee for high-risk activities. With a grade II or III pivot shift, only 15% of the patients were able to participate in such activities.—J.S. Torg, M.D.

The Arthroscopic Meniscal Repair: Techniques and Clinical Experience
Jakob RP, Stäubli HU, Zuber K, Esser M (Univ of Bern, Switzerland)
Am J Sports Med 16:137–142, March–April 1988   8–40

Ideally, conservative meniscal repair should be limited to resection of only pathologic portions of the meniscus. Because the periphery of the meniscus is well vascularized, longitudinal tears can heal. Stable healing can also be achieved with sutures that perforate the meniscus vertically. Arthroscopic meniscal surgery enables isolated tears to be sutured within the joint, usually by techniques related to specially developed instrumentation. A technique of arthroscopic meniscal repair was applied to 54 meniscal tears.

Technique.—Three curved cannulas of various radii and a specific needle of 1.2-mm thickness are used. For repair of a vertical longitudinal tear of the medial meniscus, a lateral arthroscopic approach is performed next to the patellar tendon, and a second approach just medial to the tendon is used for the probe. After arthroscopic examination, the peripheral rim is débrided until a vertical, vascularized wall is reached. This procedure induces an inflammatory reaction from the synovium and enhances vascularization of the repair. The meniscal rasp is used to abrade the upper and lower synovial attachments of the tear. A femoral distractor type AO/ASIF is used for adequate exploration. The least curved can-

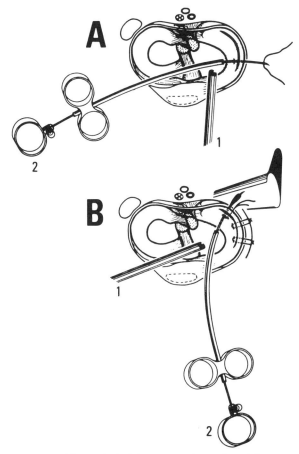

Fig 8—15.—A, for the middle one third of the meniscus, the needle with least curvature is inserted from the opposite compartment. **B,** for the posterior horn, the most curved needle is inserted from the ipsilateral compartment. A Henning retractor secures safe posterior perforation. (Courtesy of Jakob RP, Staübli HU, Zuber K, et al: *Am J Sports Med* 16:137–142, March–April 1988.)

nula is used for anterior lesions, and the more curved is used for posterior lesions. For the posterior horn the most curved cannula is inserted from the ipsilateral compartment (Fig 8–15). A nonabsorbable suture of size 0 or 00 is used for the periphery and a resorbable suture for central areas. In a 3-cm tear, 4–5 sutures are used in the upper and 3–4 sutures are used in the lower surfaces of the meniscus.

Of the 54 ruptured menisci, 42 (78%) healed without reinjury. Reruptures occurred in 12 patients, including 4 with partial anterior cruciate tear. Ten of these reruptures were treated by arthroscopic partial meniscectomy.

The type of meniscal tear most suitable for arthroscopic repair is a vertical longitudinal lesion that involves the vascularized zone. Because of possible damage to major vessels and nerves with posteriorly inserted needles, blind percutaneous introduction of the needles is cautioned against. Repair of extensive longitudinal (bucket-handle) meniscal tears can be performed with sutures placed through the collateral ligament. A combination of nonabsorbable suture for the periphery and resorbable suture for the central parts is recommended. Postoperatively, knee immobilization is recommended for 6 weeks. The repair should be examined at 4 months by arthroscopy or arthrography.

Arthroscopic Meniscal Repair With Two-Year Follow-Up: A Clinical Review
Ryu RKN, Dunbar WH IV (Orthopaedic Specialists of Santa Barbara, Calif)
Arthroscopy 4:168–173, 1988   8–41

Meniscal repair and the potential for meniscal healing are widely acknowledged concepts. A review was made of results of experience with arthroscopic meniscal repair in 31 patients. Twenty-nine patients, 15 men and 14 women (average age, 31 years), were followed for a minimum of 2 years.

Using a closed arthroscopic cannulated technique, 16 lateral and 15 medial menisci were repaired. All tears were vertical bucket-handle tears involving the posterior horn and averaged 2.5 cm in length. Of the 31 tears, 29 were either at the meniscocapsular junction (red-red zone) or within 3 cm of the peripheral attachment (red-white zone). Of the 29 patients, 16 had concomitant anterior cruciate ligament (ACL) injuries ranging from partial tears to complete disruption.

Usually a rating system based on symptoms, physical examination, and postrepair functional status, results were rated as excellent in 9 patients and good in 16, for a clinical success rate of 87%. Nine patients underwent relook arthroscopy 3 months postoperatively; healing was confirmed in 8 and a retear in 1. There were 4 reruptures, for a failure rate of 13%. Of the 7 patients who underwent stabilization procedures for ACL disruption, 6 had meniscal healing. Of the 9 untreated ACL disruptions, 8 had meniscal healing; the single failure occurred in a patient with marked instability. Among those patients with reruptures, chronic anterolateral rotatory instability was identified as a significant risk factor for rerupture. The complication rate was 13%.

Arthroscopic ACL repair remains a desirable alternative to meniscal excision. Results are excellent when proper selection and technique are implemented.

▶ These 2 reports (Abstracts 8–40 and 8–41), in addition to presenting the technique for arthroscopic meniscal repair, attempt to answer significant questions associated with the procedure. Pointed out is the proper selection of meniscal tears that would benefit from repair. Specifically, Ryu et al. (Abstract 8–41) limited their repairs to vertical tears occurring in the red-red or red-white zone and emphasize a need for perimeniscal synovial preparation. Jakob et al.

(Abstract 8–40) present essentially the same criteria with regard to selection. Both groups also point out that reattachment of a meniscus with a concomitant anterior cruciate lesion has a more doubtful prognosis. It is interesting to note that Jakob et al. make the point that refixation in middle-aged patients is probably not justified, and that serious athletes tend to reject this approach because of the prolonged immobilization, 22% risk of retear, and general pressure to return to their activity as quickly as possible. Somewhat disconcerting is that neither of these 2 articles deal with possible neurovascular complications, which would appear to be increased by virtue of their "closed" techniques.—J.S. Torg, M.D.

Arthroscopic Meniscectomy for Discoid Lateral Meniscus in Children
Hayashi LK, Yamaga H, Ida K, Miura T, (Nagoya Univ, Japan)
J Bone Joint Surg [Am] 70-A:1495–1500, December 1988   8–42

Between August 1983 and May 1986, 46 children (53 knees) were followed after undergoing total, subtotal, or partial arthroscopic meniscectomy in management of a symptomatic discoid lateral meniscus. Most were between ages 10 and 15 years. According to the classification of Watanabe et al., 46 discoid menisci tears were complete and 7 were incomplete. Each tear was identified on arthroscopic examination and confirmed after excision of the meniscal tissue.

Technique.—In the operative technique, using Metzenbaum scissors and the scissors for surgical arthroscopy, the meniscus is exposed and the segment to be resected is removed completely with a grasper (Fig 8–16). The edge is trimmed

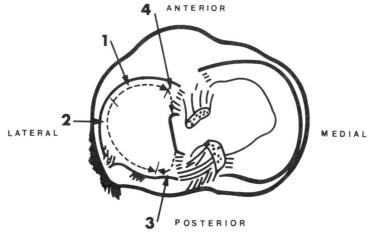

Fig 8–16.—Steps of meniscectomy by the technique of 1-piece excision. *1.* Initial incision, with scissors, into the anterior segment of the meniscus. *2.* Extension of the incision to the middle and posterior segments. *3.* Release of the posterior horn. *4.* Release of the anterior insertion and removal of the entire meniscus with the grasper. (Courtesy of Hayashi LK, Yamaga H, Ida K, et al: *J Bone Joint Surg [Am]* 70-A:1495–1500, December 1988.)

with power instruments or basket forceps when necessary. The amount of meniscal tissue excised depends on the type of meniscus and shape and extent of the tear.

The average follow-up was 31.2 months. In children who had total or subtotal meniscectomy for either type of lesion, the result was excellent; only 2 patients who had partial meniscectomy had an excellent result. The typical signs of osteoarthritic changes such as flattening of the femoral condyle, cupping of the tibia, and formation of osteophytes that are common in adults did not occur in this group of children. Longitudinal rather than horizontal tears were predominant.

The most desirable width for the rim (6–8 mm) should be retained, but it is recommended that excessive thickness of the discoid meniscus be reduced from 12 or 13 mm to 6–8 mm for complete and incomplete lesions. When the meniscus was reduced to this width, no new tears developed.

9 Injuries of the Foot and Ankle

Orthotic Treatment of Sesamoid Pain
Axe MJ, Ray RL (Wilmington Orthopaedic Consultants, Wilmington, Del; Allegheny Gen Hosp, Pittsburgh)
Am J Sports Med 16:411–415, July–August 1988   9–1

It is often difficult to distinguish between sesamoid stress fracture and sesamoiditis as the cause of pain and tenderness beneath the first metatarsal in an athlete. Surgical excision provides satisfactory results in symptomatic patients, but this treatment sidelines an athlete for a minimum of 6 weeks. An alternative treatment that alleviates pain beneath the first metatarsal on impact and push-off and enables the athlete to continue performing may be useful, even though surgery may be required later.

Four male and 6 female athletes had tenderness beneath the first metatarsal head. Two patients also had flexible cavus feet and 1 had a pronated forefoot. All patients underwent bilateral foot radiography and 1 had a bone scan. The medial sesamoid was involved in 6 patients and the lateral sesamoid in the others. Orthotic castings of both feet were made for all patients.

After being fitted with orthotics, 3 athletes had almost complete relief of symptoms, 1 had a gradual resolution of symptoms over 4 weeks, and another required 6 weeks before the pain resolved. Four football players had initial persistent pain with lateral changes of direction. These symptoms also resolved after several weeks. Two patients, a toe-dancer and a distance jogger, remained symptomatic despite orthoses, and surgery was undertaken.

▶ Although an attempt has been made to evaluate orthotic treatment of sesamoid pain, the authors have not clearly defined and segregated pain caused by sesamoid stress fractures, sesamoiditis, and symptomatic multipartite sesamoid. Certainly, the diagnosis of sesamoiditis or symptomatic bipartite sesamoid calls for implementation of conservative measures. However, I would agree with Van Hal et al. (1) that stress fractures of the great toe sesamoid are frequently refractory to conservative measures and require surgical excision.—J.S. Torg, M.D.

Reference

1. Van Hal ME, Keene JS, Clancy WG: *Am J Sports Med* 10:122–128, 1982.

Operation for Non-Union of Stress Fracture of the Tarsal Navicular

Fitch KD, Blackwell JB, Gilmour WN (Royal Perth Hosp, Perth, Western Australia)

J Bone Joint Surg [Br] 71-B:105–110, January 1989   9–2

Treatment of tarsal navicular stress fractures initially is conservative. These fractures tend to heal slowly, however, and nonunion or recurrence is not uncommon. Athletes often find the lengthy treatment and uncertainty of outcome unacceptable. A more accelerated treatment using autologous bone grafts was attempted in selected patients. Bone grafting was undertaken if the fracture was symptomatic, radiographs showed wide separation of a complete fracture, an incomplete fracture was extended, there was delayed healing, or a medullary cyst was present. After en bloc resection of the fracture surfaces, with care taken to expose the fracture fully to its distal limits, an autologous bone graft is inserted.

Of 19 fractures in 18 patients in whom the procedure was performed, 6 were complete and 12 were incomplete; 1 patient had a residual medullary cyst. Fifteen patients were available for an average follow-up of 42 months. Of these, 12 were able to resume preinjury activities within 5–12 months. Computed tomography was valuable in confirming the diagnosis (Fig 9–1), but it was rarely required postoperatively.

Recent fractures should be treated with 8–10 weeks of non-weight-bearing in a cast. If delayed union or nonunion occurs, autologous bone grafting is an effective method of management for complete fractures and fractures in which a medullary cyst develops.

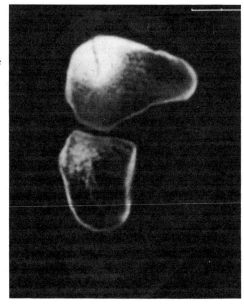

Fig 9–1.—Computed tomographic scan of a 16-year-old National Junior 800-m title holder showing an incomplete fracture with surrounding sclerosis. This fracture could not be demonstrated by standard radiographs. (Courtesy of Fitch KD, Blackwell JB, Gilmour WN: *J Bone Joint Surg (Br)* 71-B:105–110, January 1989.)

▶ The logic of the authors' approach to managing stress fractures of the tarsal navicular is, to say the least, somewhat lacking. The paper begins with an admission that previously only 6 tarsal navicular stress fractures treated surgically had been reported in the literature. Although it has been well documented that all but the rare fracture heals with non-weight-bearing with return to full activity after 6–8 weeks of treatment (1), the authors of this article state that ". . . we have adopted a more positive approach to these fractures, and tried to accelerate and augment healing by using autologous bone grafts. . .". They further admit that: "Many of our patients were not treated initially by prolonged periods of non-weight-bearing. . ." Following surgery they employ non-weight-bearing for 3–4 weeks and state that: "After a gradual return to training and sport, most patients resumed full activity six months after the operation." The point is this: surgical intervention in lieu of non-weight-bearing treatment of stress fracture of the tarsal navicular without clear documentation of nonunion significantly prolongs recovery and return to activity. However, the paper does demonstrate the efficacy of autogenous inlaid bone grafting, and the authors do conclude that ". . . we now treat recent fractures with eight to 10 weeks, non-weight-bearing in a cast. . ."—J.S. Torg, M.D.

Reference

1. Torg JS, et al: *J Bone Joint Surg [Am]* 64–A:700–712, 1982.

Computed Tomography Scan and Magnetic Resonance Imaging of Ankle Tendons: An Overview
Rosenberg ZS, Cheung Y, Jahss MH (Hosp for Joint Diseases Orthopedic Inst, New York; Beth Israel Med Ctr, New York)
Foot Ankle 8:297–307, June 1988   9–3

It is difficult to diagnose injuries to the tendon of the ankle on clinical grounds, and the pain and disability associated with this injury are often attributed to ankle sprain or bony pathology. Imaging techniques such as arthrography, tenography, ultrasonography, and xeroradiography contribute little to a definitive diagnosis. However, computed tomography (CT) and magnetic resonance imaging (MRI) reportedly are useful for imaging the various ankle tendon injuries.

Posttraumatic or postsurgical stenosing tenosynovitis results in synovial proliferation or scar tissue around a tendon. On both CT and MRI the lesion appears as a soft tissue density that obliterates the normal fat around the tendon. Scar tissue appears on CT as an area of increased density relative to fat, and as an area of low signal intensity on T1- and T2-weighted MR images.

Both CT and MRI are highly accurate in diagnosing tendon ruptures. However, the appearance on CT and MRI depends on the chronicity and extent of the rupture. Chronic partial ruptures appear on CT as increased girth of the tendon associated with decreased density and areas of radiolucency within the tendon substance itself and on T1-weighted MR images as high signal intensity areas within the tendon substance. More severe chronic partial ruptures are depicted as focal attenuation of the tendon, with the gap being replaced by either fat or fluid. A complete tendon rupture is seen on both CT and MRI as the complete absence of a portion of the tendon.

When CT and MRI are compared for efficiency, both are highly accurate in detecting various types of ankle tendon pathology. Magnetic resonance imaging is the preferred study because of its superior soft tissue contrast resolution, multiplanar capabilities, lack of beam hardening artifacts, and its lack of ionizing radiation. However, CT may serve as an excellent substitute when cost containment is a consideration, or when MRI is not available.

Magnetic Resonance Imaging in the Diagnosis of Disruption of the Posterior Tibial Tendon
Alexander IJ, Johnson KA, Berquist TH (Cleveland Clinic; Mayo Clinic, Scottsdale, Ariz; Mayo Clinic and Found, Rochester, Minn)
Foot Ankle 8:144–147, December 1987   9–4

If pain is present in an unusual site and suggestive signs are absent, it may be difficult to diagnose disruption of the posterior tibial tendon.

Woman, 44, had pain in the right lower limb for 3 years, initially in the area of the navicular tubercle. Cortisone injections were tried, and the navicular prominence was "shaved" elsewhere. Once ambulatory, the patient noted pain posterosuperior to the medial malleolus, extending along the posteromedial tibial border and aggravated by activity. Paresthesias were noted in the great toe. A bone scan showed increased uptake in the navicular area. Magnetic resonance imaging showed an inhomogeneous mass in the course of the posterior tibial tendon; the tendon was attenuated or absent distally. At exploration a heavily scarred stump of tendon was seen attached to the navicular tubercle. Tendon fibers ended within a scarred mass 5–6 cm proximal to the tip of the medial malleolus. The damaged tendon was replaced with the flexor digitorum longus tendon, and the patient was much improved after 6 months.

Magnetic resonance imaging excluded a suspected neurilemoma in this patient and clearly showed a complete tear of the posterior tibial tendon.

▶ Partial and complete ruptures of the posterior tibial tendon are lesions that occur infrequently and are a diagnostic challenge. The authors have established the role of magnetic resonance imaging in dealing with this problem.—J.S. Torg, M.D.

Rupture of Posterior Tibial Tendon: CT and MR Imaging With Surgical Correlation
Rosenberg ZS, Cheung Y, Jahss MH, Noto AM, Norman A, Leeds NE (Hosp for Joint Diseases Orthopedic Inst, New York; Beth Israel Med Ctr, New York)
Radiology 169:229–235, October 1988   9–5

Chronic rupture of the posterior tibial tendon has been recognized as a distinct clinical entity only since 1982. It is common among women older than age 50 years and usually occurs without antecedent trauma. Chronic stress and tension on the tendon as it curves around the medial malleolus is the most likely cause of this flatfoot deformity. The rupture does not respond to conservative treatment. Chronic rupture of the posterior tibial tendon is classified surgically into 3 types: Type 1 is a partially torn bulbous tendon with vertical splits and defects; type 2 is a partially torn, attenuated tendon; and type 3 is a complete rupture with a tendon gap. Computed tomography (CT) and magnetic resonance (MR) imaging are both effective for detecting this type of rupture.

The CT and MR images of 19 women and 8 men aged 43–70 years, with 32 clinically suspected posterior tibial tendon ruptures, were compared with images obtained from 23 controls aged 35–65 years. Twenty-two (69%) of the 27 patients underwent operation to repair the deformity.

The sensitivity of CT was 90%, and its specificity was 100%. The sensitivity of MR imaging was 95%, and its specificity was 100%. Computed tomography correctly depicted the tendons as ruptured in 20 of the 22 operated-on patients, for an accuracy of 91%; MR imaging was correct in 21 patients, for an accuracy of 95%. In 7 of the 22 patients, CT correctly showed the tendons as torn but incorrectly classified the type of rupture. The overall accuracy, reflecting the percentage of lesions correctly diagnosed as well as those correctly classified, was 59% for CT and 73% for MR imaging.

Magnetic resonance imaging is the method of choice for detecting ruptures of the posterior tibial tendon. Even though the differences between CT and MR imaging parameters were not statistically significant, MR imaging provided greater definition of tendon outline, vertical splits, synovial fluid, edema, and degenerated tissue. However, CT was superior to MR imaging in showing associated bone abnormalities, such as periostitis, subtalar osteoarthritis, and subtalar dislocation.

► This paper is a well-illustrated study concerning a disabling entity that often is not that well recognized either clinically or radiographically. Recognition and appropriate diagnostic procedures may facilitate the correct treatment and expedite surgical repair.—J.S. Torg, M.D.

Sliding Fibular Graft Repair for Chronic Dislocation of the Peroneal Tendons
Micheli LJ, Waters PM, Sanders DP (Children's Hosp Med Ctr, Boston)
Am J Sports Med 17:68–71, January–February 1989   9–6

Chronic recurrent subluxation of the peroneal tendons is a potentially disabling condition in the athlete. Conservative treatment is generally ineffective; however, there have been recent reports of favorable results with surgical reconstruction consisting of bone block or tenoplasty procedures, groove deepening, or periosteal reattachment. Six women and 5 men with 12 chronic dislocations of the peroneal tendons underwent a sliding fibular graft repair. In 7 patients conservative treatment had failed, and 4 had not sought treatment previously.

Technique.—A slightly curved incision is made over the lateral malleolus, and the distal 5 cm of the lateral malleolus is exposed extraperiosteally. A cortical slot graft 3 cm long and 5 mm wide is made in the cortex of the lateral malleolus. The cortical graft is elevated from its bed; the distal bed may be deepened with curettes to facilitate sliding the graft distally. The graft is then fixed in the distal position with 3.5-mm cortical AO screws.

Ten of 11 patients had no recurrent dislocations or pain and had returned to sports activities at follow-up. The average time to return to sports was 4.3 months. Patients had no functional loss of eversion or difficulty in wearing shoes. There were 3 complications: 1 patient sustained fracture of the fibular graft during a fall 1 year after full return to athletics; she was treated nonoperatively and later returned to full competition. Two patients had reexploration because of pain and swelling. One of these had an exostosis that was excised in the area of the graft, and she returned to athletic participation; the other had tenosynovitis of the peroneus brevis tendon and recurrent subluxation of the peroneal tendons.

The sliding fibular graft repair combines the advantages of bone block and groove-deepening procedures. The results are comparable to those for other procedures, with a 91% excellent result measured by lack of recurrent dislocation and return to preinjury physical activities.

▶ Although the authors report a 91% rate of excellent results, it should be noted that there was a 25% rate of significant complications. One patient had a fracture of the fibular graft within 1 year after surgery, and 2 patients required reexploration for pain and swelling, attributed in 1 to an exostosis that developed in the graft area; the other patient had recurrent subluxation.—J.S. Torg, M.D.

Injuries of the Lateral Ligaments of the Ankle Joint: Operative Treatment and Long-Term Results
Jaskulka R, Fischer G, Schedl R (Univ of Vienna)
Arch Orthop Trauma Surg 107:217–221, 1988   9–7

Optimal treatment of lesions of the lateral ligaments of the ankle is controversial. At 1 clinic fresh ligament ruptures of the ankle are treated by early surgery.

In a 4-year period, 268 patients with recent ankle ligament ruptures underwent primary surgical repair. The decision to operate immediately was based on clinical findings and positive stress radiograph. Ligament ruptures were diagnosed if the talar tilt on the injured side was at least 5 degrees more than that on the uninjured side, or if the ventral subluxability of the talus was more than 5 mm that of the uninjured side. At follow-up 2–6 years after surgery, 122 patients were available for evaluation, which consisted of physical examination and standardized and stress radiographs.

Results were good in 80% of the patients, moderate in 17%, and poor in 3%. The poor results were attributable to persistent radiologically observed instability or arthrotic joint degeneration, or both. Infection occurred in 1.5% of the patients.

Early surgical treatment for recent instability is preferred. Conservative therapy should be used only if there are serious contraindications to surgery, especially when the patient is young or athletic.

▶ There are 2 problems with this paper. First, the authors state that the indication for surgery is more than 5 degrees of talar tilt or anterior subluxation of the talus of more than 5 mm compared with the uninjured side on ventral stress. I would question the wisdom of basing an indication for a surgical procedure on a positive stress test in only 1 plane. It has been my experience that a good result can be obtained uniformly with conservative management in those ankles having 1-plane varus instability.

The second problem is that in reporting 80% of the patients treated surgically as having a good result, they state that: "In comparable control groups of patients who had undergone conservative therapy, the number of results in the 'very good' category was clearly lower." However, their report is lacking any data to support this contention. What is lacking here is a randomized study comparing conservative and surgical management of injuries of the lateral ligaments of the ankle.—J.S. Torg, M.D.

Reconstruction of the Lateral Ligaments of the Ankle for Chronic Lateral Instability
Karlsson J, Bergsten T, Lansinger O, Peterson L (East Hosp, Göteborg, Sweden)
J Bone Joint Surg [Am] 70-A:581–588, April 1988   9–8

Rupture or sprain of the lateral ligaments of the ankle is a common injury. Chronic instability is not always a severe disability, but reconstruction may be needed for some patients. Shortening and reinsertion or imbrication of the lateral ligaments of the ankle was done to correct lateral instability in 180 ankles in 176 patients. The procedure is shown in Figure 9–2.

Technique.—The ankle is opened both proximal and distal to the anterior talofibular ligament. Each ligament is divided 3–5 mm from its insertion on the fibula. The surface of the bone on the distal end of the fibula is roughened to promote ligamentous healing. Drill holes are made through the fibula, aimed about 45 degrees to the articular surface of the fibula, perforating about 10 mm deep. Holes are also drilled from the lateral aspect of the lateral malleolus about 10 mm proximal to the ligamentous insertion, aimed at the corresponding hole drilled in the roughened lateral surface of the distal part of the fibula. The distal

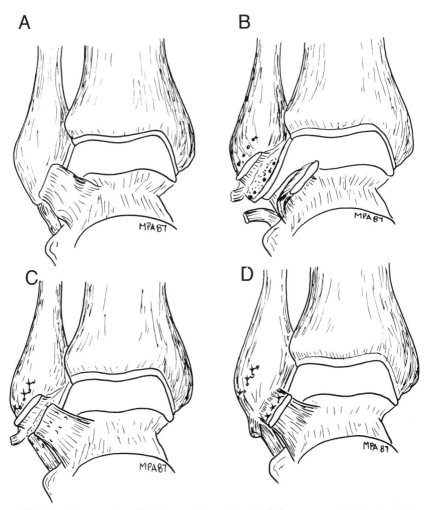

Fig 9–2.—Reconstruction of the ligaments (frontal view). **A,** before reconstruction. **B,** after the ligaments have been divided, the surface between the proximal stump of the ligaments and the anterior border of the articular surface is roughened. **C,** the ligaments are reinserted into the roughened surface with maximum tightening. **D,** imbrication is performed using the proximal stump of the ligaments. (Courtesy of Karlsson J, Bergsten T, Lansinger O, et al: *J Bone Joint Surg [Am]* 70-A:581–588, April 1988.)

stump of the ligament is fixed to the roughened surface of the fibula while the foot is held in dorsiflexion and pronation. The proximal end of the ligament is then imbricated over the distal portion. The joint capsule proximal and distal to the ligament is also imbricated, and the tendon sheaths and retinaculum are sutured.

Of 152 ankles reexamined, an excellent or good result was achieved in 132, all of which had radiographic evidence of improved mechanical stability. Contraindications to this technique include long-standing ligamentous insufficiency, generalized hypermobility of joints, and previous tenodesis.

▶ This excellent paper presents a relatively simple solution to a common problem with impressive long-term follow-up numbers. Historically, Broström (1) originally reported simple suture of the chronically unstable ankle. It is interesting to note that in this series the authors found it technically impossible to suture the ends of the ligaments directly. They also noted that in all of their patients, the ligaments were in continuity and scarred as well as elongated. Although there is an elaborate description of the technique used to obtain stress radiographs with TELOS equipment, no accompanying pre- or postoperative data based on the stress radiographs are given. Also lacking are data pertaining to parameters of pre- and postoperative joint motion, as well as discussion of rehabilitation techniques.—J.S. Torg, M.D.

Reference

1. Broström L: *Acta Chir Scand* 132:551–565, 1966.

Surgical Treatment of Lateral Ankle Instability Syndrome
Sammarco GJ, DiRaimondo CV (Univ of Cincinnati; Foot and Ankle Ctr, Cincinnati)
Am J Sports Med 16:501–510, September–October 1988   9–9

Lateral ankle instability syndrome is characterized by pain and instability resulting from ligament laxity. Anterior talofibular ligament laxity, with or without calcaneofibular laxity and other anomalies, is frequently associated with peroneus brevis tendon tears, abnormal ligament placement, tibialis posterior tendon tears, osteochondritis dissecans, arthritis, synovitis, loose bodies, and tarsal coalition. Results of surgical repair of this condition were evaluated.

Forty-three ankles were treated using a split peroneus brevis tendon graft routed through osseous tunnels in the talus, fibula, and calcaneus and resutured to the reconstructed anterior talofibular and calcaneofibular ligaments. The tunnel locations, transfer routes, and tendon reinforcement used were based on Elmslie's technique. Good or excellent results were achieved in 91% of the patients and stability was achieved in 98%. Patients were followed for 9 months to 11 years. Twenty-one patients needed additional procedures.

Thorough assessment of patients with lateral ankle instability syndrome increases the likelihood of finding associated abnormalities. If left untreated, they could adversely affect surgical outcome.

▶ Whereas Karlsson et al. (Abstract 9–8) in their report on reconstruction of lateral ligaments of the ankle for chronic lateral instability describe a relatively simple solution to a common problem with impressive long-term follow-up, Sammarco and DiRaimondo, conversely, present what appears to be a surgically complicated procedure to achieve similar results. It would seem to me that the shortest distance between two points is a straight line.—J.S. Torg, M.D.

Fractures of the Distal Part of the Fibula With Associated Disruption of the Deltoid Ligament: Treatment Without Repair of the Deltoid Ligament
Baird RA, Jackson ST (Univ of California Irvine)
J Bone Joint Surg [Am] 69-A:1346–1352, December 1987   9–10

Controversy surrounds the question of surgical or nonsurgical treatment of injuries to the ankle involving rupture of the deltoid ligament and fracture of the distal part of the fibula. After surgical repair of the ligament was discontinued in 1979, treatment at the present institution has been by stabilization of the lateral side of the ankle. After reduction of the distal fibular fracture, patients wear a long cast for 5–6 weeks and a short walking cast for the same length of time. The treatment effect was evaluated by questionnaire, personal interview, physical examination, and radiographic criteria.

Of 21 patients treated without repair of the deltoid ligament, 19 had good or excellent results after a mean follow-up of 36 months. The 2 patients whose results were only fair or poor experienced mild pain and some limitation of movement. Nevertheless, their radiographs showed normal findings.

Three patients were treated by open reduction, internal fixation of the fracture, and repair of the deltoid ligament. Only 1 of these patients reported excellent results. The other 2 had outcomes classified as poor because they complained of pain while standing.

Exploration of the medial side of the ankle is necessary only when the medial clear space remains widened after reduction of the fibular fracture. Because of the success with patients in whom the deltoid ligament was not repaired, surgeons have reduced cast time to two 4-week periods. The syndesmosis screws are left in place, however, for 12 weeks to prevent widening.

▶ This report supports the previous observations of Bonnin (1), Denham (2), Mast and Teipner (3), and deSouza (4). These earlier studies, however, presented only few data with regard to pain, function, joint motion, and roentgenographic findings. The current study is supported by data indicating that the results in these areas are acceptable.—J.S. Torg, M.D.

References

1. Bonnin JG: *J Bone Joint Surg [Br]* 47-B:609–611, 1965.
2. Denham RA: *J Bone Joint Surg [Br]* 46-B:206–211, 1964.
3. Mast JW, Teipner WA: *Orthop Clin North Am* 11:661–679, 1980.
4. de Souza LJ, et al: *J Bone Joint Surg [Am]* 67-A:1066–1074, September 1985.

Arthroscopic Treatment of Sports-Related Anterior Osteophytes in the Ankle
Hawkins RB (Fitchburg, Mass)
Foot Ankle 9:87–90, October 1988   9–11

Anterior osteophytes in the ankle are caused by an injury or by the quick, forceful dorsiflexion of the joint by dancers, runners, and high jumpers. If left untreated the osteophyte can cause damage to the articular cartilage and eventual loss of ankle function. Arthroscopic treatment for this problem was undertaken in 3 patients.

In most cases, pain and swelling are experienced during activity and the ankle returns to normal with rest. Radiographic evaluation is usually simple and accurate. A bony protuberance into the joint space confirms the presence of an osteophyte. The osteophytic bone is removed by an arthroplastic procedure consisting of excision, débridement, or abrasion. The original contour of the anterior talus or tibia should be retained to avoid impingement of the joint space. Exposure of bleeding capillary bone promotes healthy regeneration of fibrocartilage.

Rehabilitation therapy is important for restoration of motion, strength, and endurance. An 8-week period on weight-bearing crutches is recommended. Early exercise encourages regeneration of fibrocartilage and return to normal function. In two 30-year-old men and a 23-year-old woman, all active athletes, the procedure brought freedom from pain and a return to full activity.

▶ The observations and conclusion presented in this report are in keeping with my own clinical experience.—J.S. Torg, M.D.

Operative Ankle Arthroscopy: Long-Term Followup
Martin DF, Baker CL, Curl WW, Andrews JR, Robie DB, Haas AF (Hughston Orthopaedic Clinic, Columbus, Ga)
Am J Sports Med 17:16–23, January–February 1989   9–12

Ankle arthroscopy is now being recommended for a wide variety of disorders. However, the effectiveness of these procedures must be evaluated by long-term follow-up to define more precisely the role of arthroscopy in the treatment of ankle disorders. Indications, preoperative examinations, operative data, and radiographs were reviewed in 57 patients with 58 arthroscopically treated ankles who were followed for at least 1 year (average, 25 months).

Overall, good or excellent results were achieved in 64% of the ankles. Subjectively, 77% of all patients said they would have the surgery again. Fifteen percent of ankles required surgery during follow-up, but most of these were in a group with unsuccessfully treated degenerative joint disease. Results in 20 of 26 ankles with synovitis were good or excellent. Results were similar in 12 of 17 ankles with transchondral defects of the talus. Whereas good or excellent results were achieved in 4 of 7 ankles with osteophytes or loose bodies, the outcome in 3 was only fair or poor. Six of these 7 ankles had concomitant synovitis. In only 1 of 8 ankles with degenerative joint disease were good or excellent results achieved. The latter patients averaged 18 years older than the other patients in the study and degenerative joint disease was prevalent. Three patients underwent subsequent tibiotalar fusion; 1 had an arthrotomy, and 2 were considering further surgery at follow-up. The overall complication rate was 15%, with temporary paresthesias and permanent sensory loss being the most common complications. There were 2 superficial and 2 deep infections, all of which responded to treatment.

Despite a significant risk of complication, ankle arthroscopy can be recommended for selected patients.

▶ This is a good techniques paper that attempts, on the basis of a significant personal experience, to indicate the potential for ankle arthroscopy. The authors' position is conservative and cautious. Specifically, they state: "Ankle arthroscopy is in a developmental period; the effectiveness of these procedures must be evaluated with long-term followup and critical analysis of results." To be noted, there was a 15% complication rate with 2 superficial and 2 deep infections. Emphasized is a knowledge of anatomy and meticulous surgical technique on the part of the surgeon.—J.S. Torg, M.D.

10 Exercise Testing

Factor Analysis of Various Anaerobic Power Tests
Manning JM, Dooly-Manning C, Perrin DH (William Paterson College of New Jersey, Wayne; Univ of Virginia, Charlottesville)
J Sports Med 28:138–144, June 1988   10–1

Many field and laboratory anaerobic power tests have been used by physical educators, coaches, trainers, and researchers to predict anaerobic power. There appears to be no single best test or anthropometric measure to predict anaerobic power. To identify the single best test and to correlate various anthropometric and isokinetic measures with various anaerobic power tests, studies were made in 31 college-aged men.

The anaerobic power tests assessed were the vertical jump, using the Lewis formula; the Margaria-Kalamen stair climb test; the Wingate maximum anaerobic capacity and peak power test; the Cybex II isokinetic measures for knee extension and ankle plantar flexion at 180 degrees and 240 degrees per second; the 40-yard dash; and the standing long jump. Significant correlations were used in principal factor analysis, then rotated using the varimax criterion.

No single factor emerged. Unrelated aspects exist among these tests, and they do not measure similar qualities. These results concur with those of previous studies, which found that there is no single anaerobic power test that can be used to measure anaerobic power compared with maximum oxygen uptake used to obtain aerobic power.

▶ There is no easy method and no single test that predicts anaerobic power. A variety of tests must be done to determine an individual's anaerobic power.—F.J. George, ATC, PT

Relationship Between a Two Mile Run for Time and Maximal Oxygen Uptake
Mello RP, Murphy MM, Vogel JA (US Army Research Inst of Environmental Medicine, Natick, Mass)
J Appl Sport Sci Res 2:9–12, February–March 1988   10–2

It is generally thought that a best-effort run of 1–2 miles correlates reasonably well with an individual's aerobic fitness as determined by maximal oxygen uptake. Studies supporting this belief most often involve a relatively short timed run of a specific distance, or an unlimited distance run for a specific length of time. The relationship between a maximal effort 2-mile run for time and maximal oxygen uptake as measured

211

by treadmill running was investigated in 44 men aged 20–51 years and 17 women aged 20–17 years, of various fitness and activity levels.

The mean maximal oxygen uptake (VO_2 max) value was 50.4 ml/kg per minute for men, and 42 ml/kg per minute for women. The mean 2-mile run time was 14:44 ± 2:06 for men and 17:26 ± 3:01 for women. The correlation between maximal oxygen uptake and 2-mile run time was $r_m = -0.91$ for men, and $r_f = -0.89$ for women (table). Adding variables such as age, height, weight, and percent body fat produced no significant improvement in the predictability of either equation. Inclusion of body weight in the male equation, however, did increase its predictive accuracy.

These data confirm the value and validity of a timed, best-effort 2-mile

Conversion of 2-Mile Run Time to VO_2 max Values
(Eq 1 and 2)

2-Mile Run Time *	$\dot{V}O_2$ max † Male	Female
10.0	66.2	
10.5	64.5	
11.0	62.8	
11.5	61.2	
12.0	59.5	
12.5	57.8	
13.0	56.2	49.9
13.5	54.5	49.0
14.0	52.8	48.1
14.5	51.1	47.2
15.0	49.5	46.4
15.5	47.8	45.5
16.0	46.1	44.6
16.5	44.4	43.7
17.0	42.8	42.8
17.5	41.1	41.9
18.0	39.4	41.0
18.5	37.7	40.2
19.0	36.1	39.3
19.5	34.4	38.4
20.0	32.7	37.5
20.5		36.6
21.0		35.7
21.5		34.8
22.0		34.0
22.5		33.1
23.0		32.2

* Minutes	† ml·kg⁻¹·min⁻¹

*Minutes.
†ml . kg⁻¹ . minute ⁻¹.
(Courtesy of Mello RP, Murphy MM, Vogel JA: *J Appl Sport Sci Res* 2:9–12, February–March 1988.)

run to indicate the level of aerobic fitness capacity when the test is properly supervised and the participants well motivated.

▶ Every year we have difficulty deciding which method of testing we should use in our pre-season fitness test to determine cardiorespiratory endurance. It is apparent that a 2-mile timed run is a fairly accurate assessment of Vo_{2max}, especially if weight is included in the formula. The authors state that ". . . the addition of weight alone improved the shared variance from 82 percent to 89 percent."

This appears to be a valid, inexpensive, and efficient method of testing large numbers of athletes for their aerobic capacity.— F.J. George, ATC, PT

Development of a Telemetry System for Measuring Oxygen Uptake During Sports Activities
Ikegami Y, Hiruta S, Ikegami H, Miyamura M (Nagoya Univ; Nagoya Holy Spirit Junior College, Japan)
Eur J Appl Physiol 57:622–626, Spring 1988   10–3

Oxygen uptake is an excellent indicator of the intensity of physical activity. The Douglas bag method is generally used for measurement, but the procedure is time consuming and not suitable for determining continuous rapid changes during field sports. A new system for continuous measurement of oxygen uptake by means of a telemeter was developed. Oxygen uptake and pulmonary ventilation during rest and exercise were determined using a portable oxygen consumption meter (Oxylog).

Method.—The person being tested wears a face mask containing inspiratory and expiratory valves to which a turbine-type flow meter is attached. Two oxygen electrodes in the instrument measure the pressure of oxygen in the inspired and expired air. A small interface circuit is installed in the Oxylog to transmit data to a frequency-modulated biotelemeter system. Data are passed to a receiver and fed into a microcomputer system, which displays minute values of ventilation and oxygen uptake.

When the telemetry system was compared with the Douglas bag method, the 2 systems were in substantial agreement. The upper limit of 21 minutes^{-1} in measuring oxygen uptake by this system is not of sufficient range for all sports activities.

The telemetry system using the Oxylog is a practical and useful way to measure oxygen uptake during sports activities. The method is not suitable for activities lasting longer than 20 minutes.

▶ These workers adapted the PK Morgan Oxylog system by adding telemetry and found that it functions well, provided one is measuring moderate exercise activity. In a ventilatory range of 2–80 L/minute, the authors found it comparable to the Douglas Bag technique.

The advance made by these authors is in the adaptation of the telemeter, which increased the weight of the Oxylog by only 390 gm (14%), making the weight of the total package 3.5 kg. This was light enough to be carried in a backpack and enabled the wearer to play sports unencumbered: a useful modification.—J.R. Sutton, M.D.

Energy–Speed Relationship of Walking: Standard Tables
Waters RL, Lunsford BR, Perry J, Byrd R (Rancho Los Amigos Med Ctr, Downey, Calif)
J Orthopaedic Res 6:215–222, 1988   10–4

The rate of oxygen consumption during normal level walking increases with gait velocity. However, energy expenditures at different speeds and in different age groups have not been established. To provide a basis against which the energy expenditure of patients with gait disabilities could be assessed, standard reference tables were developed to show the energy expenditure of normal walking at different speeds and in different age groups for males and females.

The energy expenditure of level walking was determined in 260 normal males and females walking around a 60.5-m circular outdoor track. Participants in the study represented 4 age groups: children aged 6–12 years, teenagers, adults aged 20–59 years, and older adults aged 60–80 years. Oxygen consumption was determined using the modified Douglas Bag technique during the fourth and fifth minutes of each trial. Standard tables were developed according to age and sex and for the gait characteristics at slow, normal, and fast walking (table). Tables such as these can be used as references for assessing the energy expenditure of patients who have gait disabilities.

▶ The habitual walking pace is increasingly used as a method of estimating the maximum oxygen intake of senior citizens, particularly the frail elderly (to whom there is an understandable reluctance to suggest deliberate vigorous exercise on a treadmill or a cycle ergometer). Although Waters and associates do not discuss their results in the context of functional assessment, their findings do argue somewhat against the use of habitual walking pace as a measure of aerobic power, because the oxygen consumption while walking (12 ml/kg per minute) was essentially identical in "young" (39-year-old) adults and in those aged 60–80 years (although the latter group almost certainly had a much smaller average maximum oxygen intake). A better basis for distinction was seen when the subjects walked rapidly; "young" adults moved at a speed of 106 m/minute, compared with 90 m/minute in the elderly, and there were then parallel differences of oxygen consumption (18.4 vs 15.4 ml/kg per minute).

As might be expected, children and teenagers walked less efficiently than adults, developing higher oxygen consumptions for a given speed of movement. However, again Walters and associates found no difference in oxygen cost between "young" and old adults (perhaps because they screened out all candidates with orthopedic and medical disabilities). Certainly, there is some evidence in the literature that disabled patients (for instance, those with

Energy Expenditure of Customary Normal, Slow, and Fast Walking

Group	Heart rate (beats/min)			Rate O₂ consumption (ml/kg·min)			O₂ Cost (ml/kg·m)		
	Normal	Slow	Fast	Normal	Slow	Fast	Normal	Slow	Fast
Children (6–12 yr)									
F	118.33[b]	110.77	132.15[b]	14.70	12.28[b]	19.31	0.217	0.223	0.218
	12.11	12.53	14.54	2.90	3.06	3.71	0.040	0.058	0.035
M	111.32[b]	105.11	122.94[b]	15.82	13.64[b]	19.88	0.224	0.237	0.229
	11.12	12.62	12.07	2.06	1.88	3.32	0.030	0.035	0.039
T	114.43	107.16	126.93	15.32	12.73	19.63	0.221	0.231	0.224
	11.94	12.69	13.87	2.51	2.59	3.48	0.035	0.047	0.038
Teens (13–19 yr)									
F	102.75[b]	99.63[b]	124.11[b]	12.62	10.60	18.52	0.172	0.188	0.190
	11.65	11.74	19.25	1.66	1.28	3.33	0.015	0.037	0.026
M	90.12[b]	87.79[b]	107.84[b]	13.16	11.23	19.95	0.181	0.207	0.201
	10.13	9.04	13.59	1.89	1.48	4.68	0.025	0.049	0.028
T	96.79[c]	94.06[c]	116.93[c]	12.88[c]	10.89[c]	19.19	0.176[c]	0.197[c]	0.195[c]
	12.58	12.04	18.57	1.76	1.39	4.01	0.020	0.043	0.027
Adults (20–59 yr)									
F	103.21[b]	88.83	127.34	12.05	7.54	17.43	0.155	0.218	0.175
	12.09	11.80	19.66	2.43	2.18	3.67	0.024	0.066	0.025
M	96.10[b]	85.33	122.08	12.04	8.43	19.23	0.148	0.186	0.174
	13.28	13.65	18.76	2.04	1.87	5.00	0.021	0.038	0.030
T	99.41	86.97[c]	124.39[c]	12.05[c]	8.02[c]	18.44	0.151[c]	0.201	0.174
	13.14	12.84	19.19	2.21	2.03	4.54	0.022	0.055	0.028
Seniors (60–80 yr)									
F	105.85[b]	95.09[b]	120.40	11.88	8.95	14.36[b]	0.166	0.184	0.169
	11.25	10.84	16.03	1.69	1.52	2.55	0.018	0.043	0.020
M	97.15[b]	86.83[b]	116.04	12.21	9.16	17.09[b]	0.160	0.188	0.176
	12.70	13.27	16.61	2.25	1.45	3.34	0.019	0.029	0.024
T	102.75	92.22[c]	118.80[c]	12.00	9.02[c]	15.36[c]	0.164[c]	0.185[c]	0.171
	12.43	12.30	16.26	1.89	1.48	3.14	0.018	0.039	0.021

a: Mean and 1 SD
b: Significant (P < .05) difference between male and female patients.
c: Significant (P < .05) difference between preceding value in younger age group.
(Courtesy of Waters RL, Lunsford BR, Perry J, et al: J Orthopaedic Res 6:215–222, 1988.)

chronic obstructive lung disease) use short and mechanically inefficient pace-lengths when walking.— R.J. Shephard, M.D., Ph.D.

Effect of Carotid Palpation on Postexercise Heart Rate: Validity of Palpation Recovery Technique to Estimate Actual Exercise Heart Rate

Boone T, Edwards CA (Univ of Southern Mississippi, Hattiesburg)
Ann Sports Med 4:29–31, 1988   10–5

Carotid palpation is commonly used to monitor the heart rate during and after dynamic aerobic exercise. Although it has long been known

216 / Sports Medicine

	Exercise Data for 20 Healthy College Women		
Protocol	Heart rate (beats/min^{-1})	F-ratio	Prob- ability
Phase II (Treatment I)			
EHR	157.65 ± 12.31		
PEP	154.55 ± 15.96	4.43	.04 [†]
PESC	146.30 ± 16.65	4.15	.05 [†]
Phase III (Treatment II)			
EHR	154.60 ± 12.18		
PENP	153.25 ± 13.55	5.22	.03*

*EHR, exercise heart rate; PEP, postexercise palpation; PESC, postexercise subject count; PENP, postexercise nonpalpation. Values are mean ± SD.
†$P < .05$.
(Courtesy of Boone T, Edwards CA: Ann Sports Med 4:29–31, 1988.)

that pressure on the carotid artery decreases the heart rate, the potential danger of carotid palpation in either underestimating the actual exercise heart rate or in stimulating the carotid sinus has only recently been recognized. The immediate postexercise heart rate as determined by carotid palpation can mislead the exerciser by being lower than the actual heart rate during exercise and jeopardize the individual's safety.

Twenty healthy college women aged 18–31 years were studied to determine the effect of carotid palpation on the postexercise heart rate. After a familiarization session the women exercised on a treadmill while connected to an electrocardiograph (ECG). After the first exercise routine the women determined their postexercise heart rate by palpating their carotid artery for 10 seconds while counting heart beats. At the same time the postexercise heart rate was determined by using a continuous ECG strip for 10 seconds. After the second exercise routine the postexercise heart rate was determined while the woman stood motionless.

Means and standard deviations for heart rate responses are shown in the table. There was a statistically significant difference between the actual exercise heart rate and the postexercise palpated heart rate. The heart rate decreased significantly while the women palpated the carotid artery. The difference between the postexercise palpated heart rate and the postexercise count by each individual was also significant.

In light of the importance of the individualized exercise heart rate when monitoring exercise intensity, the use of manual carotid palpation as a substitute for either the radial artery or electrically recorded heart rate should be considered a questionable procedure.

▶ There have been various papers discussing the extent to which carotid palpation leads to a slowing of the exercise heart rate. Much undoubtedly depends on how hard a person compresses the sinus, and, unfortunately, Boone and Edwards do not indicate what instructions their subjects were given in the technique of palpation. Another factor that has led to some confusion is the difference between a statistically significant slowing and a clinically significant slowing of heart rate. In the present report the combination of postexercise measurement and carotid palpation slowed the heart rate from 157.7 to 154.6 beats per minute, hardly an important change from the viewpoint of exercise prescription. More serious was the error made by the subject in counting the rate—a 10-second count yielded an average figure of 146.3 beats per minute. The Canada Fitness survey has also found systematic underreporting of exercise heart rates when these are palpated by the exerciser (1). The errors become smaller as a subject is trained in pulse counting; if the answer is important to the safety of exercise, the patient should either use a cheap electronic monitor or be required to practice counting until readings of an acceptable accuracy are obtained.—R.J. Shephard, M.D., Ph.D.

Reference

1. Shephard RJ: *Fitness of a Nation.* Basel, Karger Publishing, 1986.

Comparison of Dipyridamole-Handgrip Test and Bicycle Exercise Test for Thallium Tomographic Imaging
Huikuri HV, Korhonen UR, Airaksinen KEJ, Ikäheimo MJ, Heikkilä J, Takkunen JT (Oulu Univ Central Hosp, Oulu, Finland)
Am J Cardiol 61:264–268, February 1988   10–6

Myocardial perfusion scintigraphy with thallium-201 in conjunction with symptom-limited exercise is useful in assessing coronary artery disease (CAD). However, poor exercise performance can reduce the test's sensitivity. Combining isometric handgrip exercise with intravenously administered dipyridamole further increases coronary blood flow. Findings on single-photon emission computed thallium tomography (Tl-SPECT) using this stress method were compared with those of conventional dynamic exercise testing in the evaluation of CAD.

Seventy-three patients with angina pectoris and 20 with atypical chest pain who had undergone coronary angiography were studied. Perfusion defects were found in 78 of 81 patients with angiographically significantly CAD by Tl-SPECT using combined dipyridamole-handgrip stress testing, for a sensitivity of 96% (table). In 9 of 12 patients without CAD, thallium images were normal, for a specificity of 75%. Thirty-five patients with CAD were reassessed by Tl-SPECT using a dynamic cycle ergometer exercise stress test. The sensitivity of this test was 94%. Multiple thallium defects were seen in 86% of the patients with multivessel CAD by the dipyridamole-handgrip test and in only 64% of patients by the cycle ergometer exercise test. Noncardiac adverse effects occurred in 18% of patients undergoing dipyridamole infusion. Cardiac symptoms were less common during the dipyridamole-handgrip test (15%) than during the cycle exercise (76%).

These findings suggest that the dipyridamole-handgrip test is a useful

Accuracy of Thallium Tomographic Imaging Using 2 Different Stress Methods in Relation to Location of Individual Coronary Arterial Stenosis

Coronary stenosis (≥70%)		LAD	LC	RCA
Thallium defects/stenosed vessels				
Sensitivity				
Dipyridamole-handgrip test	(n = 93)	55/58 (95%)	32/48 (67%)	42/48 (88%)
Dipyridamole-handgrip test	(n = 35)*	24/24 (100%)	11/16 (69%)	20/22 (91%)
Bicycle exercise test	(n = 35)*	22/24 (92%)	8/16 (50%)	17/22 (77%)
Specificity				
Dipyridamole-handgrip test	(n = 93)	26/35 (74%)	39/45 (87%)	39/45 (87%)
Dipyridamole-handgrip test	(n = 35)*	9/11 (82%)	16/19 (84%)	10/13 (77%)
Bicycle exercise test	(n = 35)*	9/11 (82%)	18/19 (95%)	10/13 (77%)
Predictive accuracy				
Dipyridamole-handgrip test	(n = 93)	81/93 (87%)	71/93 (76%)	81/93 (87%)
Dipyridamole-handgrip test	(n = 35)*	33/35 (94%)	27/35 (77%)	30/35 (86%)
Bicycle exercise test	(n = 35)*	31/35 (89%)	26/35 (74%)	27/35 (77%)

LAD, left anterior descending coronary artery; LC, left circumflex coronary artery; RCA, right coronary artery.
*Patients studied by thallium imaging using both dipyridamole-handgrip test and bicycle exercise test.
(Courtesy of Huikuri HV, Korhonen UR, Airaksinen KEJ, et al: Am J Cardiol 61:264–268, February 1988.)

alternative stress method for thallium perfusion imaging, especially in detecting multivessel CAD.

▶ Considerable progress has been made in evaluating myocardial function during submaximal exercise. Nevertheless, there remain substantial difficulties in applying echocardiography and nuclear cardiography during vigorous and maximal endurance effort, and, unfortunately, it is only as maximum effort is approached that many of the problems associated with deficient coronary vascular perfusion (such as a limitation of ejection fraction) come to light.

The movements of the trunk that disturb measurements of cardiac function during cycle ergometry are largely avoided by adoption of a simple isometric handgrip test; unfortunately, however, the latter test may not place a maximal stress on the coronary vascular circulation. It is thus useful to combine the isometric exercise test with administration of a substantial dose of the coronary vasodilator dipyridamole. The sensitivity of this approach is somewhat better than that of cycle ergometry, whereas the specificity of the 2 procedures is very comparable.— R.J. Shephard, M.D., Ph.D.

Reciprocal Change, Exercise-Induced ST Segment Depression, and Coronary Anatomy: Are They Related in the Post-Infarct Patient?
Murray DP, Tan LB, Salih M, Weissberg P, Murray RG, Littler WA (Univ of Birmingham; East Birmingham Hosp, England)
Clin Sci 74:621–627, June 1988   10–7

The significance of ST segment depression in leads remote from the site of acute myocardial infarction, the so-called reciprocal change, is controversial. A prospective study was conducted to assess the relationship of reciprocal changes in the electrocardiogram at the time of myocardial infarction to ST segment changes on a predischarge exercise test and to correlate these changes with findings at coronary angiography. The series included 125 postinfarct patients.

Eighty-three patients had reciprocal changes, 90 had exercise-induced ST depression, and 72 had both. Patients with reciprocal changes had larger myocardial infarctions, determined by peak enzyme release and ejection fraction, than patients without this finding. Multivessel disease was significantly more common among patients with reciprocal changes and those with exercise-induced ST depression than in patients without these findings. The exercise test was more sensitive and had a higher predictive accuracy than reciprocal change. In both tests the anterolateral leads were significantly more sensitive but less specific than the inferior leads in classifying patients.

Although both tests yielded information on coronary anatomy in postinfarct patients, the exercise test was a better predictor of coronary anatomy than reciprocal change. Thus the presence or absence of reciprocal change alone should not be relied on when evaluting patients for further investigation after myocardial infarction.

▶ The suggestion that, relative to catheterization findings, exercise-induced ST segmental depression is a better diagnostic sign than reciprocal change is a fairly heavy condemnation of reciprocal change as a measure of coronary vascular disease; based on an interpretation of exercise-induced ST segmental depression, the study of Murray and associates yielded 17 false among 90 positive results, with 8 false of 35 negative results. Because the decision to allow cardiac catheterization was based on the exercise test results, there may have been some bias of patients in favor of ST segmental depression; however, there was little evidence that a search for reciprocal change added to a diagnosis based on ST depression alone.

Argument continues concerning the physiologic basis of reciprocal change. Some authors maintain it is an electrical consequence of voltage change at the infarct site (1), whereas others suggest that it reflects ischemia caused by residual disease in vessels not contributing to the original infarct (2).— R.J. Shephard, M.D., Ph.D.

References

1. Marriot HJL: *Practical Electrocardiography.* Baltimore, Williams & Wilkins, 1977.
2. Gibson RG, et al: *Circulation* 66:732–741, 1982.

Jogging in Place: A Valid Alternative to Multistage Exercise Testing
Papazoglou NM, Kolokouri-Dervou ES, Viaros PA, Vassiliou SV, Korkodilos GA
(Third Social Security Hosp, Athens)
Am J Cardiol 61:1146–1147, May 1, 1988   10–8

The treadmill exercise test is commonly used to detect and evaluate coronary artery disease. Monitored jogging in place was assessed as a simpler, faster type of electrocardiograph exercise test in a series of 100 patients with chest pain symptoms; all performed the Bruce protocol on the treadmill as well as jogging in place. Both exercises were done at the patient's maximum capacity. A 3-channel electrocardiograph measured the treadmill results and a 1-channel device recorded results of the jogging test. Blood pressure was determined before exercise and at peak.

Peak heart rate, systolic blood pressure, and peak double product were all significantly higher with jogging in place. Discordant rates were always in favor of the jogging test, but the 2 tests gave highly similar results regarding ST segment depression (table). At least 100% of the expected maximal heart rate was obtained in 47% of the jogging tests and in 23% of the treadmill tests. Based on these results, jogging in place, monitored with a 1-channel electrocardiograph, is a valid test that may be especially valuable in mass screening for coronary artery disease.

▶ The likelihood of detecting a coronary vascular abnormality increases as the intensity of effort is increased, and many authors regard 85% of the maximum heart rate as a minimum standard for an acceptable stress test. In normal office practice, a portable electrocardiograph is often available, but a treadmill is much less likely to be "on site." It is thus interesting that in terms of developing an appropriate peak heart rate and blood pressure, 2 minutes of jogging in place seems as effective as a Bruce treadmill test.

Diagnostic Parameters in the Two Compared Exercise Tests

Exercise Parameter	Concordant Result		Discordant Positivity		Total Paired Comparison
	Positive	Negative	J I P	B T P	
ST↓ ≥1 mm	18	70	10	2	100
Chest pain	23	64	12	1	100
Arrhythmia	10	59	28	3	100

*BTP, Bruce treadmill protocol; JIP, jogging in place, ST ↓, ST segment depression.
(Courtesy of Papazoglou NM, Kolokouri-Dervou ES, Viaros PA, et al: *Am J Cardiol* 61:1146–1147, May 1, 1988.)

Before all treadmills are consigned to the scrap heap, however, let us note some advantages of the treadmill approach: One not only defines a double-product at which ST depression occurs but also gains an impression of the corresponding effort tolerance; indeed, there is an approximate relationship between the final speed of walking or jogging and the symptom-limited maximal oxygen intake. This can be helpful in exercise prescription.—R.J. Shephard, M.D., Ph.D.

Evaluation of Criteria Associated With Abdominal Fitness Testing
Robertson LD, Magnusdottir H (Portland State Univ, Portland, Ore)
Res Q Exer Sport 58:355–359, December 1987   10–9

Recently, concern has been expressed over the efficacy of current fitness tests to determine either the performance level or health status of test participants. Although the sit-up test is almost universally described as a test of abdominal strength and endurance, there is still dissatisfaction with it. A modified curl-up test was compared with the standardized modified sit-up test. Twenty volunteers, aged 21–37 years, participated. To perform the curl-up test, participants curled their heads and upper backs and slid fingers forward 7.62 cm to touch a frame. To perform the sit-up test, participants curled up to touch forearms to thighs.

There was an unexplained variance between sit-up and curl-up scores of almost 60%. This lack of association was attributed to predetermined differences in dynamic abdominal and hip flexor muscle activity and active range-of-motion differences in trunk flexion between each test. Angular displacement of the trunk was greater for women than for men in the curl-up test.

Comparisons between 2 tests suggest that the large percentage of unexplained variance between test scores may be accounted for by differences in abdominal and hip flexor muscle activity within each test and by differences in the angular displacement of the trunk required for both tests. These results and previous data suggest that the curl-up test may be a more sensitive test than the sit-up test when evaluating dynamic muscular function of the abdominals in young, healthy adults.

▶ We have been searching many years for the best way to strengthen the abdominal muscles and the best way to test this strength. The authors have described a modififed curl-up test that appears to be a better method of testing abdominal strength. A few years ago we modififed our method of doing sit-ups, which closely approximates this test. We call them curl-ups now, not sit-ups, and they are done in the following manner:

1. The athlete lies supine with the knees bent and the feet flat on the floor (hook-lying position).
2. The arms are folded across the upper chest.
3. The low back is flat (pelvic tilt).
4. A curl-up or partial sit-up is done and held for a count of 6 (when doing

this type of sit-up, the shoulders come off the floor only about 12 in. The chin is brought to the chest in a curling motion).—F.J. George, ATC, PT

Assessment of Technical Accuracy of the Cybex II Isokinetic Dynamometer and Analog Recording System
Bemben MG, Grump KJ, Massey BH (Univ of Illinois, Urbana-Champaign)
J Orthop Sports Phys Ther 10:12–17, July 1988   10–10

The Cybex II isokinetic dynamometer is often used to evaluate muscular strength, power, and endurance in various performance and health-related areas such as physical therapy, rehabilitative medicine, and exercise physiology. The technical accuracy of the analogue torque recordings of the Cybex II was evaluated.

The Cybex calibration T-Bar was set at "C," which gave a lever arm 2.5 ft in length and produced a distal force of 2.4 lb with the bar horizontal to the floor. The accuracy of the dynamometer velocities was assessed using a system of photoelectric cells and timers. The accuracy of peak torque recordings was checked using an equation for calculating true peak torque. The effect of analogue recorder damping setting on the recorded peak torque and the angle of the lever arm at which peak torque was recorded was assessed at 4 velocities, 6 experimental loads, and 5 damping settings.

The Cybex II controlled the velocity of movement at all settings of the machine. The damping characteristics of the analogue recorder affected the accuracy of the torque recordings, however. The damping setting of 4 produced the most accurate peak torque recordings and angle of occurrence for peak torque, irrespective of load or speed.

The damping setting used for calibration should be the same as that used in testing, not varied depending on range of motion or body part tested, as has been recommended by the manufacturer. The Cybex II can be used at all velocity settings for isokinetically exercising and conditioning selected muscle groups. It is suitable for clinical work and research in which there is an interest in peak torque and lever arm angle at peak torque, but only when used at lower velocities and higher damping settings.

▶ After reading this article I contacted the Cybex company and asked for their comments regarding the recommendation of this study, i.e., to use a damping of 4 on all tests. Following is their response: "Our consistent position is that damping values should be chosen as specified by the manufacturer's instructions for each joint tested. The referenced article uses *swinging* weights as the torque input. This is like dropping weights on a scale to calibrate the scale. Our calibration instructions state that you should manually assist the calibration T-Bar to smoothly engage the resistance mechanism by starting on the far side of vertical. Then it's OK. The body, soft tissue, seat, shin pad, etc. connection between human subject and Cybex arm is not properly simulated by free swinging heavy weights on a long slender bar. Users should follow the manufacturer's instructions for use of test devices and that includes calibration and damping among other—positioning, stabilization, warm-up, motivation, etc., etc.)".—F.J. George, ATC, PT

Normative Strength Values for Knee, Shoulder, Elbow, and Ankle for Females Ages 9-73 as Determined by Isokinetic Testing

Weldon G, Snouse SL, Shultz S (Women's TRACC Sportsmedicine Clinic, Los Angeles)
Athletic Training 23:325–331, Winter 1988   10–11

TABLE 1.—Isokinetic Knee Extension in Females (Ft Lb Torque)

Range of Weight (lbs)	9 - 12 (18) 27.0-88.5		13 - 18 (76) 39.0-150.0		19 - 30 (449) 34.5-195.0		31 - 45 (570) 35.5-163.0		46 - 60 (147) 26.5-146.0		Over 60 (22) 35.0-75.55	
(Sample Size) (Torq. Range)	Mean	SD	Mean	SD	Mean	SD	Mean	SD	Mean	SD	Mean	SD
0.0 - 59.9	*29.8	2.8	*39.0	0.0								
60.0 - 69.9	*41.8	7.4	*52.5	0.0								
70.0 - 79.9	*41.5	5.0										
80.0 - 89.9	63.3	16.7	68.0	2.0	68.6	12.9	*66.8	23.3	*33.5	0.0		
90.0 - 99.9	63.7	15.6	74.3	11.1	70.6	14.2	64.7	20.6	56.0	14.5		
100.0 - 109.9	*66.5	0.0	79.2	15.2	80.2	12.7	73.3	14.1	*64.7	10.5		
110.0 - 119.9			89.3	19.4	91.9	22.0	74.5	19.1	56.7	14.4		
120.0 - 129.9			98.2	22.5	97.9	21.3	80.7	18.9	68.0	15.4		
130.0 - 139.9			109.1	18.8	101.3	24.0	82.3	15.6	74.5	17.8	50.7	7.4
140.0 - 149.9			130.9	19.2	111.5	25.4	88.7	21.5	75.1	20.8	54.9	10.3
150.0 - 159.9			*122.5	6.0	119.0	31.2	96.6	20.8	79.4	20.5	55.8	11.9
160.0 - 169.9			*88.2	10.2	120.1	20.9	97.4	24.1	79.5	14.2	*67.0	0.0
170.0 - 179.9					113.1	26.6	108.9	21.9	*77.4	27.8	*59.0	7.0
180.0 - 189.9					*77.8	22.3	86.3	16.5	86.4	4.2	*63.8	10.3
190.0 - 199.9			*149.0	0.0	104.4	28.7	116.1	22.2	80.2	19.2		
200.0 - 209.9			*131.0	0.0	*123.5	29.3	95.2	11.0	*86.0	0.0		
210.0 - 219.9			*131.5	0.0	*100.8	40.8	92.5	27.4	*70.5	0.0		
220.0 - 229.9							*94.8	17.3				
230.0 - 239.9					*130.5	0.0	*91.3	19.3				
240.0 - 249.9					*125.5	0.0	*109.5	0.0				
250.0 - 259.9												
260.0+							*115.5	0.0	*82.0	0.0		

*Fewer than 5 individuals.
(Courtesy of Weldon G, Snouse SL, Shultz S: *Athletic Training* 23:325–331, Winter 1988.)

TABLE 2.—Isokinetic Knee Flexion in Females (Ft Lb Torque)

Range of Weight (lbs)	9 - 12		13 - 18		19 - 30		31 - 45		46 - 60		Over 60	
(Sample Size)	18		76		449		570		147		22	
(Torq. Range)	16.5-61.0		27.0-103.5		25.0-138.0		15.0-129.0		13.0-107.0		20.5-54.5	
	Mean	SD	Mean	SD	Mean	SD	Mean	SD	Mean	SD	Mean	SD
0.0 - 59.9	*17.3	.8	*27.0	0.0								
60.0 - 69.9	*23.2	6.3	*37.5	0.0								
70.0 - 79.9	*29.8	2.3										
80.0 - 89.9	43.6	11.4							*23.5	0.0		
90.0 - 99.9	37.8	6.4					*50.3	.3	35.5	8.0		
100.0 - 109.9	*44.0	0.0	42.0	9.0	45.1	8.2	39.5	10.4	*42.5	7.8	30.7	6.1
110.0 - 119.9			47.2	8.2	48.8	13.1	49.4	9.1	36.7	10.8	36.3	6.5
120.0 - 129.9			50.2	13.7	50.4	10.9	49.5	11.2	44.1	11.2	42.4	5.9
130.0 - 139.9			56.0	8.6	59.0	14.2	52.5	12.6	48.4	10.2	*34.5	0.0
140.0 - 149.9			58.6	12.9	64.0	14.3	52.4	11.3	50.8	11.1	*41.0	13.0
150.0 - 159.9			72.5	14.0	63.6	16.5	58.9	14.5	53.6	12.9	*41.5	11.5
160.0 - 169.9			80.3	16.8	73.0	20.1	62.0	16.8	51.3	10.4		
170.0 - 179.9			*66.5	1.0	75.9	20.8	64.6	19.1	*55.6	20.8		
180.0 - 189.9			*62.2	10.4	78.5	18.0	70.8	15.3	55.4	6.7		
190.0 - 199.9			*93.5	0.0	68.6	21.9	53.2	9.4	54.0	12.8		
200.0 - 209.9			*90.5	0.0	*43.7	11.0	74.6	20.8	*46.0	0.0		
210.0 - 219.9			*68.0	0.0	63.9	16.2	54.7	9.5	*38.5	0.0		
220.0 - 229.9					*77.0	13.7	60.5	16.7				
230.0 - 239.9					*72.5	21.0	*62.0	4.0				
240.0 - 249.9					*83.0	0.0	*52.0	14.9				
250.0 - 259.9					*83.5	0.0	*80.5	0.0				
260.0+							*66.0	0.0	*66.5	0.0		0.0

*Fewer than 5 individuals.
(Courtesy of Weldon G, Snouse SL, Shultz S: *Athletic Training* 23:325–331, Winter 1988.)

Increasing isokinetic evaluation and exercise has created a need for normative data. Few data can be found for females in general, specifically for women older than 30 years of age. There is also a need for norms related to age and body weight for persons in 5 reciprocal joint motions. A study was done on 1,282 females aged 9–73 years. Data were collected using a Cybex II Isokinetic Dynamometer. Peak torque was obtained at 60 degrees per second or 30 degrees per second in 5 reciprocal joint motions.

Joint motion mean peak torque values increased with increasing age.

The highest peak values were noted among women aged 19–30 years. Beyond the age of 30 years torque values progressively and incrementally declined with increasing age. Torque values also increased with increasing weight until reaching women who weighed 220 lb or more (Tables 1 and 2).

Testing was done to develop normative strength data for a healthy female population. The norms established can be used to develop strength training and rehabilitation programs.

▶ This is a very ambitious study with almost 1,300 participants from whom data were obtained. The figures and tables that this study produced will be very beneficial in determining norms and developing guidelines in our screening and rehabilitation programs.—F.J. George, ATC, PT

11 Respiratory Function

Metabolic, Thermoregulatory, and Psychophysiological Responses During Arm and Leg Exercise
Pivarnik JM, Grafner TR, Elkins ES (Univ of Houston)
Med Sci Sports Exerc 20:1–5, February 1988   11–1

The metabolic, thermoregulatory, and psychophysiologic responses during arm and leg exercise at a given submaximal power output were determined in different environmental conditions. Oxygen consumption ($\dot{V}O_2$), rectal and skin temperatures, heart rate, and rating of perceived exertion were measured in 8 healthy men who performed four 60-minute exercise bouts at room temperature (23 C, relative humidity, 75%) and in the heat (33 C, relative humidity, 57%). Power output was 75 W for all experiments.

Exercise $\dot{V}O_2$ averaged 1.54 L/minute in all experiments and was equivalent to 60% of arm and 37% of leg peak values. Rectal temperature increased by an average of 0.43 C regardless of exercise mode or ambient temperature (Fig 11–1). Similarly, skin temperature was increased in all experiments, but final skin temperatures were 1.2 C higher when exercising in the heat, regardless of whether the arms or legs were used. Heart rate and rating of perceived exertion were increased signifi-

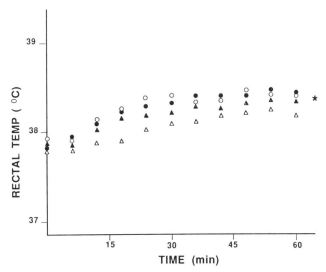

Fig 11–1.—Average rectal temperatures during inside arm *(open triangles)* and leg *(open circles)* and outside arm *(solid triangles)* and leg *(solid circles)* exercise. *Significant increase in temperatures by end of exercise in all conditions. Average SE across all conditions is 0.09 C. (Courtesy of Pivarnik JM, Grafner TR, Elkins ES: *Med Sci Sports Exerc* 20:1–5, February 1988.)

cantly when exercise was performed with the arms rather than the legs. When arm exercise was performed in the heat, the heart rate was greater by 6 beats per minute than when performed at room temperature.

Exercise performed at a given absolute power output with arms or legs results in a similar energy expenditure and temperature, but the greater relative exercise intensity in arm work results in a higher heart rate and rate of perceived exertion. The similar increases in rectal temperature in all experiments indicate that core temperature is controlled by absolute heat production, regardless of mode of exercise and ambient temperature.

▶ Heat elimination under hot and humid conditions is a particular problem for paraplegic patients because they lack the normal sympathetic mechanisms of heat dissipation. Studies of cycle ergometer exercise have suggested that the increase in core temperature during vigorous exercise is proportional to the fraction of maximal oxygen intake that is used; if this principle gave rise to a greater rise in core temperature when one performs a given task with the arms rather than the legs, then the paraplegic would be in double jeopardy on a hot day. The paper of Pivarnik et al. confirms earlier work by Sawka and associates (1) in showing that despite the lower peak oxygen intake during arm exercise, the rise in core temperature is similar when a given oxygen consumption is developed by the arms rather than the legs. Nevertheless, arm exercise tends to cause a higher heart rate than leg exercise, and there is thus less cardiac reserve to accommodate the effects of a rising core temperature.

Those organizing track events are now more conscious of the hazards of heat than was the case a few years ago, although battles must still sometimes be fought with television crews who wish to film competitions in mid-afternoon (when direct radiant heat from the sun tends to be maximal, and there is much reflected heat from the track). On a hot and sunny summer day, dangerous hyperthermia can develop even in an able-bodied person within as little as 30 minutes of all-out exertion, and the wheelchair competitor who completes a marathon run in 2 hours is at considerable risk.—R.J. Shephard, M.D., Ph.D.

Reference

1. Sawka MN, et al: *Eur J Appl Physiol* 52:230–234, 1984.

Acute Altitude Exposure and Altered Acid-Base States: I. Effects on the Exercise Ventilation and Blood Lactate Responses
McLellan T, Jacobs I, Lewis W (Defence and Civil Inst of Environmental Medicine, Downsview, Ont)
Eur J Appl Physiol 57:435–444, March 1988   11–2

The cause-and-effect relationship proposed in 1973 between the exercise ventilatory and lactate responses has been challenged by many researchers under various environmental and experimental conditions. The hypoxic stimulus of acute altitude exposure was used to examine the relationship between the exercise ventilatory and blood lactate responses. A dissociation between the relative exercise intensity, which represented a ventilation and lactate "threshold," was reported at the residential locations of natives living at low and moderate altitudes. Compared with ground level conditions, in natives accustomed to low altitudes, the lactate threshold occurred at a higher relative exercise intensity after acute altitude exposure. The influence of acute altitude exposure alone or combined with metabolic acid-base manipulations on the exercise ventilatory and blood lactate responses was investigated.

Four men performed a 4-minute, 30-W incremental test to exhaustion at ground level and a 4-minute, 20-W incremental test during 3 acute exposures to a simulated altitude of 4,200 m: normal after 0.2 gm/kg^{-1} ingestion of sodium bicarbonate; and after 0.5 gm per day^{-1} ingestion of acetazolamide for 2 days before exposure. The $\dot{V}_E.\dot{V}_{O_2}{}^{-1}$ increased progressively through the incremental tests at acute altitude; the minimum value was not related to a change in the blood lactate response. The $\dot{V}_E.\dot{V}_{CO_2}{}^{-1}$ decreased initially to reach a minimum value at the same power output for each altitude trial and was related to a lactate threshold defined by a log-log transformation (Fig 11–2). This was not affected by the changed acid-base states. The relative exercise intensity corresponding to both a δ lactate of 1 mM and absolute lactate of 4 mM was significantly increased during acetazolamide therapy.

These findings suggest that strong relationships exist between the ventilatory and blood lactate responses during acute altitude exposure and

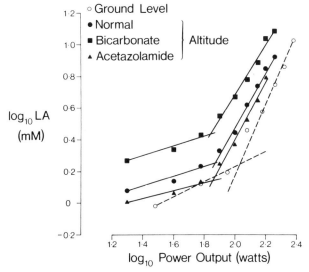

Fig 11–2.—An example of the log-log transformation used for the absolute blood lactate (LA), power output relationship observed at ground level and for the 3 altitude trials. The intersection of the regression lines represents the power output that defines the "lactate threshold" for each condition. (Courtesy of McLellan T, Jacobs I, Lewis W: *Eur J Appl Physiol* 57:435–444, March 1988.)

changed acid-base states. Unless the acid-base status is known, the use of an absolute or δ lactate value to compare submaximal exercise should be interpreted cautiously.

▶ The concept of a ventilatory indication of the anaerobic threshold, originally proposed by Wasserman and associates (1), was attractive to those who wished to carry out exercise tests on large populations without making tedious analyses of blood lactate concentrations. However, as the noninvasive method has been used more widely, the tenuous nature of the relationship between a disproportionate increase in ventilation and accumulation of lactate in the working muscles has been increasingly recognized. Among other variables, the relationship is influenced by the pattern of exercise adopted (particularly the rate of increase of workload), the volume of active muscle relative to the total blood volume, the rate of efflux of lactate from the working muscles, the rate of metabolism of lactate locally and elsewhere in the circulation, and the buffering capacity of the blood. Even if all of these variables can be controlled, it may be quite difficult to determine a unique "breakpoint" in the curve relating ventilation to oxygen consumption or work rate.

In the present study the impact on these relationships of high altitude respiratory alkalosis, bicarbonate ingestion, and acetazolamide administration was examined. In all of the conditions examined there were substantial discrepancies between the ventilatory threshold (ventilation vs. oxygen consumption) and the lactate threshold (log/log plot). Thus, at ground level, respective fractions of maximal oxygen intake were 44.3% and 48.2%; at altitude, 35.6% and 51.9%; after bicarbonate treatment, 32.8% and 50.5%; and after administration of acetazolamide, 33.7% and 52.4%; further, individual values showed a coefficient of variation of at least 10% around these averages.

These findings reinforce earlier doubts about the value of ventilatory threshold determinations. Although no useful breakpoint could be found in the relationship of ventilation to oxygen consumption, ventilation did show a minimum when plotted against carbon dioxide output; this value was quite closely related to the lactate threshold ($r = .78$), and it was uninfluenced by either alkalotic or acidotic manipulation while at altitude. This finding can be compared with the observations of Kowalchuk et al. (2) at sea level, where the intensity of exercise needed to increase the blood lactate level by 1 mM was increased by acidosis, but the ventilatory threshold was unchanged. McLellan and associates point out that because of effects attributable to differences of pCO_2 and the effects of the drugs administered, a blood lactate increment of 1 mM does not have the same impact on blood hydrogen ion concentrations and ventilatory patterns in the several experiments. Another factor in lactate accumulation is the balance between lactate accumulation and clearance, which is influenced by the rate and distribution of blood flow (variables that are probably quite susceptible to changes in the degree of alkalosis or acidosis, whether occasioned by drug treatment or exposure to altitude).—R.J. Shephard, M.D., Ph.D.

References

1. Wasserman K, et al: *J Appl Physiol* 35:236–243, 1973.
2. Kowalchuk JM, et al: *J Appl Physiol* 57:1558–1563, 1984.

Exercise Responses in Patients With an Enzyme Deficiency in the Mitochondrial Respiratory Chain

Bogaard JM, Busch HFM, Scholte HR, Stam H, Versprille A (Erasmus Univ, Rotterdam)

Eur Resp J 1:445–452, May 1988   11–3

The mechanisms behind the threshold of anaerobic metabolism may be complex. Mitochondrial enzyme deficiencies may cause a rate limitation of mitochondrial oxidative phosphorylation that decreases the threshold at which anaerobic glycolysis begins to contribute to the energy-delivering metabolic processes. Findings in 6 patients with mitochondrial enzyme deficiency and symptoms of early fatigue during exercise were compared with those in 14 controls during exercise-ergometer testing. Metabolic, ventilatory, and cardiologic variables were measured.

The mean maximal heart rate and mean change in blood lactate level were not significantly different between groups. However, in patients the early occurring lactate threshold caused carbon dioxide flux to the lungs, resulting in a much sharper increase in respiratory exchange rate than in

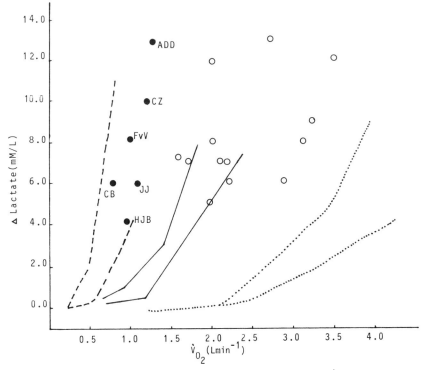

Fig 11–3.—Change in blood lactate (with respect to resting condition, at $\dot{V}O_{2max}$. Patients with mitochondrial myopathy *(black dot)*; control group *(white dot)*. Ranges for patients with heart disease *(broken line)*, sedentary normal persons *(solid line)*, and well-trained individuals *(dotted line)*. (Courtesy of Wasserman K, Whipp BJ: *Am Rev Respir Dis* 112:219–249, 1975. From Bogaard JM, Busch HFM, Scholte HR, et al: *Eur Resp J* 1:445–452, May 1988.)

controls. For patients there was no threshold in the mean respiratory exchange response, which showed an early and abrupt increase at low workloads. Patient responses were similar to those in patients with heart disease (Fig 11–3).

Patients with a mitochondrial enzyme deficiency have a severely limited exercise performance. Exercise response compares with that of patients with severe cardiovascular impairment. Exercise testing can reveal metabolic disturbances and can be valuable in the diagnosis of neuromuscular disorders.

▶ The low anaerobic threshold observed in conditions such as heart disease and anemia has been interpreted as evidence of a deficient oxygen delivery to the working tissues. However, authors such as George Brooks (1) have repeatedly hammered home the message that blood concentrations of lactate depend on many factors in addition to tissue oxygen supply, including the overall rate of metabolism in the muscle, the rate of diffusion of lactate from the muscle to the bloodstream, and the rate of removal of lactate from the blood by the liver and other tissues.

Normally, the level of mitochondrial enzymes is not a significant determinant of lactate accumulation. Although training increases aerobic enzyme activity, the main purpose of the change in enzyme function seems to divert metabolism from glycogen to fat. However, there are specific if rare biochemical disorders, as in the example here (a sixfold reduction of NADH-CoQ reductase activity), that apparently limit the local rate at which lactate can be metabolized, thereby reducing the anaerobic threshold.

The exercise response of such patients is severely restricted. Maximal oxygen intake was only half of the anticipated value in the present sample and the anaerobic threshold was seen at even lower absolute oxygen consumption. A plot of ventilation against oxygen consumption may be helpful in diagnosis and, at least in some patients, the clinical condition improves in response to administration of riboflavin.—R.J. Shephard, M.D., Ph.D.

Reference

1. Brooks G: *Med Sci Sports Exerc* 17:22–31, 1985.

Increased Exercise Ventilation in Patients With Chronic Heart Failure: Intact Ventilatory Control Despite Hemodynamic and Pulmonary Abnormalities
Sullivan MJ, Higginbotham MB, Cobb FR (Duke Univ; Durham VA Med Ctr, NC)
Circulation 77:552–559, March 1988   11–4

In patients with acute pulmonary edema a rapid increase in pulmonary capillary wedge pressure leads to interstitial fluid accumulation, decreased lung compliance, and obstructive airway physiology. It is the primary factor causing dyspnea. The role of increased intrapulmonary vascular pressures in causing ventilatory anomalies and dyspnea in stable ambulatory patients with chronic heart failure has not been defined clearly. A study was conducted to determine the hemodynamic, metabolic, and pulmonary factors associated with the increased ventilatory drive in congestive heart failure and the relationship between peak exercise drive and exertional dyspnea.

Sixty-four ambulatory patients with chronic heart failure and 38 age-matched healthy controls performed exercise on a bicycle. Compared with controls, ventilation and the ratio of ventilation to carbon dioxide production ($\dot{V}e/\dot{V}CO_2$) and pulmonary capillary wedge pressure were increased in patients at rest and during exercise. The ratio of pulmonary deadspace to tidal volume also was elevated in those with heart failure at rest and during exercise and was closely related to $\dot{V}e/\dot{V}CO_2$. Peak exercise $\dot{V}e/\dot{V}CO_2$ did not correlate with pulmonary vascular pressures but was related inversely to cardiac output (Fig 11–4).

Neurohumoral ventilatory control mechanisms are intact in patients with chronic heart failure and act to maintain normal partial pressure of carbon dioxide in arterial blood levels in the face of increased pulmonary deadspace. Activation of abnormal reflexes by hemodynamic derangements during exercise are not important in determining ventilation in patients with chronic heart failure. The correlation between decreased cardiac output and increased ventilation in the patient group suggests that

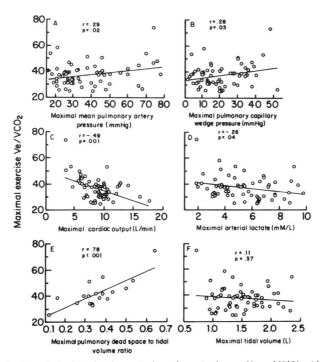

Fig 11–4.—The relationship of peak exercise hemodynamics, lactate, Vt, and Vd/Vt with $\dot{V}e/\dot{V}CO_2$ in patients with chronic heart failure. $P < .005$ is considered indicative of a statistically significant difference. (Courtesy of Sullivan MJ, Higginbotham MB, Cobb FR, et al: *Circulation* 77:552–559, March 1988.)

attenuated pulmonary perfusion may play a role in causing exercise hyperpnea in the presence of chronic heart failure by producing ventilation perfusion abnormalities and thereby increasing physiologic pulmonary deadspace.

▶ The pattern of resting ventilation in patients with cardiac failure caused by rheumatic heart disease was explored many years ago (1). In this early paper it was demonstrated that pulmonary congestion was associated with an unusually shallow breathing pattern, and it was hypothesized that the cause was the increased pulmonary compliance associated with pulmonary edema. More recently, Weber et al. (2) suggested that the same pattern of shallow ventilation persists during exercise, giving rise to early dyspnea of effort. Other possible factors contributing to respiratory distress are an increase of deadspace ventilation (caused by both the shallow breathing and coexisting pulmonary disease), a reflex hyperventilation (3), and an early accumulation of lactate as a result of poor circulation to the working muscles (4). In normal exercise the component of deadspace attributable to a poor matching of ventilation with perfusion is lessened as cardiac output increases. The present authors suggest as a further hypothesis that the limited increase of cardiac output in patients with chronic heart failure contributes to increased deadspace ventilation. The earlier observations of an increased frequency of breathing were confirmed for rest and submaximal effort, but (probably because the peak work rate was much lower in the diseased subjects), the peak ventilatory frequency was similar in patients with chronic heart failure and in controls.—R.J. Shephard, M.D., Ph.D.

References

1. Shephard RJ, Venner A: *Br Heart J* 18:241–247, 1956.
2. Weber KT, et al: *Circulation* 65:1213, 1982.
3. Ingram RH, McFadden ER: *Prog Cardiovasc Dis* 19:109, 1976.
4. Rubin SA, Brown HV: *Am Rev Respir Dis* 129:563, 1984.

Dichotomous Airway Response to Exercise in Asthmatic Patients
Rubinstein I, Zamel N, Rebuck AS, Hoffstein V, D'Urzo AD, Slutsky AS (Univ of Toronto)
Am Rev Respir Dis 138:1164–1168, November 1988   11–5

Exercise-induced airway narrowing in patients with asthma has been well documented. To define the precise site and caliber of affected airways, the airway cross-sectional area in patients with asthma and healthy controls was measured after exercise. Fourteen nonsmoking patients with asthma and 8 nonsmoking controls underwent treadmill exercise testing for 6 minutes. Forced vital capacity and forced expiratory volume in 1 second (FEV_1) were measured before and after exercise. The airway cross-sectional area was measured using the acoustic reflection technique.

After exercise, the normal persons had no significant change in FEV_1 or bronchial area but a significant increase was noted in the intrathoracic tracheal area. After exercise patients with asthma had a 37% decrease in FEV_1 and a 36% decrease in bronchial area. However, the extrathoracic and intrathoracic tracheal areas increased significantly.

In normal persons exercise is associated with significant dilation of the intrathoracic trachea; but in patients with asthma, exercise results in significant bronchoconstriction and tracheal dilation.

▶ Using the elegant acoustic reflection technique, these authors have confirmed structurally the previously documented physiologic changes during exercise-induced asthma, i.e., airway bronchoconstriction, together with tracheal dilatation.—J.R. Sutton, M.D.

12 Cardiac Function and Cardiac Disease

Contributions of Epidemiology to Exercise Science and Cardiovascular Health
Paffenbarger RS Jr (Stanford Univ)
Med Sci Sports Exerc 20:426–438, October 1988   12–1

Epidemiology, the study in human populations of frequencies and distributions of disease in terms of time, place, and personal characteristics, has much to contribute to exercise science and cardiovascular health. Comparison and contrast are key to the epidemiologic method; however, epidemiologic analyses of physical activity and cardiovascular health must often be based on circumstantial evidence to assess cause-and-effect relationships. Study procedures must meet rigid epidemiologic standards: statistical association, temporal sequence, persistence, consistency, dose-response relationship, independence, specificity, alterability, repeatability, and confirmation of findings.

Measurement and contrast are used to determine whether physically active persons have a lower incidence of cardiovascular disease than do sedentary persons. Based on these principles current evidence suggests that exercise induces protective benefits against coronary heart disease, enabling most individuals to approach their potential longevity.

▶ This material was presented as the Joseph B. Wolffe Memorial Lecture at the American College of Sports Medicine 35th Annual Meeting on May 25, 1988. It is an excellent primer on the basic principles of epidemiology that are not necessarily limited to exercise or cardiovascular health. The interested reader is referred to the original article.—J.S. Torg, M.D.

A Mail Survey of Physical Activity Habits as Related to Measured Physical Fitness
Kohl HW, Blair SN, Paffenbarger RS Jr, Macera CA, Kronenfeld JJ (Inst; of Aerobics Research, Dallas; Stanford Univ; Univ of South Carolina, Columbia)
Am J Epidemiol 127:1228–1239, June 1988   12–2

The relationship between reported exercise behavior and true exercise behavior was studied by using physical fitness as a marker for true exercise behavior. A cross-sectional study was done comparing responses to physical activity questions on a mail survey with maximal treadmill test performance at a clinic visit. The study included 12,225 respondents to a health status survey conducted in 1982 by the Institute for Aerobics Research in Dallas. From this population 375 males (mean age, 47 years) having a clinical examination within 60 days of the return of their questionnaire served as subjects.

The men completed a maximal physical fitness assessment using a modified Balke and Ware protocol. One section of the questionnaire addressed leisure time activity on which the subjects recalled quantitatively their exercise participation for varying periods of time. Hours of exercise participation were converted to estimate energy expenditure, and indices of physical activity participation were created. Individual contributions of the physical activity indices in predicting physical fitness were determined by multiple regression analyses.

Variables that were significant predictors of physical fitness were the run-walk-jog index, frequency of sweating, and age. The 3-month leisure time index and 7-day activity index did not add to the predictability of physical fitness. For the 3 significant variables, the multiple correlation coefficient was 0.65 in predicting physical fitness.

Exercise behavior can be estimated efficiently and inexpensively in large populations by using a mail survey with simple questions. However, research for investigating ways to partition physical fitness into its activity and genetic components is necessary to enable measurement of those components in future studies.

Relation of Cardiovascular Fitness and Physical Activity to Cardiovascular Disease Risk Factors in Children and Adults

Sallis JF, Patterson TL, Buono MJ, Nader PR (Univ of California, San Diego, La Jolla)
Am J Epidemiol 127:933–941, May 1988   12–3

The relationships between physical activity, cardiovascular fitness, and cardiovascular disease risk factors were assessed in families recruited from elementary schools in San Diego, Calif. The families consisted of 268 adults (88 men, 180 women) and 290 children (148 boys, 142 girls). Cardiovascular fitness was assessed by a cycle ergometer submaximal graded exercise test. Physical activity was measured by a 7-day physical activity questionnaire from which caloric expenditure was derived and by self-rating of activity. Blood pressure, high-density lipoprotein (HDL) cholesterol concentration, the ratio of HDL to low-density lipoprotein (LDL), and body mass index were all considered risk factors.

In both adults and children, fitness was significantly correlated with all risk factors. When adjusted for body mass index, the correlation between most fitness-risk factors was no longer significant. Energy expenditure was correlated with none of the risk factors in adults and children, except for body mass index and the HDL/LDL ratio in women and the HDL/LDL ratio in girls. The simple activity rating was more strongly correlated with risk factors. In 3 of the 4 subgroups activity rating was associated with body mass index and either HDL cholesterol level or the HDL/LDL ratio.

Cardiovascular fitness is consistently correlated with cardiovascular disease risk factors, whereas measures of physical activity are only weakly correlated with risk factors. In this sample of families, relationships between measures of cardiovascular fitness, physical activity, and cardiovascular disease risk factors are similar in children and adults, thus reinforcing recommendations for increased activity and fitness in childhood to enhance cardiovascular risk profiles.

▶ These 2 studies (Abstracts 12–2 and 12–3) were included because they represent excellent examples of the application of epidemiologic techniques to the study of fitness habits. In the first study an enormous population base was sampled by questionnaire; in the second, assessments were made on subjects sampled from schools. One of the important lessons of these papers is the painstaking care necessary to ensure that those sampled are truly representative of the population under study.—J.R. Sutton, M.D.

Resistive Training Can Reduce Coronary Risk Factors Without Altering $\dot{V}o2_{max}$ or Percent Body Fat

Hurley BF, Hagberg JM, Goldberg AP, Seals DR, Ehsani AA, Brennan RE, Holloszy JO (Washington Univ; Univ of Maryland, College Park)
Med Sci Sports Exerc 20:150–154, April 1988   12–4

Aerobic exercise training reduces the relative risk for coronary artery disease (CAD) by improving glucose metabolism and lipoprotein-lipid profiles and lowering blood pressure. Substantial increases in oxygen uptake capacity ($\dot{V}o_{2\ max}$) and reductions in body weight are necessary, however, to achieve these benefits. Resistive training reportedly has favorable effects on lipoprotein-lipid profiles, glucose metabolism, and blood pressure, independent of improvement in oxygen uptake capacity ($\dot{V}o_{2\ max}$). To clarify this further, lipoprotein-lipid profiles, the plasma glucose level, and insulin responses during an oral glucose test, as well as blood pressure, were determined before and after 16 weeks of high-intensity resistive training in 11 healthy, untrained middle-aged men (mean age, 44 years).

Body weight, percentage of body fat, or $\dot{V}O_{2max}$ did not change significantly after training. However, the training program resulted in a 10% increase in high-density lipoprotein (HDL)-cholesterol, a 43% increase in HDL_2-cholesterol, a 5% reduction in low-density lipoprotein (LDL)-cholesterol, and an 8% decrease in LDL-cholesterol/HDL-cholesterol ratios. Furthermore, the training program resulted in significantly lower glucose-stimulated plasma insulin concentrations and lower supine diastolic blood pressure. No such changes occurred among sedentary controls.

These data suggest that, despite the absence of an effect in $\dot{V}o_{2\ max}$, body weight, or body composition, high-intensity resistive training improves plasma lipoprotein-lipid profiles, reduces the insulin response to glucose ingestion, and lowers diastolic blood pressure in middle-aged men.

▶ Our obsession with aerobic forms of exercise and training programs, coupled with the substantially high blood pressure responses during resistance training, has meant that resistance training is rarely used in cardiac rehabilitation programs. This same thinking has extended to preventive programs. However, this report by Hurley and colleagues indicates that benefits might accrue to several coronary risk factors including lipoproteins, plasma glucose, insulin, and blood pressure. Although it supports other work of a similar nature, further studies are required to substantiate these effects and also to attempt to define mechanisms. Nevertheless, for those engaged in conducting preventive programs, the inclusion of resistance training regimes in an overall activity program may well be justifiable on the basis of a reduced coronary risk profile as well as improvement in the tone and strength of muscles.—J.R. Sutton, M.D.

Exercise-Related Sudden Death: What Autopsy Findings Reveal About Its Causes in Conditioned Persons Over Age 30 Years
Waller BF (Indiana Univ, Indianapolis)
Postgrad Med 83:273–282, June 1988   12–5

The incidence of premature sudden death among athletes is low. However, because of the much-publicized sudden deaths of prominent athletes and the increased popularity of vigorous exercise in the United States, there is a need to identify the causes of such phenomena. The postmortem cardiac findings in 72 conditioned middle-aged individuals (aged 30 years and older) who died suddenly or shortly after vigorous physical activity were investigated. Of these, 24 were personally examined by the author and 48 were reported previously by others. The majority of these individuals had no symptoms of heart disease, but most of the 24 examined by the author had at least 1 coronary risk factor, such as hypertension, increased total serum cholesterol level, or family history of cardiac disease.

Overall, coronary artery abnormalities accounted for 70 (97%) of 72 exercise-related sudden deaths. Coronary atherosclerosis accounted for 96% of all deaths, congenital coronary anomalies for 1%, and hypertrophic cardiomyopathy for the remaining 3%. No person had fatal valvular or aortic structural abnormalities.

The cardiovascular system should be the focus of any evaluation for healthful exercise in patients older than 30 years. A prescription for healthful exercise for middle-aged athletes should include cardiovascular screening, concentrating on coronary atherosclerosis, and prompt evaluation of new symptoms, especially those suggestive of myocardial ischemia.

▶ Although we are not told what percentage of all national acute cardiac deaths were entered into this registry, the overwhelming cause of death (97%) was atherosclerotic coronary artery disease. This is in complete contrast to findings in those under 30 years of age whose deaths are caused predominantly by congenital lesions. Such lesions include congenital anomalies of the coronary arteries, weakness of the aorta (as in Marfan's syndrome), hypertrophic cardiomyopathies, and valvular lesions.

Also, occasionally, the over-30-year-old athlete may succumb to a congenital cardiac abnormality, but there seems little doubt that ischemic disease on the basis of coronary atherosclerosis is the major culprit.—J.R. Sutton, M.D.

Cardiac Fatigue After Prolonged Exercise

Douglas PS, O'Toole ML, Hiller WDB, Hackney K, Reichek N (Hosp of the Univ of Pennsylvania; Baptist Mem Hosp, Memphis; Univ of Tennessee, Memphis)
Circulation 76:1206–1213, December 1987   12–6

Extreme exercise creates a variety of health hazards, although myocardial dysfunction is generally not considered one of them. However, with

Prolonged Exercise: Physical, Echographic, and Doppler Results

	Before race	Finish	Recovery
Physical characteristics			
Body weight (pounds)	154.4	148.6	—
Heart rate (beats/min)	59±9	89±11[B]	61±9
	(38–79)	(64–110)	(44–79)
Systolic blood pressure (mm Hg)	128±12	123±15	122±15
	(105–148)	(90–160)	(100–155)
Echographic variables			
Cavity dimension, diastole (cm)	5.4±0.6[A]	5.1±0.6	5.2±0.6
Cavity dimension, systole (cm)	3.3±0.5	3.3±0.4	3.2±0.4
Wall thickness, diastole (cm)	1.0±0.2	1.0±0.2	1.0±0.2
Wall thickness, systole (cm)	1.6±0.3	1.5±0.2[A]	1.7±0.2
Fractional shortening (%)	39±5	35±5[A]	40±4
Wall stress ($\times 10^3$ dynes/cm^2)	61±17	61±16	49±10[A]
Rate of cavity enlargement (dD/dt/D)	2.5±0.4	2.5±12	2.6±0.5
Rate of wall thinning (−dh/dt/h)	9.5±2.7	10.1±3.0	8.3±4.1
Doppler variables — mitral flow			
Early velocity (cm/sec)	69±16	68±16	70±14
Late velocity (cm/sec)	38±12	51±19[B]	36±9
Velocity ratio	1.9±0.6	1.5±0.6[B]	2.0±0.4
Doppler variables — aortic flow			
Peak velocity (cm/sec)	101±22	98±25	105±20
Flow velocity integral	20.7±5.2	16.9±6.4	19.3±4.8
Heart rate × flow velocity integral	1232±414	1565±682[B]	1161±303

[A] $p < .05$ vs. both other determinations.
[B] $p < .01$ vs. both other determinations.
(Courtesy of Douglas PS, O'Toole ML, Hiller WDB, et al: *Circulation* 76:1206–1213, December 1987.)

increased participation by athletes in ever-more grueling exercise, clear delineation of the cardiac response is becoming more important. The effects of prolonged exercise on systolic and diastolic left ventricular function were determined in 21 athletes before, at the finish, and during recovery after the Hawaii Ironman Triathlon.

Two-dimensionally guided M-mode echocardiograms were digitized for wall thickness, cavity dimension, fractional shortening, and peak rates of wall thinning and cavity enlargement. Pulsed Doppler left ventricular inflow recordings were examined for peak early and late velocities and their ratio.

In the athletes studied the left ventricular diastolic dimension was diminished at the finish of the race and remained diminished after 1 recovery day. Fractional shortening dropped at the race finish, although systolic blood pressure remained the same and rose to 40% after recovery. Return to prerace shortening values after recovery occurred despite 2 continued decrease in diastolic size. Peak circumferential shortening did not alter significantly.

When assessed in individual athletes, decreases in fractional shortening were correlated with increases in systolic cavity size but not with reductions in diastolic size. The stress–shortening relationship was displaced downward at the race finish but returned to prerace values after 1 recovery day despite persistent reduction in cavity size. The left ventricular filling pattern was changed at the finish of the race, with later an increased inflow velocity and a decreased ratio of early to late velocities. Peak rates of cavity enlargement and wall thinning remained unchanged. All functional variables returned to baseline values during recovery (table).

Prolonged intensive exercise may result in changes in systolic and diastolic left ventricular performance. The rapid reversal of all the noted alterations suggested cardiac "fatigue."

▶ It has been known for a number of years that some species such as dogs can be exercised on the treadmill until they literally die of fatigue. However, physiologists have tended to argue that the upright posture preserves humans from this fate; if cardiac function begins to deteriorate, the person simply collapses, putting an end to excessive exercise. The paper by Douglas and associates nevertheless provides evidence that really gruelling events can have at least a temporary adverse effect on human myocardial function. The hawaii triathlon demands 2.4 miles of swimming, 112 miles of cycling, and 26.2 miles of running, the whole being completed in about 10½ hours. Not only was myocardial contractility impaired by triathlon participation, but a delay in early diastolic filling suggested some slowing of ventricular relaxation. Fortunately, in the healthy contestants who were examined, normal function was restored within 24 hours of competition. Relative to M-mode echocardiography, Doppler measurements are apparently more sensitive to changes in early diastolic filling. The mechanism leading to disturbance of myocardial function remains puzzling. The present group of athletes had no acidosis or electrolyte abnormalities, no ischemic electrocardiographic changes, and no elevation of cardiac subfraction creatine kinase and lactic dehydrogenase enzymes, so that it is difficult to blame either metabolic disturbances or local injury.—R.J. Shephard, M.D. Ph.D.

Left Ventricular Dysfunction After Prolonged Strenuous Exercise in Healthy Subjects

Seals DR, Rogers MA, Hagberg JM, Yamamoto C, Cryer PE, Ehsani AA (Washington Univ)
Am J Cardiol 61:875–879, Apr 15, 1988   12–7

Whether strenuous exercise can cause left ventricular (LV) dysfunction in healthy persons is still debated. A study was done to examine whether LV dysfunction can occur after prolonged exhausting exercise in young healthy persons and to characterize the metabolic and hormonal changes concurrent with changes in LV function.

Twelve men (mean age, 26 years) participated. They exercised on a treadmill at a mean of 69% of maximal O_2 uptake until exhaustion at 170 minutes. Hemodynamic variables were determined before and 10 minutes after the exercise.

The baseline systolic blood pressure dropped from 124 to 113 mm Hg after exhausting exercise. Left ventricular end-diastolic diameter, measured by echocardiography, dropped from 51 to 47 mm but LV end-systolic diameter did not change. Both LV fractional shortening and the mean velocity of circumferential fiber shortening decreased despite a lower end-systolic wall stress after exercise (Fig 12–1). A repeat course of exercise of the same intensity but of a shorter duration resulted in in-

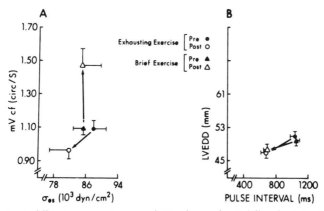

Fig 12–1.—**A,** different responses in mean velocity of circumferential fiber shortening *(mVcf)* after prolonged exhausting and brief exercise at comparable heart rates. Despite a lower end-systolic wall stress, mVcf decreased after strenuous exercise to exhaustion (consistent with depressed contractile state). In contrast, the contractile state was enhanced after brief exercise of the same intensity (relative to $\dot{V}O_{2max}$), characterized by a large increase in mVcf at comparable levels of wall stress. **B,** at comparable heart rates (pulse interval), the changes in left ventricular end-diastolic dimension (LVEDD) were similar between the 2 bouts of exercise. (Courtesy of Seals DR, Rogers MA, Hagberg JM, et al: *Am J Cardiol* 61:875–879, Apr 15, 1988.)

creases in LV fractional shortening and mean velocity of circumferential fiber shortening and a decrease in LV end-diastolic diameter at heart rates comparable to those attained after prolonged exhausting exercise.

Prolonged strenuous exercise can result in impaired LV function in healthy young men. Thus, engaging in prolonged strenuous exercise without supervision is not advisable in a high-risk population.

▶ Young adults seem determined to run ever longer distances—the marathon run has been outshone by the Comrades marathon, and 100-km runs are not unknown. It is thus appropriate to inquire whether there is truth in the legend of Pheidippides, who reputedly died of exhaustion shortly after completing the original run announcing the victory of the Athenians over Darius and the Persians at Marathon in 494 BC.

There seems little argument that there is a progressive "drift" of circulatory function if endurance exercise is continued at the same intensity for 30–60 minutes, but much of this change can be explained by a progressive rise of core temperature, peripheral vasodilatation, and a reduction in venous return to the heart (a diminution of ventricular pre-load) (1). Nevertheless, Niemela et al. (2) did find some evidence of reversible changes in left ventricular function after a 100-km event, and there continue to be occasional reports of pulmonary edema developing after prolonged exertion (3).

Many of the findings in the present study could be attributed to a decrease in preloading, but the decreased velocity of circumferential shortening despite a reduced afterload point to deterioration of myocardial function in response to 170 minutes of exhausting exercise. The intensity of effort producing this change (70% of maximum oxygen intake) is surprisingly low. The mechanism is unclear, although one suggestion advanced by Seals et al. is a reaction to an increased concentration of circulating fatty acids. It would seem important to repeat studies of this sort on postcoronary patients who are eager to exercise at 70% to 80% of their maximum oxygen intake for 4–5 hours in marathon competitions. If indeed there is a depression of myocardial function, it should be much more striking in the postcoronary sample.—R.J. Shephard, M.D. Ph.D.

References

1. Saltin B, Stenberg J: *J Appl Physiol* 19:833–838, 1964.
2. Niemela KO, et al: *Circulation* 70:350–356, 1984.
3. McKechnie JK, et al: *S Afr Med J* 56:261–265, 1979.

Exercise-Induced Hypotension as a Manifestation of Right Ventricular Ischemia
Rich MW, Keller A, Chouhan L, Fischer K (Jewish Hosp, St Louis)
Am Heart J 115:184–186, January 1988   12–8

In the setting of ischemic heart disease, exercise-induced hypotension is a highly specific sign of advanced multivessel or left main coronary disease with or without left ventricular dysfunction. A woman experienced symptomatic exercise-induced hypotension resulting from right ventricular ischemia.

Woman, 55, had dizziness and presyncope accompanied by palpitations and diaphoresis after moderate exertion. On a thallium stress test, the patient achieved a maximum heart rate of 112/minute and a blood pressure of 150/80 mm Hg. At 12 minutes of exercise the patient complained of severe dizziness and near syncope. Her blood pressure dropped to 90 mm Hg. No murmurs or gallop were noted on cardiac auscultation. The exercise 12-lead electrocardiogram showed anterolateral ST segment depression and prominent ST segment elevation in lead V_{4R}. These changes persisted for several minutes and then gradually resolved. Thallium images showed a small area of reperfusible ischemia in the inferior wall of the left ventricle and marked ischemia of the right ventricle. Cardiac catheterization revealed normal wall motion, total proximal occlusion of the right coronary artery with a large acute marginal branch and 2 smaller right ventricular branches, and normal left coronary circulation. The patient remained symptom free after successful transluminal angioplasty of the right coronary artery. A follow-up thallium stress test revealed no evidence of ischemia.

Although uncommon, right ventricular ischemia should be considered in the differential diagnosis of a patient with exercise-related dizziness or syncope in the absence of other causes of exertional hypotension.

▶ This is an interesting case report highlighting a most unusual mechanism for exercise-induced hypotension. Unless a patient is taking medication, the most common causes of hypotension during exercise are left ventricular dysfunction on the basis of left ventricular aneurysm, left main stem disease, or severe multivessel disease. Postexercise hypotension is quite common but, of course, this usually reflects venous pooling; although syncope may ensue, it is unusual for this to signify myocardial dysfunction. Now we must also consider right ventricular ischemia.—J.R. Sutton, M.D.

Comparative Effects of *Alpha*-1 and *Alpha*-2 Adrenoceptors in Modulation of Coronary Flow During Exercise
Strader JR, Gwirtz PA, Jones CE (Texas College of Osteopathic Medicine, Forth Worth)
J Pharmacol Exp Ther 246:772–778, August 1988   12–9

During increased myocardial performance coronary blood flow increases, primarily because of vasodilation after the increased demand for oxygen. When exercise is submaximal sympathetic α-adrenergic vasoconstriction that opposes metabolic dilation exists in the coronary vasculature. The adrenoceptor subtype involved in this sympathetic vasoconstriction is controversial, and evidence has been reported that implicates both α_1- and α_2- adrenoceptors. To clarify this issue, 15 dogs were subjected to graded exercise and at peak exercise received injections of either the α_1-antagonist prazosin or the α_2-antagonist yohimbine. Effects on both coronary flow and cardiac contractile function were assessed before and after treatment with the antagonists.

As expected, exercise resulted in increase in heart rate, left ventricular pressure, rate of change in segment length, systolic shortening and rate of shortening, and coronary blood flow. When prazosin was injected, circumflex blood flow increased as did both regional and global contractile function. When yohimbine was injected, no changes occurred in any recorded parameter.

These experiments suggest that coronary vasoconstriction during exercise is mediated primarily by α_1-adrenoceptors, and that α_2-adrenoceptors have little involvement in this sympathetic, exercise-induced coronary vasoconstriction. Other reports implying mediation of this effect by α_2-adrenoceptors all involved artificial cardiac sympathetic stimulation. It is possible that at high levels of sympathetic stimulation, α_2-adrenoceptors mediate coronary constriction, whereas α_1-adrenoceptors mediate constriction caused by lower levels of stimulation.

▶ This paper gives further insight into the autonomic control of coronary circulation by examining the effects of 2 α-adrenergic receptor-blocking agents. By their choice of α-adrenergic receptor antagonists, these authors concluded that, at least in dogs, myocardial blood flow, even during maximum exercise, is far from maximum. The reserve in coronary blood flow, however, would ordinarily be unobtainable, as some α-adrenergic constrictor tone is maintained. It should be emphasized that these observations apply to normal dogs and not to humans with coronary vascular disease, although in patients with coronary artery spasm, Prinzmetal's angina, the use of β-adrenergic blocking agents is contraindicated because it leaves unapposed the α constrictor tone.—J.R. Sutton, M.D.

Norepinephrine Spillover to Plasma During Steady-State Supine Bicycle Exercise: Comparison of Patients With Congestive Heart Failure and Normal Subjects
Hasking GJ, Esler MD, Jennings GL, Dewar E, Lambert G (Alfred Hosp; Baker Med Research Inst, Prahan, Vic, Australia)
Circulation 78:516–521, September 1988   12–10

Elevated plasma concentrations of norepinephrine in patients with congestive heart failure result from reduced plasma clearance and increased spillover of norepinephrine to plasma. To determine the relative contributions of plasma clearance of norepinephrine and norepinephrine release to increased plasma concentrations of norepinephrine during exercise in normal persons and patients with congestive heart failure, 6 patients with clinical evidence of left ventricular failure and 9 normal controls underwent infusion with tritiated norepinephrine before supine bicycle exercise. The patients and controls exercised at 50% of maximum voluntary exercise capacity.

In patients with congestive heart failure, the mean plasma concentration of norepinephrine rose from 385 pg/ml to 2,200 pg/ml. The mean concentration in the controls increased from 208 pg/ml to 882 pg/ml. In both groups the increased concentration was caused by an increase in norepinephrine spillover to plasma; there was no change in plasma clearance of norepinephrine. In the patients the mean cardiac spillover increased from 80 ng/minute to 528 ng/minute, and the mean renal spillover rose from 146 ng/minute to 418 ng/minute during exercise. In normal persons the mean cardiac spillover increased from 5 ng/minute to 73 ng/minute and the mean renal spillover rose from 76 ng/minute to 275 ng/minute.

There was no evidence of a reduced reserve for overall or regional sympathetic stimulation in patients with congestive heart failure. In these patients, reduced reflex responses apparently are caused by end-organ refractoriness rather than inadequate stimulation.

▶ This is the latest in the very elegant studies from this Melbourne-based group. Using the combination of organ-specific venous catheterization, arterial catheterization, and the infusion of tritiated norepinephrine, they have given new insights into catecholamine dynamics.

The specific details of this study suggest that patients with cardiac failure have impaired cardiac responsiveness to norepinephrine.—J.R. Sutton, M.D.

A Randomized Double-Blind Comparison of Diltiazem and Nifedipine in Stable Angina
Klinke WP, Kvill L, Dempsey EE, Grace M (Royal Alexandra Hosp, Edmonton, Alta; Nordic Labs Inc, Kirkland, PQ)
J Am Coll Cardiol 12:1562–1567, December 1988   12–11

All calcium channel blockers share basic properties, but there is considerable variation in their effects on the coronary vasculature. The efficacy and safety of 2 calcium channel blockers—nifedipine and diltiazem hydrochloride—were evaluated in 21 patients with stable angina. A 2-week placebo period was followed by random assignment to 1 of the 2 drugs. After 3 weeks the patients were given the alternate treatment after a placebo washout of 1 week. The trial was completed with a final week of placebo treatment. Patients underwent treadmill exercise testing at each phase of the trial.

There were no significant differences between treatments in relation to ST depression responses to exercise, time to onset of angina, heart rate, or systolic or diastolic blood pressure. However, patients treated with nifedipine reported 37 adverse effects, whereas only 9 adverse effects were reported with diltiazem treatment. Two patients treated with nifedipine had to be withdrawn from the study before crossover. Seven of 22 patients taking nifedipine had edema, as did only 1 of 22 taking diltiazem. Seven patients experienced dizziness with nifedipine, but none of those taking diltiazem were so affected. Rash was the most common adverse effect associated with diltiazem treatment. Three patients experienced severe adverse effects with nifedipine therapy; 1 had severe effects with diltiazem. Further, whereas 37% of nifedipine-treated patients required a reduction in dosage, this was necessary in only 6% of diltiazem-treated patients. Both drugs reduced the number of angina attacks, diltiazem significantly more so than nifedipine. In addition, diltiazem was better tolerated.

▶ This nicely designed study demonstrates the clear clinical superiority of diltiazem over nifedipine in this patient population. In patients with chest pain on effort, drug side effects need to be minimized as they increase anxiety in the patient, relatives, and physicians, as well as having the real potential for significant harm. Although this study cannot be generalized to other patient groups, diltiazem is probably the best tolerated of the calcium channel blocking agents in a variety of clinical settings. However, in comparison with β-adrenergic blocking agents, there is much greater variability in the actions of the calcium channel blockers.—J.R. Sutton, M.D.

Exercise Capacity Prior to Myocardial Infarction Relates Inversely to Enzyme Activity During Infarction
Berglund B, Mogensen L (Karolinska Hosp, Stockholm)
Int J Cardiol 19:120–122, April 1988   12–12

Exercise testing shortly after acute myocardial infarction is standard medical practice and gives important diagnostic and prognostic information. It is not known whether physical exercise capacity measured before

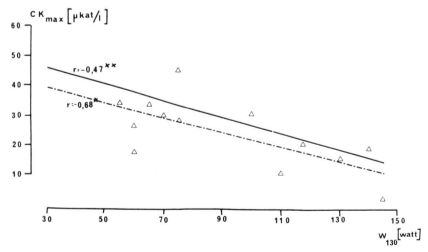

Fig 12–2.—Relationship between maximal creatinine kinase activity (CK_{max}) during acute myocardial infarction and the physical working capacity at heart rate of 130 beats per minute (W_{130}) before infarction. *Solid line* shows the relationship for all 35 patients. *Broken line* shows the relationship for the 13 patients *(triangles)* who sustained infarction within 12 months after exercise testing. *Asterisk: P <* .05; *double asterisk: P < .01.* (Courtesy of Berglund B, Mogensen L: *Int J Cardiol* 19:120–122, April 1988.)

infarction has any implications for the size of a myocardial infarction. Exercise capacity measured before infarction was related to enzyme activity during subsequent infarction in consecutive patients.

Of 512 men who sustained an acute infarction, 35 (mean age, 59 years) had previously performed an exercise test. Exercise testing had been performed using electrically braked cycle ergometers. The tests were interrupted because of general fatigue in 32 men, general fatigue and insignificant chest discomfort in 2, and hypertension in 1. Patients with preceding exercise testing did not differ significantly from the total group in age or major clinical features. Patients with higher physical exercise capacity before infarction had lower serum creatinine kinase activity, suggesting smaller infarcts (Fig 12–2).

Thus exercise capacity determined before infarction was related to enzyme activity during subsequent infarction. Exercise capacity was inversely related to enzymic activity during the infarction.

▶ Although there are many practical difficulties in examining the value of regular physical activity in reducing the mortality from ischemic heart disease, the best of the more recent epidemiologic studies suggest such an effect. In general, it appears that the number of fatal, rather than nonfatal, infarctions is reduced by regular exercise. The present paper shows a lesser increase in enzyme readings (and thus presumably a smaller infarct) in those with a higher level of aerobic fitness before the clinical incident. The authors looked at and excluded the possible confounding effects of age and body mass, but nevertheless caution that the sample (35 of 512 nonfatal infarcts) is hardly representative. There is the further difficulty that the favorable test score before infarction might reflect an inherited advantage rather than a response to regular physical activity. However, the findings are sufficient to encourage more research of this type, particularly as an increased proportion of the supposedly healthy population undergoes exercise testing.—R.J. Shephard, M.D. Ph.D.

Survival With Painless Strongly Positive Exercise Electrocardiogram
Dagenais GR, Rouleau JR, Hochart P, Magrina J, Cantin B, Dumesnil JG (Laval Univ, Quebec)
Am J Cardiol 62:892–895, November 1988   12–13

Approximately one third of positive electrocardiograms (ECGs) in patients with coronary artery disease (CAD) occur without documentation of chest pain. Reports have indicated that the survival of patients with painless positive ECGs during exercise-testing is better than, or as good as, survival in patients with exercise-induced angina. A study was conducted to verify whether the 6-year survival of patients with painless strongly positive ECGs varied according to exercise duration.

The series included 179 patients who terminated exercise because of angina and 119 patients who stopped exercise testing because of dyspnea or fatigue. All patients had horizontal or downsloping ST depression of at least 2 mm during treadmill exercise testing.

Eighteen deaths occurred in 119 patients without angina. Of these, 16 were caused by CAD and 8 occurred suddenly. Thirty-six of 179 patients with exercise-induced angina died; 33 deaths were caused by CAD and 13 were sudden deaths. The mean overall 6-year survival rate was 85% of patients without angina and 80% of those with angina. Patients without angina had a significantly longer duration of exercise and a higher maximal heart rate and systolic blood pressure during exercise. Survival decreased with decreasing duration of exercise in both groups. In patients achieving stage IV the survival rate was of 100% in the angina group and 97% in the group who had no pain. In those who accomplished only stage I, the mean survival rate was 44% in the angina group and 60% in the group without angina.

Patients with exercise-induced painless strongly positive ECGs die of causes similar to those causing death in patients with induced angina. The survival rate in both groups varies according to the duration of exercise.

▶ Silent myocardial ischemia is a difficult condition to diagnose, monitor, and treat. Yet this study suggests that in those with strongly positive exercise ECGs (more than 2 mm ST depression), exercise performance is a good indicator of prognosis. All things being equal, the implication is that performance time, myocardial function, and prognosis are linked, and if performance is excellent, so is prognosis. By contrast, a strongly positive exercise test in a patient with a poor performance augurs poorly, irrespective of the presence or absence of angina. Such patients require aggressive treatment.—J.R. Sutton, M.D.

Low-Fat Diet and Regular, Supervised Physical Exercise in Patients With Symptomatic Coronary Artery Disease: Reduction of Stress-Induced Myocardial Ischemia
Schuler G, Schlierf G, Wirth A, Mautner H-P, Scheurlen H, Thumm M, Roth H, Schwarz F, Kohlmeier M, Mehmel HC, Kübler W (Univ of Heidelberg, West Germany)
Circulation 77:172–181, January 1988   12–14

Reduction in consumption of dietary fat, weight reduction in overweight patients, and regular physical exercise are part of nearly all rehabilitation programs for patients who are recovering from myocardial infarction or have symptomatic coronary artery disease. Studies in laboratory animals have shown that such a regimen enhances capillary density in muscle fibers recruited during training and increases maximal arteriovenous oxygen; it also halts the progression of coronary atherosclerosis because of normalization of serum levels of lipoprotein.

To assess the effects of physical exercise and normalization of the serum level of lipoprotein on stress-induced myocardial ischemia in a clinical setting, 36 men with (mean age, 51 years) who had angiographically documented coronary artery disease and mild hypercholesterolemia were

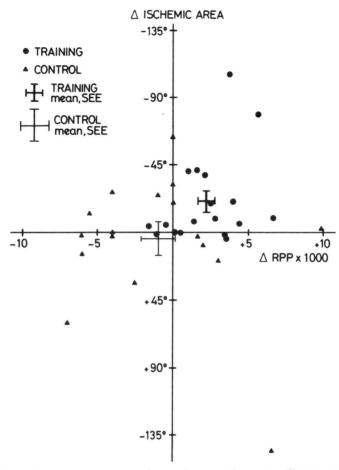

Fig 12–3.—Change in rate-pressure product vs. change in ischemic area. Change in rate-pressure product in observation period is plotted against change in ischemic area. *Closed circles* denote patients taking part in intervention; *closed triangles* denote control patients. In the intervention group the ischemic area decreased significantly despite improvement in the rate-pressure product. In the control group the ischemic area tended to increase, whereas the rate-pressure product remained essentially unchanged. (Courtesy of Schuler G, Schlierf G, Wirth A, et al: *Circulation* 77:172–181, January 1988.)

studied. Half of the patients received a low-fat, low-cholesterol diet plus regular, supervised physical exercise at high intensity for 12 months. The other 18 received only the usual medical care from their private physicians.

At the end of the 12-month study, the serum levels of lipoproteins in the 18 patients in the intervention group had been lowered to ideal and their physical work capacity was improved by 21%. The maximum achievable rate-pressure product increased significantly (Fig 12–3). No significant effect on high-density lipoproteins was noted, probably because of the low-fat, high-carbohydrate diet. Stress-induced myocardial ischemia in these patients was decreased by 54% despite higher myocardial oxygen consumption. In the 18 control patients no significant changes were seen in the serum levels of lipoproteins, physical work capacity, maximal rate-pressure product, or stress-induced myocardial ischemia.

Regular physical exercise at high intensity, lower body weight, and normalization of serum levels of lipoproteins may alleviate compromised myocardial perfusion during stress.

▶ It has been increasingly recognized that exercise training can increase myocardial perfusion in patients with coronary vascular narrowing, not by reversing the atherosclerotic lesions or by enhancing the development of a collateral vascular supply, but, rather, by extending the diastolic phase of the cardiac cycle, when most of the myocardial perfusion occurs. Previous evidence of this phenomenon was a lessening of ST segmental depression, not only at the same external power output but also at the same rate-pressure product (if this was reached by means of a higher blood pressure and a lower heart rate). The present report, based on scintigraphy, adds another dimension to such evidence, and lengthening of the diastolic phase seems a more likely explanation of the 53% reduction of myocardial ischemia than the low-fat diet and collateral development suggested by Schuler et al.

No increase of high-density lipoprotein (HDL)-cholesterol was seen over the course of the study. The authors attribute this to the low-fat diet, but a further factor may be an insufficient dose of exercise. Patients were loaned cycle ergometers and expected to carry out 30 minutes of exercise per day. However, the only check on compliance was the ultimate increase in physical work capacity, which was attributable as much to an increase in maximum heart rate (i.e., a symptom-limited gain) as to a true increment of endurance. The threshold for an increase of HDL-cholesterol is the equivalent of 18–20 km of jogging per week, and although more moderate bouts of exercise may improve physical work capacity, they do not seem to increase HDL-cholesterol, irrespective of the fat content of the diet.—R.J. Shephard, M.D. Ph.D.

Exercise Training After Anterior Q Wave Myocardial Infarction: Importance of Regional Left Ventricular Function and Topography
Jugdutt BI, Michorowski BL, Kappagoda CT (Univ of Alberta, Edmonton)
J Am Coll Cardiol 12:362–372, August 1988   12–15

Exercise training may shorten the duration of convalescence after acute myocardial infarction; however, survivors of anterior Q wave infarction are at increased risk of complications. Even mild exercise might be harmful to patients with incompletely healed Q wave infarcts. To determine whether the extent of left ventricular dysfunction and the degree of shape distortion can predict outcome, the effects of a standard low-level exercise program on left ventricular function were studied in survivors of moderate-sized Q-wave infarcts.

Left ventricular dysfunction and the degree of shape distortion were measured by 2-dimensional echocardiography before and after 12 weeks of a low-level exercise program starting 15 weeks after infarction in 13 patients (7 in group 1 and 6 in group 2), and 12 weeks apart in 24 controls without training. At the end of training, the functional class score had increased in group 2 from 2.25 to 2.67 but had not changed in group 1. Further discrimination of groups 1 and 2 was provided by an initial asynergy (akinesia, dyskinesia, or both) more or less than 18%. Compared with group 1, group 2 had greater initial asynergy, expansion index, and peak shape distortion index, but lower ejection fraction and thinning ratio.

These variables did not change after training in group 1. However, in group 2, training caused a significant increase in asynergy, expansion index, and peak shape distortion associated with a decrease in thinning ratio and ejection fraction. Initial values for tested variables were similar in control groups but did not change over the 12 weeks.

Patients with 18% or greater left ventricular asynergy on initial echocardiography had more shape distortion, expansion, and thinning before exercise training and functional and topographic deterioration was demonstrated with training. Two-dimensional echocardiography could be useful in differentiating those patients who might respond adversely to exercise training after acute myocardial infarction.

▶ This study is particularly important to those who conduct rehabilitation programs for postcoronary patients. The application of 2-dimensional echocardiography to assess left ventricular function and derive indices of "asynergy" is the integral aspect of this study and showed a relationship to outcome after a training program. Those with poor scores of "asynergy" deteriorated in terms of both New York Heart Association score and left ventricular function following the training program, although no relationship with trainability was found.

Caution must be exercised in interpreting and applying the results of this study. The numbers were small, and although impairment in left ventricular function was apparently demonstrated, left ventricular function was presumably not limiting, as all participants were able to increase their work performance. In addition, by design, this was not a long-term outcome study, and a longer-term follow-up would be required to assess the real clinical importance of the findings. Nevertheless, the findings do suggest that we need to direct our universal enthusiasm for cardiac rehabilitation programs in such a way that they are tailored to the individual patient.—J.R. Sutton, M.D.

Calcium Antagonists and Skeletal-Muscle Function in Man
Lehnhard RA, Lehnhard HJ, Kirby TE, Muir WW (Ohio State Univ)
J Cardiopulmonary Rehabil 8:45–49, Feb 20, 1988   12–16

Calcium antagonists affect cardiac muscle and vascular smooth muscle by inhibiting the normal influx of calcium through the muscle-cell membrane during depolarization, thereby prolonging late-phase repolarization of the action potential in cardiac muscle and causing vasodilation in vascular smooth muscle. To determine whether the calcium antagonists verapamil, nifedipine, and diltiazem affect skeletal muscle strength or endurance, or anaerobic or aerobic power, 8 healthy men aged 19–26 years were given 6 separate treatments of calcium antagonists plus 2 administrations of placebo in a randomized, double-blind trial.

Treatments included 2 dosage levels of verapamil, 80 mg and 120 mg 4 times daily; nifedipine, 10 mg and 20 mg 4 times daily; and diltiazem, 90 mg and 120 mg 4 times daily. During each drug treatment and while receiving placebo, the knee extension/flexion strength and endurance of the men were assessed by using an isokinetic dynamometer. Anaerobic power was determined using a cycle ergometer, and aerobic capacity was measured while the men exercised on the treadmill. No significant differences between treatments for any of the tests of skeletal muscle function were observed, but further study may be warranted. These findings support those of other investigations of the specific cardiac and smooth muscle effects of this class of drugs in man.

▶ Calcium antagonists are used with ever-increasing frequency in the treatment of a variety of cardiac conditions, including angina, myocardial ischemia, supraventricular arrhythmias, hypertension, congestive failure, and hypertrophic cardiomyopathy. However, it is often overlooked that normal calcium transport is also essential to skeletal muscle function. There is evidence from isolated skeletal muscle preparations that calcium channel blockers inhibit the inward current of calcium ions, thereby modifying excitation-contraction coupling and potentiating twitch, tetanus, and contractures (1). However, the present experiments (admittedly on healthy persons) showed no influence of clinically approved doses of verapamil, nifedipine, or diltiazem on the isokinetic performance of the knee extensors and flexors.—R.J. Shephard, M.D. Ph.D.

Reference

1. Gonzalez-Serratos H, et al: *Nature* 298:292–294, 1982.

Regional Distribution of Cardiac Output at Rest and During Exercise in Patients With Exertional Angina Pectoris Before and After Nifedipine Therapy
Thomson A, Fletcher PJ, Harris PJ, Freedman B, Kelly DT (Royal Prince Alfred Hosp, Sydney; Univ of Sydney)
J Am Coll Cardiol 11:837–842, April 1988   12–17

The magnitude and distribution of cardiac output change markedly from rest to exercise, mostly because of the increase in exercising muscle blood flow. Antianginal medications with vasodilating properties may not only increase cardiac output but may also alter its distribution. To determine whether nifedipine alters the distribution and the magnitude of the cardiac output response to exercise, the short-term effects of sublingually administered nifedipine, 20 mg, at rest and during exercise were assessed in 10 men with stable angina pectoris controlled by metoprolol.

Effects of Nifedipine on Leg Hemodynamic and Metabolic Responses to Exercise in 10 Patients*						
	Leg Flow (liters/min)	Leg $\dot{V}O_2$ (ml/min)	FVR (dynes·s·cm^{-5}·10^2)	O_2ext (%)	Lactate (mmol/liter)	Lact Prod (mmol/min)
Control						
Rest	0.34 ± 0.04	29 ± 3	294 ± 36	42.6 ± 2.4	0.52 ± 0.09	−0.01 ± 0.04
30 W	2.54 ± 0.21	282 ± 14	40 ± 3	56.6 ± 3.3	1.34 ± 0.18	0.80 ± 0.32
50 W	2.96 ± 0.24	372 ± 27	35 ± 3	61.2 ± 3.2	1.93 ± 0.38	1.13 ± 0.51
Max	4.67 ± 0.47	672 ± 80	23 ± 2	70.8 ± 3.1	6.50 ± 0.72	3.89 ± 0.90
Nifedipine						
Rest	0.57 ± 0.11 [†]	40 ± 9	164 ± 29 [‡]	35.0 ± 3.5	0.55 ± 0.10	0.04 ± 0.05
30 W	2.44 ± 0.28	285 ± 40	36 ± 3	59.2 ± 4.4	1.57 ± 0.24	1.00 ± 0.40
50 W	3.04 ± 0.37	374 ± 37	29 ± 3	63.2 ± 3.4	2.09 ± 0.36	0.65 ± 0.51
Max	4.36 ± 0.58	651 ± 76	21 ± 3	75.9 ± 2.7	7.68 ± 0.96	5.78 ± 0.99 [†]

*Data are mean ± SEM. FVR, iliofemoral vascular resistance; Lactate, iliofemoral venous lactate; Lact Prod, iliofemoral lactate production; O_2ext, iliofemoral oxygen extraction; and Max, maximal.

[†] $P < .05$ vs. corresponding level during control exercise test.

[‡] $P < .01$ vs. corresponding level during control exercise test.

(Courtesy of Thomson A, Fletcher PJ, Harris PJ, et al: J Am Coll Cardiol 11:837–842, April 1988.)

At rest, nifedipine significantly reduced iliofemoral vascular resistance from a mean of 294 to 165 dynes·s·cm^{-5}·10^2 and significantly increased iliofemoral blood flow from a mean of 0.34 L/minute to 0.57 L/minute. Systemic vascular resistance was reduced from 19 to 13 dynes·s·cm^{-5}·10^2, and cardiac output increased significantly from 4.7 L/minute to 5.8 L/minute. The mean arterial pressure decreased significantly and the heart rate rose significantly. During maximal upright cycle ergometer exercise when nifedipine was given, iliofemoral vascular resistance and leg blood flow were unaltered compared with control values, cardiac output remained significantly increased, and systemic vascular resistance remained significantly decreased (table). The proportion of cardiac output distributed to the working lower limbs was significantly lowered at all exercise levels.

Nifedipine therapy caused a redistribution of cardiac output by vasodilating nonexercising vascular beds without changing the locally mediated vasodilation in exercising muscle. In patients with coronary artery disease undergoing nifedipine treatment, an increase in exercise tolerance is caused by relief of myocardial ischemia rather than increased peripheral oxygen delivery.

▶ Because of a blocking of calcium channels in vascular smooth muscle, agents such as nifedipine reverse the normal exercise-induced vasoconstriction in nonexercising vascular beds. The end result is a tendency to increased oxygen extraction in the exercised tissues (1), with greater sensations of leg fatigue. The present study confirms the concept of increased flow to inactive tissues by direct measurement of iliofemoral flow, cardiac output, and total systemic vascular resistance. Although total vascular resistance during exercise was substantially reduced, the flow to active muscles (increased at rest) was apparently unchanged by the calcium blocker during exercise; the usual clinical dose of nifedipine seems unable to augment exercise-induced vasodilatation. Exercise tolerance was nevertheless increased; the arterial blood pressure was reduced, presumably reducing myocardial ischemia. Certainly, electrocardiography showed less ST segmental depression after administration of the calcium channel blocker, and the average maximum heart rate was boosted from 124/minute to 139/minute.—R.J. Shephard, M.D. Ph.D.

Reference

1. Choong CYP, et al: *Circulation* 71:787–796, 1985.

"Effort" Thrombosis (Paget-Schroetter's Syndrome) Secondary to Martial Arts Training
Zigun JR, Schneider SM (Univ of Pittsburgh)
Am J Sports Med 16:189–190, March–April 1988   12–18

Effort-induced thrombosis, or Paget-Schroetter's syndrome, usually involves the upper extremities and can be attributed to sports activities or manual labor. A man trained in martial arts sustained deep venous thrombosis in the lower extremity secondary to "kick punching."

Man, 20, had a 2-week history of pain and a 5-day history of swelling in the right calf and thigh. The symptoms had started with an aching pain in his right buttock. He had begun martial arts instruction 10 years previously and had taken up the specific discipline of "kick punching" 3 years earlier. He practiced daily. He denied contact trauma, and his family history was significant for deep vein thrombosis. Impedance plethysmography and Doppler studies were characteristic of deep venous thrombosis in the posterior tibial, popliteal, and femoral distribution. The patient was hospitalized, and anticoagulant therapy was started. The pain and swelling subsided, and he was discharged in improved condition.

▶ Venous thrombosis in young, active, and otherwise healthy individuals is uncommon, unsuspected, and often undiagnosed. However, the condition is well described in runners, cyclists, skiers, soccer players, and high-altitude climbers. The classic Virchow triad of stasis, vessel wall injury, and changes in blood viscosity apply equally to this group of individuals as to the general population. The reason for including this case report is not because of any especially unusual features of this presentation or mechanism of occurrence, but because of the potentially fatal or severe consequences if venous thrombosis is not diagnosed or treated. In the past 12 months I have seen 2 athletes in whom the condition was not diagnosed until death caused by a pulmonary embolism had occurred in 1 of them, and chronic pulmonary hypertension and incipient right heart failure had occurred in the other. These complications are preventable if the diagnosis is made early and treatment with anticoagulants begun.—J.R. Sutton, M.D.

Hemodynamic, Ventilatory and Metabolic Effects of Light Isometric Exercise in Patients With Chronic Heart Failure
Reddy KH, Weber KT, Janicki JS, McElroy PA (Univ of Chicago)
J Am Coll Cardiol 12:353–358, August 1988   12–19

Patients with chronic heart failure often report breathlessness with light isometric exercise, but the pathophysiology of this response is unknown. It was hypothesized that the inability to increase systemic blood flow adequately during isometric exercise would lead to lactate production followed by enhanced carbon dioxide production as a result of lactic acid buffering by bicarbonate; this in turn would increase ventilatory drive and minute ventilation.

Twenty patients with chronic heart failure and abnormal ejection fractions and 17 normal controls underwent 6 minutes of light isometric forearm exercise. Metabolic, hemodynamic, and ventilatory responses were measured.

During exercise the cardiac index increased by 58% in controls, whereas it remained the same in patients. However, the cardiac index rose 44% above baseline in patients during recovery but remained 20%

higher than the resting value in controls. Mixed venous lactate concentrations increased above resting levels in patients with heart failure, and blood lactate concentrations remained elevated at 90 seconds of recovery. Venous lactate concentrations in the nonexercising arm were unaltered.

In patients with heart failure, light isometric forearm exercise represents an anaerobic contraction accompanied by lactate production. The subsequent increase in carbon dioxide production causes a disproportionate increase in oxygen uptake and minute ventilation during recovery that may manifest as breathlessness.

▶ This is an intriguing study of important clinical hemodynamic and respiratory findings in patients with chronic heart failure. The selection of "normals" who are very different in age complicates the comparison somewhat, but the central observations stand, although the mechanisms may be more complicated than the authors imply:

1. The markedly increased lactate in the patients may be the result of several factors that the authors mentioned. But they fail to consider the possible impairment of hepatic and nonexercising muscle metabolism of lactate in the patients.

2. Regarding the mechanism of breathlessness in these patients, at least 2 additional factors need to be considered: (1) Because the patients were sick and older, they may well have weaker respiratory muscles; (2) as the patients had increases in pulmonary capillary wedge pressure, their lungs would certainly be less compliant and interstitial pulmonary edema may develop in the course of exercise.

Despite these reservations, the fundamental observations are of considerable interest.—J.R. Sutton, M.D.

Hemodynamic Effects of Alcohol at Rest and During Upright Exercise in Coronary Artery Disease
Kelbaek H, Heslet L, Skagen K, Christensen NJ, Godtfredsen J, Munck O, Bülow K (Herlev Hosp; Univ of Copenhagen; Herlev)
Am J Cardiol 61:61–64, Jan 1, 1988   12–20

Whether moderate amounts of alcohol cause clinical symptoms in patients with ischemic heart disease is a matter of controversy. To study the hemodynamic effects of alcohol, a number of parameters in 28 men with coronary artery disease (CAD) were measured.

The patients, none of whom drank alcohol daily, were divided into 2 groups. Eighteen were given 80-proof whiskey and water after a period of submaximal bicycle exercise designed to bring about a 30% to 40% increase in heart rate. The 10 controls followed the same testing and exercise schedule but drank nonalcoholic juice.

Alcohol did not cause deterioration in cardiac symptoms in any of the patients. The mean systemic arterial blood pressure at rest showed a

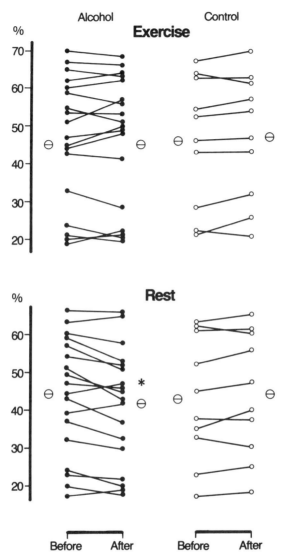

Fig 12–4.—Left ventricular ejection fraction at rest and during exercise before and after alcohol in-gestion in patients with coronary artery disease. *Circles* indicate mean values. *P < .05. (Courtesy of Kelbaek H, Heslet L, Skagen K, et al: *Am J Cardiol* 61:61–64, Jan 1, 1988.)

5.2% reduction. Pulmonary artery pressure, pulmonary artery wedge pressure, heart rate, and stroke volume index were unchanged. Alcohol caused a small but significant decrease in left ventricular (LV) ejection fraction at rest (Fig 12–4).

A moderate amount of alcohol produces no hemodynamic changes during mild exercise. In patients with CAD, there is a small reduction in

LV emptying and a slight lowering of systemic arterial blood pressure at rest. A moderate amount of alcohol should not cause clinical symptoms in patients with CAD.

▶ Patients who have sustained a myocardial infarction may ask for advice on their drinking habits. Orlando et al. (1) suggested that the angina threshold was reduced by a moderately heavy dose of alcohol, with a corresponding increase in ST segmental depression. The present experiments were not carried to the point of angina, but the subjects were moderately intoxicated, as in the experiments of Orlando and associates, by a dose of alcohol (0.9 gm/kg) equivalent to 4–5 drinks, taken simultaneously. As might be anticipated from the cutaneous vasodilatation, there was some reduction in the resting arterial blood pressure and cardiac ejection fraction, but during moderate exercise these effects were counterbalanced, presumably by reflex vasoconstriction, so that there were no hemodynamic changes relative to those in controls.

Occasional moderate doses of alcohol probably do not harm the postcoronary patient greatly, although the reduction in the ejection fraction is not an encouraging sign in a person who already has marginal ventricular function. Other factors to consider in advising the "postcoronary" patient are that the patient may be depressed, with an increased tendency to abuse alcohol, and that the possible long-term effect of heavy alcohol usage is a ventricular cardiomyopathy, compounding the infarct.—R.J. Shephard, M.D. Ph.D.

Reference

1. Orlando J, et al: *Ann Intern Med* 84:652–655, 1976.

Response to Exercise After Withdrawal From Chronic Alcoholism
Moskowitz RM, Parent MG, Marshall RC, Barnett CA, Errichetti AJ (Martinez VA Med Ctr, Martinez, Calif; Univ of California, Davis)
Chest 93:1190–1195, June 1988   12–21

Various techniques reveal cardiac abnormalities among chronic alcoholics who do not have overt heart failure. A study was conducted to document early evidence of alcoholic cardiomyopathy and to assess changes in exercise response after abstinence. Twelve asymptomatic alcoholic men (group 1) underwent maximal upright bicycle exercise radionuclide ventriculography 2–6 days after they stopped drinking; 6 of these men had similar testing 2–4 weeks later (group 1A). Six controls (group 2) repeated exercise testing without isotope study.

The left ventricular ejection fraction (LVEF) response in group 1 (12 men) was normal; the LVEF at similar workloads did not differ in group 1A. Unlike control group results, the linear regression line relating double product to exercise group 1A was higher at first exercise, probably because of the effects of alcohol withdrawal (Fig 12–5).

The radionuclide left ventriculographic findings in these patients do not support the concept of a preclinical alcoholic cardiomyopathy made appar-

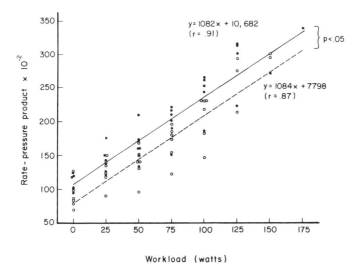

Fig 12–5.—Relationship between exercise workload and rate-pressure product in group 1A 2–6 days and 2–4 weeks after withdrawal from alcohol. *Solid line,* regression line for the first test; *dashed line,* regression line for the second test. There was a statistically significant difference between the 2 lines. *Filled circles,* first exercise test; *open circles,* second exercise test. (Courtesy of Moskowitz RM, Parent MG, Marshall RC, et al: *Chest* 93:1190–1195, June 1988.)

ent by exercise. Exercise early after alcohol withdrawal is associated with an increased myocardial oxygen demand at any given workload.

▶ Cardiomyopathy is a well-recognized complication of alcoholism; pathologic findings, in the absence of overt symptoms of heart failure, include lengthening of systolic time intervals, ventricular enlargement, and impaired myocardial contractility (particularly when presented with an increase of cardiac afterload). The present group of 12 alcoholics showed less evidence of impaired cardiac function than found in some previous series, but this is probably attributable to less advanced disease. Although they had been heavy drinkers (80 gm/day) for 5–15 years), there was only equivocal evidence of impaired hepatic function. In the first 6 days of detoxification, the rate/pressure product was increased at a given power output; the authors attributed this finding to increased secretion of catecholamines during the early phases of detoxification (1). If confirmed, this would be an indication for a cautious approach to exercise in the early days of detoxification.—R.J. Shephard, M.D. Ph.D.

Reference

1. Clark LT, Friedman HS: *Alcoholism* 9:125–130, 1985.

Exercise Test in Patients With Sarcoidosis: The Importance of Repolarization Disturbances
Thunnell M, Pjerle P, Karp K, Stjernberg N (Univ Hosp, Umeå, Sweden)
Acta Med Scand 223:69–73, 1988   12–22

Myocardial sarcoidosis, which is symptomless in most patients, has been identified as a major cause of sudden death in young persons. Electrocardiographic (ECG) abnormalities have been reported in 30% to 50% of patients with sarcoidosis, including conduction disturbances, arrhythmias, and repolarization disturbances. One study found that functional ST-T changes were normalized by β-blockade, but those of organic origin continued. In 29 patients with sarcoidosis, all of whom had repolarization disturbances in the exercise ECG, testing was done to determine if these disturbances persisted after β blockade, thus indicating an organic myocardial lesion. None of the patients had hypertension or known cardiovascular diseases. Within 1 month of the first examination, patients performed repeated exercise during β blockage with intravenously administered propranolol.

Before β blockade 13 patients had slightly abnormal ST-T changes in the ECG at rest and 5 had abnormal ST-T changes. After β blockade, 3 patients had abnormal ST-T changes as well as abnormal ST-T changes in their exercise ECG that persisted after β blockade. However, 9 patients with normal ECG at rest after β blockade had ST-T abnormalities that persisted with exercise ECG after β blockade. Thus those having normal ECG findings at rest after β blockade may have persistent ST-T abnormalities in the exercise ECG after β blockade.

Exercise ECG with β blockade is a simple way of establishing suspicion of organic myocardial lesions if ECG abnormalities in the ST-T region are present in those patients with sarcoidosis. Careful follow-up is recommended in patients with sarcoidosis who have persistent abnormal ST-T changes in the exercise ECG after β adrenergic blockade.

▶ Myocardial involvement is surprisingly frequent in sarcoidosis; for example, Silverman et al. (1) found a cardiomyopathy in 27% of autopsies. Prompt diagnosis is important, because the overall prognosis is poor, but at an early stage in the disease process corticosteroid therapy may be effective. If ST-T wave changes are seen in the exercise ECG, a repeat test after β-blockade may prove a useful diagnostic tool, although further comparison of the proposed test against subsequent autopsy evidence would be reassuring; at present, we have little beyond Furberg's suggestion (2) that β blockade reverses functional changes while leaving organic changes unaltered.—R.J. Shephard, M.D. Ph.D.

References

1. Silverman KJ, et al: *Circulation* 58:1204–1211, 1978.
2. Furberg C: *Acta Med Scand* 181:21–32, 1967.

Cardiorespiratory Responses to Exercise Training After Orthotopic Cardiac Transplantation
Kavanagh T, Yacoub MH, Mertens DJ, Kennedy J, Campbell RB, Sawyer P (Toronto Rehabilitation Ctr; Harefield Hosp, Middlesex, England)
Circulation 77:162–171, January 1988   12–23

The actuarial survival rates after cardiac transplantation are now 78% for the first 2 years after operation and more than 60% for the first 5 years. Because there have been no reports of the effect of long-term endurance-type exercise training on cardiorespiratory function in these patients, the functional status of 36 men, all orthotopic cardiac transplant recipients, was assessed at entry and at the end of a 16-month exercise training program.

The men were aged 21–57 years at enrollment in the program. The average time between transplantation and initial assessment was 7.4 months. All patients were taking cyclosporine and azathioprine. Their initial status was compared with that of 45 age-matched healthy men who were physically active but not athletic. Noninvasive evaluation consisted of assessment of body composition and cycle ergometer testing.

The average weekly training distance in the patient group was 24 km. Eight highly compliant patients progressed to 32 km or more per week, including 1 patient who finished the 42-km Boston marathon 15 months after undergoing heart transplantation. At initial assessment the patients had a lesser lean body mass and a lower percentage of body fat than controls. After training the patients had increased their body mass by 4 kg without a significant increase in body fat, implying an increase in lean mass. Patients had a higher resting heart rate and higher systolic and di-

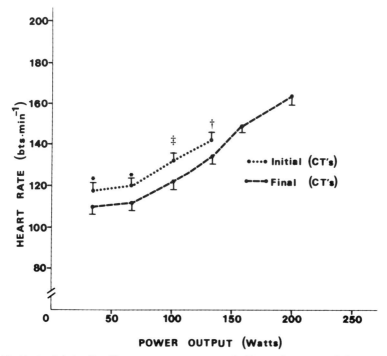

Fig 12–6.—Relationship of heart rate to power output in highly compliant patients before and after conditioning. Number = 8; mean ± SD. *$P < .05$; †$P < .01$; ‡$P < .001$. (Courtesy of Kavanagh T, Yacoub MH, Mertens DJ, et al: *Circulation* 77:162–171, January 1988.)

astolic blood pressure than controls. Peak power output, peak heart rate, peak oxygen intake, and absolute anaerobic threshold were lower, and the peak ventilatory equivalent higher, than normal. Cardiac output was slightly above normal at rest.

After training most test values approached those of healthy age-matched controls. The resting heart rate in all patients was reduced, with the greatest reduction occurring in those who were highly compliant. The peak heart rate was significantly increased in both highly compliant and moderately compliant patients, but the final resting heart rates remained higher and final peak heart rates were lower than those in controls.

The average relationship of submaximal heart rate to midrange power output showed a small reduction in the group as a whole. However, there was no change in the 28 moderately compliant patients, whereas the effect was large in the 8 highly compliant patients (Fig 12–6).

Exercise rehabilitation in cardiac transplant patients is justified because of its ability to increase working capacity.

▶ The Toronto Rehabilitation Centre team previously surprised the world when substantial groups of "postcoronary" patients completed a succession of marathon events, some in times as short as 3 hours, 17 minutes. The regular training required as a preliminary to such an event has certain medical advantages, including a progressive increase in high-density lipoprotein-cholesterol (1), very substantial increases in maximal oxygen intake (2) and correction of myocardial ischemia during exercise (3). However, the main argument in favor of such a dramatic gesture is the boost in mood given to both the participants in the event and other patients enrolled in the rehabilitation program.

The Toronto group, in collaboration with colleagues at Harefield Hospital in England, have now embarked upon a similar program of rehabilitation for patients who have successfully undergone cardiac transplantation, and 1 such patient has already progressed to the point of completing the Boston marathon distance, albeit at a conservative speed.

The process of training is inevitably somewhat different in a patient who has a denervated heart. Nevertheless, the report by Kavanagh and associates shows that substantial favorable changes can be induced by regular exercise, probably as a result of changes in the sensitivity of the heart to circulating catecholamines (an increase in the number or sensitivity of catecholamine receptors) (4–5).—R.J. Shephard, M.D. Ph.D.

References

1. Kavanagh T, et al: *Arteriosclerosis* 3:250, 1983.
2. Shephard RJ: *Ischemic Heart Disease and Exercise*. Chicago, Year Book Medical Publishers, 1982.
3. Kavanagh T, et al: *Med Sci Sports* 5:34, 1973.
4. Lurie KG, et al: *J Thorac Cardiovasc Surg* 86:195, 1983.
5. Mohanty PK, et al: *J Am Coll Cardiol* 7:419, 1986.

13 Blood Pressure

Blood Pressure Regulation During Cardiac Autonomic Blockade: Effect of Fitness
Smith ML, Hudson DL, Graitzer HM, Raven PB (Texas College of Osteopathic Medicine, Fort Worth)
J Appl Physiol 65:1789–1795, October 1988   13–1

Endurance-trained men maintain better blood pressure control that do untrained men. The roles of both the sympathetic and parasympathetic nervous systems in fitness-related differences in blood-pressure regulation were investigated. Cardiovascular responses to progressive lower-body negative pressure were studied during unblocked and fully blocked conditions in 10 endurance-trained men and 10 untrained men. Blockade conditions included β_1-adrenergic blockade with metoprolol tartrate, parasympathetic blockade with atropine sulfate, and complete blockade with metoprolol and atropine. Blood pressure, heart rate, forearm blood flow, and cardiac output were measured at rest and at -16 and -40 torr lower-body negative pressure. At each stage, forearm and peripheral vascular resistance and stroke volume were calculated from these measurements. Blood pressure was maintained equally in the trained and untrained men during complete and atropine blockade.

During unblocked and metoprolol and unblocked conditions, the decrease in systolic and mean pressure from 0 to -40 torr was greater in trained than in untrained men. Systolic and mean pressures did not differ significantly between groups during either atropine or complete blockade conditions. Baseline to -16 torr changes were similar between groups under all blockade conditions.

Reduced blood pressure control during unblocked conditions in the trained men was attributable to attenuated vasoconstrictor and chronotropic responses. Elevated baseline parasympathetic activity in highly trained persons may restrict reflex cardiac responses that, accompanied by an attenuated vasoconstrictor response lead to attenuated blood pressure control during steady-state hypotensive stress.

▶ This paper furthers our understanding of the cardiovascular characteristics of the trained state and the importance of the autonomic nervous system in regulation of blood pressure and heart rate. It is well known that the trained person has a lower resting and submaximal exercise heart rate. Such individuals have a lower intrinsic heart rate when all autonomic influences are removed by dual (para- and sympathetic) pharmacologic blockade. In addition, in both animals and man, parasympathetic activity is enhanced in the trained state.

We have recently learned that trained individuals do not maintain their blood pressure as well as the untrained do (1) in response to lower body negative pressure (LBNP).

The authors of the present paper consider, as with the chronotrophic changes in trained individuals, blood pressure regulation might also represent some change in autonomic regulation. By using a combination of parasympathetic, sympathetic, and dual pharmacologic blockade, they conclude that the observed responses to LBNP resulted primarily from enhanced parasympathetic activity in the trained state.—J.R. Sutton, M.D.

Reference

1. Raven PB, et al: *J Appl Physiol* 56:138–144, 1984.

Intra-arterial and Cuff Blood Pressure Responses During Incremental Cycle Ergometry
Robinson TE, Sue DY, Huszczuk A, Weiler-Ravell D, Hansen JE (Harbor-UCLA Med Ctr, Torrance, Calif, Univ of California, Los Angeles)
Med Sci Sports Exerc 20:142–149, April 1988   13–2

The mean blood pressure during exercise has been estimated by the traditional calculation of diastolic pressure plus one third of the pulse pressure, but this formula has not been validated during rapid incremental exercise or in older persons. Brachial intra-arterial blood pressure (systolic and diastolic) and cuff blood pressure (systolic and fourth-phase and fifth-phase diastolic) were measured simultaneously during 1-minute incremental cycle exercise in 13 middle-aged men (mean age, 55 years). Intra-arterial blood pressure also was measured in 9 younger men (mean age, 24 years).

In middle-aged men brachial intra-arterial systolic and diastolic measurements were consistently higher than cuff measurements during rest, exercise, and recovery. On average the mean intra-arterial systolic pressure exceeded the cuff systolic pressure by 10–11 mm Hg, and the mean intra-arterial diastolic pressure exceeded the fourth- and fifth-phase cuff diastolic pressures by 5 mm Hg and 13 mm Hg, respectively. During incremental exercise intra-arterial systolic and diastolic pressures and cuff systolic and fourth-phase diastolic pressures increased with increasing exercise intensity, but fifth-phase cuff diastolic pressure decreased. In both middle-aged and young men the average intra-arterial blood pressures increased in a relatively linear fashion from rest to maximal exercise.

During exercise the pulse pressure fractions that best estimated electronic mean pressure were 2/5 pulse pressure plus diastolic pressure using the intra-arterial pressures and 1/2 pulse pressure plus fourth- or fifth-phase diastolic pressure using cuff values (Fig 13–1). In contrast, during exercise the traditional calculation, using either intra-arterial phasic or first- and fourth-phase cuff pressures, was significantly lower than the electronic mean pressure.

Brachial intra-arterial blood pressure measurements are consistently higher than cuff measurements in middle-aged men. Both intra-arterial

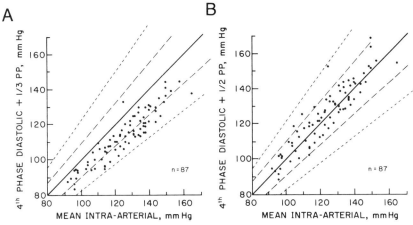

Fig 13–1.—Comparison of traditional (**A**) and suggested (**B**) cuff calculation of mean pressure with brachial intra-arterial electric mean pressure during rest and cycle incremental exercise in older men. *Solid lines*, lines of identity. *Long dashed lines* and *short dashed lines*, ±10% and 20% error, respectively. (Courtesy of Robinson TE, Sue DY, Huszczuk A, et al: *Med Sci Sports Exerc* 20:142–149, April 1988.)

and cuff fourth-phase diastolic pressure increase with increasing exercise intensity. The calculation 2/5 pulse pressure plus diastolic pressure using intra-arterial phasic pressures and 1/2 pulse pressure plus fourth- or fifth-phase diastolic pressure using cuff pressures, best approximate the peripheral mean pressure.

▶ In the average clinical exercise test, and in many simpler experimental investigations, it is necessary to rely on sphygmomanometer readings of blood pressure. Such readings are important in terms of detecting an excessive exercise-induced rise of pressure, or a failure of the blood pressure to rise (a serious indication of ventricular dysfunction, calling for early cessation of an exercise test), or an unusual peripheral resistance (as may develop in patients with congestive heart failure). Unfortunately, it is extremely difficult to measure the diastolic pressure during vigorous exercise, and many authors have been content to measure the systolic reading, assuming that the diastolic value shows little change during dynamic exercise.

The traditional formula for estimating the mean blood pressure (diastolic plus 1/3 pulse pressure) was based on resting readings. Nevertheless, if the pressures are measured by an intra-arterial catheter, this classic formula approximates to the true (electronically detected) mean throughout a progressive exercise test, the alternative estimate (diastolic plus 2/5 pulse pressure) being only marginally better. The assumption of a "constant" diastolic pressure is also not greatly violated, the increment being only 7–8 mm Hg during heavy exercise.

Comparisons with the cuff pressure depend in part on the reference level for the catheter vs. the cuff (particularly in the sitting position), in part upon the sphygmomanometer technique (surprisingly, the authors make no mention of sphygmomanometer calibration or random zero recording gauges), and in part on peripheral magnification of the pulse wave. The last factor is probably the most important, as the authors advanced their intra-arterial catheter in a peripheral direction. At their site of measurement, the cuff systematically underestimated the arterial systolic reading, and for this reason the intra-arterial figure was best approximated by (diastolic plus 1/2 pulse pressure). However, at other points in the vascular system the mean pressure might still best be specified by the traditional cuff formula.—R.J. Shephard, M.D. Ph.D.

Changes in Erythrocyte Sodium and Plasma Lipids Associated With Physical Training
Hespel P, Lijnen P, Fagard R, M'Buyamba-Kabangu J-R, Van Hoof R, Lissens W, Rosseneu M, Amery A (Univ Hosp St Raphaël-Gasthuisberg; Univ of Leuven; AZ St Jan, Brugge, Belgium)
J Hypertension 6:159–166, February 1988   13–3

Many abnormalities in the handling of sodium and potassium by the red blood cells of hypertensive patients have been reported. Accumulating evidence suggests that certain environmental factors (e.g., physical training) can alter monovalent cation transport in the human erythrocyte. The effect of physical training on the intracellular concentrations and transmembrane fluxes of sodium and potassium in the human red blood cell was investigated in 30 middle-aged volunteers before and after physical training.

In the first 4 months of the study half of the persons underwent a 3-hour-a-week training program, whereas the others served as controls.

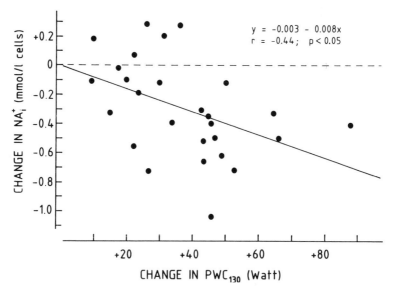

Fig 13–2.—Relationship between the training-induced change in the intraerythrocyte Na^+ concentration (Na^+_i) and the increase in physical working capacity (PWC_{130}; n = 27). (Courtesy of Hespel P, Lijnen P, Fagard R, et al: *J Hypertension* 6:159–166, February 1988.)

After 4 months the control group also underwent a training period. In both experimental groups, the intraerythrocyte Na^+ concentration was reduced; the magnitude of this reduction was related to the increase achieved in physical working capacity (Fig 13–2). After training the activity of the erythrocyte Na^+-Li^+ countertransport system was reduced in both groups, whereas Na^+,K^+ cotransport activity was increased. The training intervention had no effect on erythrocyte ouabain-sensitive ^{86}Rb uptake or the calculated rate constant for ouabain-sensitive Na^+ efflux. The plasma concentrations of high-density lipoproteins HDL_2- and HDL_3- cholesterol significantly increased in both groups during training. However, these changes were not significantly correlated with the observed training-induced alterations in erythrocyte transmembrane cationic fluxes.

Physical training reduced the intraerythrocyte Na^+ concentration. There were no significant associations between training-induced changes in plasma lipids and erythrocyte sodium balance.

▶ It is now well recognized that regular physical activity can induce a small (5–10 mm Hg) but therapeutically useful decrease in systemic blood pressure in both normal adults and hypertensive patients. Some influence of physical training on sodium transport might thus be anticipated, and it is not surprising that Hespel and associates discovered a relationship between decreases of intracellular sodium ion concentrations and increased physical work capacity. Conceivably, training-induced changes in plasma lipids could modify the composition of the red blood cell membrane and thus modify its permeability; however, in the present experiments, correlations with HDL_2-cholesterol concentrations were weak and statistically insignificant. Alternatively, the primary effect of training could be upon the concentration of hormones such as aldosterone, with a secondary impact on tissue mineral concentrations.— R.J. Shephard, M.D. Ph.D.

Exaggerated Blood Pressure Response to Exercise in the Detection of Hypertension
Jetté M, Landry F, Sidney K, Blümchen G (Univ of Ottawa, Ont; Laval Univ, Québec City; Laurentian Univ, Sudbury, Ont; Herzklinik Roderbirken, Leichingen, West Germany)
J Cardiopulmonary Rehabil 8:171–177, 1988   13–4

Traditionally, the detection of hypertension has been with measurements obtained when a person is at rest. Recent studies have suggested that an exaggerated blood pressure response to exercise could prove useful in detecting those individuals who are susceptible to hypertension in later years. Thus these individuals could be treated before hypertension occurs at rest and before any organ damage has occurred.

One study (table) showed that up to one third of individuals who are apparently normotensive at rest but in whom an excessive increase in blood pressure occurs during exercise testing are likely to have sustained

Characteristics of Retrospective Exercise Hypertension Studies

Author	Dahms et al.[9]	Davidoff et al.[12]	Dlin et al.[11]	Jackson et al.[13]	Wilson and Mayer[10]
Subjects	56 males	721 males	150 males	114 males	2746 m./f.
Age (yrs)					
Mean	—	41	24.8	—	43.7
Range	26-62	30-59	—	—	25-65
Exercise mode	Treadmill	Bicycle erg/treadmill	Bicycle erg	Treadmill	Treadmill
Exercise hypertension criteria	BP >225/90 mmHg to max WL	SBP >200 and/or DBP >90 mmHg to 70% age predicted max HR	SBP >200 and/or inc. in DBP of 10 mmHg to submax WL	SBP >230 and/or DBP >110 mmHg to 90% of age predicted max HR	SBP >225 mmHg to max WL
Follow-up	Approximately 5 yrs	Mean: 5.6 yrs (min = 6 mos)	Mean: 5.8 yrs (3-14 yrs)	2-4 yrs	Mean: 32 mos
Prevalence	38%	33%	5%	23%	10%
Sensitivity	90%	17%	100%	46%	24%
Specificity	80%	95%	5%	88%	24%
Predictive value EH	73%	62%	11%	52%	21%
Predictive value NHT	93%	70%	100%	85%	91%
Relative risk	10	2.1	—	3.5	2.3

(Courtesy of Jetté M, Landry F, Sidney K, et al: *J Cardiopulmonary Rehabil* 8:171–177, 1988.)

resting hypertension within 5 years. In another study, using data from the 1981 Canada Fitness Survey, age and gender-specific mean blood pressure responses to the Canadian Aerobic Fitness Test (CAFT), a standardized submaximal step-test of aerobic fitness, were used to develop criteria for an exaggerated blood pressure response and to calculate the prevalence of exercise hypertension in Canada. It was estimated that in as many as 176,298 Canadian adults aged 20–69 years sustained resting hypertension could have developed since being tested in 1981.

Moderate levels of exercise should be used to detect exercise hypertension rather than maximal exercise, because it is easier to measure and more comfortable for the patient, and the effects of psychological factors associated with physical stress are better observed at this level of effort. The results of these studies show the value of using an exaggerated blood pressure response to exercise as a valid indicator of the future development of sustained hypertension. However, further studies are indicated.

▶ The idea of using a submaximal exercise test to bring to light individuals who are susceptible to hypertension appears to be sound; other authors are using a cold-pressor test with the same idea. On the other hand, the question of instituting pharmacologic treatment to counter a possible future risk of hypertension is very controversial. At most, it would seem justifiable to recommend improvements of life-style (such as control of obesity, cessation of smoking, increase of physical activity, and a stress-relaxation), with perhaps careful annual measurements of blood pressure.— R.J. Shephard, M.D. Ph.D.

Exercise Testing in Patients With Aortic Stenosis
Atwood JE, Kawanishi S, Myers J, Froelicher VF (Long Beach VA Med Ctr, Calif)
Chest 93:1083–1087, May 1988   13–5

Effort syncope in patients with aortic stenosis (AS) has been recognized. Recent guidelines provided by the American Heart Association and American College of Cardiology list moderate to severe AS as a contraindication to exercise testing.

Man, 68, complaining of syncope, was assessed in an emergency room and was exercise tested despite history of syncope and a systolic murmur. After 4 minutes of exercise the ST segments were depressed, and at 6 minutes the patient became diaphoretic and dyspneic with frequent premature atrial contractions. The exercise test was stopped, and the patient lost consciousness as he was stepping off the treadmill. After revival he was referred to the cardiology department where cardiac catheterization disclosed a 52-mm Hg mean aortic valve gradient and a valve area of 0.8 cm. The patient's left ventricular end–diastolic pressure was 17 mm Hg. Although his coronary arteries had mild irregularities, no significant stenosis was observed. After catheterization the patient underwent aortic valvular replacement. He was asymptomatic at a follow-up examination. In this instance, inadequate attention was given to warning signs. Possible contributions to a po-

Summary of Nine Studies of Exercise Testing in Aortic Stenosis

	Halloran	Chandramouli	Aronow	Whitmer	James	Barton	Niemala	Kveselis	Linderholm	Nylander
N	31	44	19	23	65	11	14	12	20	91
Mean age	(8-17)	(5-19)	(35-56)	11	12	12 (6-20)	46±5	13±3	58±14	65 (52-78)
Mode	Bike	Treadmill	Treadmill	Bike	Bike	Treadmill	Bike	Bike	Bike	Bike
Mean value area (cm²)	1.22±.74	*	*	*	*	*	1.0±.6	.60±.16	*	(.48-1.63)
Mean valve gradient (mm Hg)	16<50 15>50	(10-112)	(53-80)	86 (30-225)	(<30 to <70)	38 (14-80)	*	59±18	57±23	(18-64)
Maximal heart rate (beats/min)	(160-200)	*	*	*	(183-194)	182	150±17	180±17	*	*
Exercise capacity	*	*	*	1702 kg/m†	(3,596-5,893 Kg/m)†	*	520 kg/min	800 kg/min	500 kg/min	*
Angina	0%	0%	0%	(0-29%)	6%	9%	0%	0%	35%	29%
>1.0 mm ST depression	48%	27%	37%	(71-100%)	(38-89%)	54%	*	100%	X = 1.33 ± .8	
Abnormal Blood pressure response	*	*	*	*	(0-32%)	63%	*	*	58%	

Parentheses denote range, dependent on subgrouping.
*Not available.
†Total work.
(Courtesy of Atwood JE, Kawanishi S, Myers J, et al: *Chest* 93:1083–1087, May 1988.)

tentially disastrous outcome included an initial heavy workload of the Bruce protocol, infrequent blood pressure monitoring, continuation of the test despite a blunted blood pressure response, and physician inexperience. A review of the literature (table) revealed the rarity of complications associated with exercise testing when it is done with appropriate caution and monitoring.

▶ This case report indicates the importance of taking seriously both a history of effort-induced syncope and the monitoring of blood pressure. In the case reported, the decline of pressure (142/90 mm Hg at rest, 140/88 at 1 minute of exercise, 132/84 mm Hg at 3 minutes) was not dramatic, although it was at clear variance with the anticipated rise of pressure. Swedish authors have perhaps the greatest experience in testing older adults with aortic stenosis. Linderholm et al. (1) carried out exercise tests on more than 500 such individuals (average age, 58 years) without complications. Nylander et al. (2) described details of the hemodynamics in such individuals; 29 of 76 patients had a drop in systolic pressure of 10 mm Hg or more, and a further 33 patients had less than the anticipated 10-mm Hg increment per 30 W increase of power output on the cycle ergometer. Recent literature suggests that if a careful watch is kept upon not only blood pressure but also cardiac rhythm, exercise testing can be carried out safely in both children and older adults with aortic stenosis. However, it is not a procedure to be commended to the inexperienced.— R.J. Shephard, M.D. Ph.D.

References

1. Linderholm M, et al: *Acta Med Scand* 218:181–188, 1985.
2. Nylander E, et al: *Br Heart J* 55:480–487, 1986.

14 Immune Function

Infections in Sport
Sharp JCM, Girdwood RWA, Watt B, Walker E, Fegan KE, Cossar JH (Ruchill Hosp, Glasgow; Stobhill Gen Hosp, Glasgow; City Hosp, Edinburgh; West Kilbride, Ayrshire)
Br J Sports Med 22:117–121, September 1988   14–1

The widening scope of athletic competitions has increased the likelihood that almost every kind of human infection may be acquired through participation in sports. Herpes, viral hepatitis, and acquired immunodeficiency syndrome (AIDS) are of particular concern. Other viral infections recently identified include the Coxsackie group of enteroviruses, which are known to be associated with myalgic encephalomyelitis.

Infections acquired by person-to-person contact included impetigo, erysipelas, herpes simplex, and tinea barbae. To prevent the spread of these infections, the athlete should maintain a responsible attitude, and medical and paramedical personnel should be on the alert for these diseases. Staphylococcal skin infections can be treated with topical antiseptics such as chlorhexidine and povidone iodine. Newly acquired cuts should be treated with topically applied antiseptics. Erysipelas should be treated with systematically administered antibiotics.

Infections may also be spread through contact with towels, clothing, and shower facilities. *Pseudomonas* folliculitis is associated with whirlpool baths. Infection occurs when the skin is macerated, often from excessive immersion, and the water is contaminated with *Pseudomonas aeruginosa*. Adequate chlorination of the water is essential for prevention. *Legionella micdadei* has also been identified in the water at sports complexes.

The transmission of AIDS through normal sporting activities is unlikely. Overall good hygiene should be maintained, especially when managing wounds. Sexual exposure should be avoided.

Various viruses, but particularly the Coxsackie virus, appear to be implicated in postviral fatigue syndrome. Because the illness seems to affect high achievers, a link between stress and susceptibility has been suggested. Treatment includes rest and the avoidance of caffeine, alcohol, and aspirin. Anxiolytics, antidepressants, and analgesics may be beneficial, but these should be prescribed cautiously because the illness has a long course and these drugs can be habit forming. Prevention includes avoiding exercise during active viral illness.

▶ This article's strength is its scope; it covers a wide range of infections that potentially can occur in athletes. Its weakness is its uncritical acceptance of the "postviral fatigue syndrome," otherwise known as the chronic fatigue syndrome. In 1985 the chronic fatigue syndrome sprang forth Athena-like with a pseudoepidemic in a Nevada resort community. Initially, but erroneously, linked to the Epstein-Barr virus, the cause of this age-old blend of largely subjective features continues to elude researchers but increasingly seems likely to be depression, anxiety, or another mind-body connection (1).

Do athletes contract more infections, or fewer? (see the 1988 YEAR BOOK OF SPORTS MEDICINE, pp 152–153). It may depend on the amount of habitual exercise they engage in. Prudent exercisers seem convinced that they get fewer infections, but epidemiologic surveys have suggested more frequent upper respiratory infections in hard-training Danish orienteers and marathoners in South Africa and Los Angeles. The investigators who studied the Los Angeles marathoners have shown that exhaustive endurance exercise perturbs immune function in diverse ways (2). Many other groups are now reporting similar research, but the various exercise-induced changes in immune function are modest, short-lived, and contradictory, so their biological importance is yet uncertain.

The guidelines for prevention of AIDS in athletes have recently been reviewed (3).— E.R. Eichner, M.D.

References

1. Eichner ER: *Phys Sportsmed* 17:142–160, 1989.
2. Nieman DC, et al: *Med Sci Sports Exerc* 21:651, 1989, abstract.
3. Calabrese LH, Kelley D: *Phys Sportsmed* 17:127–132, 1989.

Endogenous Opioids and the Exercise-Induced Augmentation of Natural Killer Cell Activity
Fiatarone MA, Morley JE, Bloom ET, Benton D, Makinodan T, Solomon GF (VA Med Ctr; Sepulveda, Calif; Univ of California, Los Angeles; VA Med Ctr, West Los Angeles)
J Lab Clin Med 112:544–552, 1988   14–2

Eight healthy young women aged 21–39 participated in a test of the hypothesis that the release of endogenous opioids during the stress of acute exercise may mediate natural killer (NK) cell augmentation. If β-endorphin or other endogenous opioids are involved in the stimulation of NK activity after exercise, then β-endorphin stimulation would be reduced after exercise, naloxone would decrease the rise in NK activity after exercise, and naloxone would attenuate the reduced β-endorphin stimulation that occurs after exercise. The 8 women were submitted to a maximal cycle ergometer test after in vivo administration of a saline placebo or naloxone hydrochloride (100 μk/kg), an opioid antagonist, in a randomized, crossover design, blind protocol.

A dramatic increase in NK activity, as well as an increase in the percentage of lymphocytes bearing the NK cell surface markers Leu 11a and Leu 19, accompanied exercise after the placebo injection. Before exercise significant in vitro stimulation of NK activity was observed with β-endorphin. However, after exercise, β-endorphin had a nonsignificant inhibitory effect. In the presence of naloxone in vivo, the rise in NK activity after exercise was not significant. After exercise, naloxone did not prevent the rise in Leu 11+ or Leu 19+ cells. Exercise no longer completely blocked the in vitro β-endorphin stimulation of NK cells when naloxone was given beforehand.

That the endogenous opioid system plays a significant role in the immunomodulating effects of exercise is suggested by an inability to stimulate NK cells by β-endorphin after exercise, as well as the ability of naloxone to lessen both the rise in NK activity and the diminished opioid responsiveness of NK cells after exercise.

▶ There has been a rapid explosion of knowledge concerning interactions between exercise and immune function in the past 5 years. Natural killer cells are one important aspect of immune function, being a heterogeneous subpopulation of lymphocytes having the capacity to mediate the destruction of abnormal cell variants (malignant and virus-infected cells) in vivo. As such, they form an important line of defense against both infection and malignant disease. Psychological stress tends to reduce NK cell function, but the acute response to exercise is generally an increase of NR cell activity (1). Many substances that could influence killer-cell activity are released during exercise, including catecholamines, cortisol, interleukin-1, and interferon. However, the present data point to an important role for the β-endorphins.

It seems important to encourage further research on the reactions of the immune system to chronic exercise. If this also boosts killer-cell activity, it might provide a useful measure to inhibit tumor growth, and there is already encouraging animal work supporting such a hypothesis (2).—R.J. Shephard, M.D. Ph.D.

References

1. Brahmi Z, et al: *J Clin Immunol* 5:321–328, 1985.
2. Deuster PA, et al: *Med Sci Sports Exerc* 17:385–392, 1985.

Effect of Acute Physical Exercise on Lymphocyte Subpopulations in Trained and Untrained Subjects
Oshida Y, Yamanouchi K, Hayamizu S, Sato Y (Nagoya Univ; Aichi Med Univ, Nagakute; Aichi Prefectural Univ, Nagoya, Japan)
Int J Sports Med 9:137–140, April 1988   14–3

Acute physical exercise and stress influence the immune function. Physical training is generally thought to be beneficial in preventing and treating disease, although this has not been proved. A study was conducted to investigate the difference in cellular immunity between untrained persons and well-trained athletes after acute physical exercise by using a monoclonal antibody specific for lymphocyte surface antigens and by measuring lymphocyte transformation induced by phytohemagglutinin (PHA).

Five untrained men and 6 male athletes were studied before, immediately after, and 24 and 72 hours after acute physical exercise at 60% of

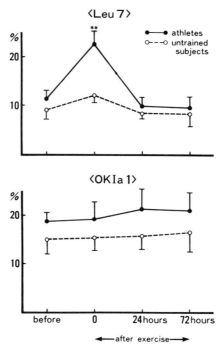

Fig 14–1.—Changes in the percentages of Leu 7 and OKIa1 positive cells in untrained persons and athletes before and after exercise. *Double asterisk, P < .01*; significantly different from preexercise level in the same group. (Courtesy of Oshida Y, Yamanouchi K, Hayamizu S, et al: *Int J Sports Med* 9:137–140, April 1988.)

maximal oxygen uptake for 2 hours. Exercise resulted in a significant rise in the number of white blood cells, lymphocytes, and neutrophils in both groups. Immediately after exercise the percentage of cells positive for OKT 3 or OKT 4 decreased significantly in both groups, whereas that of cells positive for OKT 8 markedly increased in the athletes only. Neither group had any change in the percentage of OK1a1-positive cells. In both groups the response of lymphocytes to PHA immediately after exercise was significantly decreased compared with before and 24 and 72 hours after exercise. The level of Leu 7-positive cells rose significantly immediately after exercise in the athletes but not in the untrained men (Fig 14–1).

These findings suggest that an increase in Leu 7-positive cells provide an added host defense capacity in trained athletes during periods of stress that impair T-lymphocyte function. Further research is warranted to explain the reduction in OKT-3- and OKT-8-positive cells and the increase in lymphocyte transformation induced by PHA in untrained persons 72 hours after exercise.

▶ Several pieces of evidence suggest that the immediate effect of a prolonged and stressful bout of exercise on the immune system is negative. There is less proliferation of lymphocytes in response to mitogens (1), there are changes in natural killer activity (2), and rejection of implanted tumors is delayed (3). However, the impact of repeated bouts of heavy exercise is more complex. If the athlete is in an optimal state of training, it appears that there may be enhanced resistance to the immunosuppressive effects of acute exercise and possibly beneficial effects on the response to other forms of stress. In contrast, if the athlete has persisted with an exercise program to the point of overtraining, the immune responses may be poorer than in a novitiate. Further research is hampered by the complexities of the immune cells, which are only just becoming appreciated, and other complications such as exercise-induced changes in plasma volume, sequestration of cells, and variations in total lymphocyte count. There may be increases in the total lymphocyte count but, at the same time, a decrease in the fraction of killer cells, as in the present experiments.

An intriguing possibility, raised in the discussion of the present paper, is that the lymphocytes carry receptors for β-endorphins, which are known to be released in very prolonged bouts of exercise; such compounds apparently have a biphasic action, increasing the cytotoxicity of killer cells (4) but at the same time suppressing the proliferation of lymphocytes (5). There is no suggestion in the present data that quite vigorous training (2-hour sessions at 60% of maximum oxygen intake) has any negative effect on overall immune function.—R.J. Shephard, M.D. Ph.D.

References

1. Laudenslager ML, et al: *Science* 221:568–570, 1983.
2. Riley V: *Science* 212:1100–1109, 1981.
3. Shavit Y, et al: *Science* 223:188–190, 1984.
4. Mathews PM, et al: *J Immunol* 130:1658–1662, 1983.
5. Gilman SC, et al: *Proc Nat Acad Sci USA* 79:4226–4230, 1982.

Exercise-Induced Changes in Populations of Peripheral Blood Mononuclear Cells

Deuster PA, Curiale AM, Cowan ML, Finkelman FD (Uniformed Services Univ of the Health Sciences, Bethesda, Md)
Med Sci Sports Exerc 20:276–280, June 1988   14–4

Evidence suggests that stress can influence the immune response. Changes in the populations of peripheral blood lymphocytes might serve to modify an individual's susceptibility to disease and cancer. Natural killer (NK) cells and antibody-dependent killer cells may play physiologic roles in immune surveillance. A study was conducted to determine the effects of maximal exercise on changes in the expression and distribution of peripheral blood B lymphocytes, T lymphocytes, and NK cells as determined by monoclonal antibodies that react with each cell type.

The effects of maximal treadmill exercise were studied in 20 healthy men (mean age, 32 years). The percentage and absolute number of peripheral blood mononuclear cells reacting with specific monoclonal antibodies that bind to B cells, T cells, and NK cells were enumerated by a

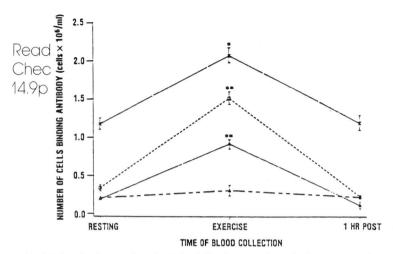

Fig 14–2.—Absolute number of peripheral blood mononuclear cells that reacted with monoclonal antibodies specific for T lymphocytes, B lymphocytes, and NK cells before, immediately after, and 1 hour after maximal treadmill exercise. Mean values ± SE are presented. *Asterisk, P* < .001; *double asterisk, P* < .0001. (Courtesy of Deuster PA, Curiale AM, Cowan ML, et al: *Med Sci Sports Exerc* 20:276–280, June 1988.

fluorescence-activated cell sorter in samples obtained before, immediately after, and 1 hour after a bout of exercise to exhaustion.

Maximal exertion effected a decrease in the percentage but no change in the absolute number of peripheral blood B cells (Fig 14–2). In addition, a small, transient increase in the number of peripheral blood cells reacting with surface markers associated with T lymphocytes and a striking, transient increase in lymphocytes having NK phenotype activity were noted.

These data indicate that maximal exertion effects no change in the number of peripheral blood B cells, a relatively small and transient increase in the number of peripheral blood T cells, and a striking transient increase in the number of peripheral blood subsets that have the NK phenotype. Whether this mobilization of cells with the NK phenotype during exercise has any physiologic function during physical stress has yet to be determined.

▶ Sports physicians who travel with national teams spend much of their time treating minor respiratory infections, but it has never been clear how the blame for such disorders should be apportioned. Is the athlete confronting a host of unfamiliar microorganisms for which no immunity has been accumulated? Are defenses lowered by the stress of travel and shifting of circadian rhythms? Is the athlete more anxious than the average member of the general public about a slight sore throat, because an entire career hinges on a superlative performance within 24 hours?

One intriguing possibility is that exercise itself influences immune function, perhaps by imposing a high level of stress on the competitor. Until recently, there has been surprisingly little research concerning the impact of vigorous activity on immune function. Now evidence is accumulating that overtraining may cause some suppression of immune function. The duration of this suppression is generally too brief to have much impact of susceptibility to infection and is certainly unlikely to influence the risk of cancer. On the other hand, it may serve as a useful measure of overtraining, as reported by T. Verde and associates at the 1989 meeting of the American College of Sports Medicine.—R.J. Shephard, M.D. Ph.D.

Operation Everest II: Alterations in the Immune System at High Altitudes
Meehan R, Duncan U, Neale L, Taylor G, Muchmore H, Scott N, Ramsey K, Smith E, Rock P, Goldblum R, Houston C (Univ of Texas, Galveston; NASA, Johnson Space Ctr, Houston; Univ of Oklahoma; US Army Research Inst of Environmental Medicine, Natick, Mass; Arctic Inst of North America, Washington, DC)
J Clin Immunol 8:397–406, September 1988   14–5

Epidemiologic evidence suggests that hypoxia caused by exposure to high altitudes may impair immune competence. Alterations in the immune system at high altitudes were investigated using a hypobaric chamber that simulated an ascent from sea level to 25,000 ft. In a 4-week period, 7 healthy men underwent this progressive hypobaric hypoxia. In vivo and in vitro variables were obtained during decompression chamber exposure.

Protein synthesis in mononuclear cells was reduced at extreme altitudes. Mononuclear cell subset analysis by flow cytometry showed an increase in monocytes without changes in T cells or B cells. Phytohemagglutinin-stimulated thymidine uptake also was reduced. At 25,000 ft, in vitro phytohemagglutinin-stimulated interferon production and natural killer cell cytotoxicity was unchanged statistically, but there were larger interindividual differences. At higher altitudes, plasma IgM and IgA levels were increased, but IgG levels were not. Pokeweed mitogen-stimulated in vitro IgG, IgA, and IgM secretions were unchanged, as were the IgA and lysozyme levels and serum antibodies to nuclear antigens.

During exposure to severe hypoxemia, T cell activation is apparently reduced, whereas B cell function and mucosal immunity are not. Exposure to hypobaric hypoxia may be a useful stimulus to activate the neuroendocrine system and to identify mechanisms responsible for immune alterations during stress.

▶ Altitude buffs will be interested in the continuing saga from the studies "Operation Everest II." Although most of the immune functions appear to remain intact, that of T cell activation was reduced at extreme simulated altitude, a finding of unknown biological importance.—J.R. Sutton, M.D.

15 Body Fluids

Sweat Iron Loss of Male and Female Runners During Exercise
Lamanca JJ, Haymes EM, Daly JA, Moffatt RJ, Waller MF (Florida State Univ, Tallahassee)
Int J Sports Med 9:52–55, February 1988   15–1

Iron depletion is fairly common among distance runners, particularly women. A possible explanation for low iron stores in runners is excessive iron loss through sweating. The iron concentration in sweat, sweat rate, and sweat iron loss in male and female distance runners during exercise was investigated.

Participants were 8 female and 9 male collegiate cross-country runners. Sweat samples were collected from the arm with polyethylene bags. Total sweat loss was calculated by weighing the athletes before and after running. The average time of sweat collection was 42 minutes for men and 39 minutes for women. The sweat rate in men was significantly greater than that in women; however, the sweat rate per km was not significantly different. Women had a significantly greater iron concentration in sweat than men had. The rate of iron loss in sweat was not significantly different between groups. The iron concentration in sweat was inversely related to the rate of sweating (table).

Although men lose more total sweat than women do, the higher iron concentration in the women's sweat leads to similar rates of iron loss. In female runners, iron loss in sweat coupled with a low dietary iron intake may result in a negative iron balance.

▶ There is considerable controversy concerning the iron content of sweat. One factor influencing results is the method of sample collection. The arm bags used by Lamanca and associates have the drawback of creating a very humid microenvironment, which can macerate the skin while at the same time cause

Sweat Iron Loss by Male and Female Runners (Mean ± SD)		
	Males (*n*=9)	Females (*n*=8)
Sweat iron concentration, (mg/l)	0.179± 0.011	0.417± 0.024
Sweat rate/BSA, (g/m^2/h)	717.5 ±145.9	460.1 ±142.9
Sweat rate/km, (g/m^2/km)	57.1 ± 11.1	49.5 ± 17.3
Sweat iron loss, (mg/h)	0.210± 0.130	0.276± 0.140
Arm sweat rate, (g/m^2/h)	66.0 ± 20.6	24.3 ± 11.0
Exercise time, (min)	41.9 ± 6.4	38.6 ± 5.0

(Courtesy of Lamanca JJ, Haymes EM, Daly JA, et al: *Int J Sports Med* 9:52–55, February 1988.)

the openings of the sweat glands to become blocked. Moreover, there is no guarantee that the concentration of the sweat found over the arm is representative of that over the trunk or elsewhere on the body. There is also the problem that the sweat sample may become contaminated by desquamated epidermal cells that have a high mineral content.

The figure found by Lamanca et al. for women (0.417 mg of iron per L of sweat) is rather similar to the whole body figure of 0.450 mg/L that we reported for male runners using a gauze pad collection method (1). There may be some contamination of these samples by cells, but the iron must be replaced whether in sweat or in cells; losses of this order, repeated on a daily basis, could contribute to anemia in an endurance athlete.—R.J. Shephard, M.D. Ph.D.

Reference

1. Shephard RJ, et al: In Ricci G, Venerando A (eds): *Nutrition, Dietetics and Sport.* Minerva Medica, 1978.

Iron, Copper, and Zinc Concentrations in Human Sweat and Plasma: The Effect of Exercise
Aruoma OI, Reilly T, MacLaren D, Halliwell B (Univ of London; Liverpool Polytechnic, England)
Clin Chim Acta 177:81–87, September 1988   15–2

There is interest in the effects of exercise and training on the human body's metabolism of essential metals such as chromium, iron, zinc, and copper. Several hypotheses have been advanced to explain sports anemia, including the possibility that it results from increased loss of iron in urine and sweat. The iron, copper, and zinc concentrations in blood plasma were analyzed in male athletes before and immediately after intensive exercise.

Twelve healthy men performed 30 or 40 minutes of hard exercise on a cycle ergometer. The ambient temperature was 21C and the relative humidity was constant. After exercise, sweat samples were collected from body sites and analyzed.

All of the men had elevated hemoglobin concentrations and decreased plasma volumes immediately after exercise. Sweat samples from different sites on the same man contained different concentrations of zinc, copper, and iron. Sweat samples obtained from the abdomen generally had greater concentrations of metals than did sweat from other sites. Losses of copper and zinc in sweat from all sites tended to be greater than losses of iron, but there was considerable individual variation. Plasma zinc, iron, or copper levels increased in some men, decreased in others, and remained virtually unchanged in still others.

Because of individual differences, no general conclusion was possible regarding the biologic significance of loss of metals in sweat in relation to whole-body metal metabolism. A mild acute-phase response may account for lowered zinc and elevated copper levels in the plasma of athletes.

▶ This research continues the focus on whether "sports anemia" results from increased loss of iron in sweat. The term "sports anemia," however, is an imprecise misnomer. It is imprecise because true anemias can develop in athletes that may be unrelated to their sport. It is a misnomer because the most common cause of "anemia" in athletes is a false anemia caused by exercise-induced expansion of baseline blood plasma that dilutes a normal or even elevated amount of hemoglobin.

This study showed only modest sweat losses of iron, copper, and zinc, and plasma changes in these metals were mild and inconsistent. Athletes sweat more than "couch potatoes" do, but the extra iron lost is not great and generally would not deplete iron stores in the face of normal dietary iron intake. For example, in one study of men in a sauna, the iron content in sweat was so low that one would have to sweat 50 L to lose 1 mg of iron (1). In contrast, as reported in the article reviewed in Abstract 15–1, when sweat from the arm was collected from collegiate cross-country runners during a training session, the iron content was about tenfold higher than in the sauna study. Even here, however, the athlete would have to sweat 5L to lose 1 mg of iron. Conceivably, however, iron loss in sweat may contribute to iron deficiency in women runners who have marginal iron stores and a low dietary iron intake. Another potential drain of iron stores in individual athletes is exercise-related gastrointestinal bleeding (see the 1988 YEAR BOOK OF SPORTS MEDICINE, pp 128–133).—E.R. Eichner, M.D.

Reference

1. Brune M, et al: *Am J Clin Nutr* 43:438–443, 1986.

Iron Deficiency in Female Athletes: Its Prevalence and Impact on Performance
Risser WL, Lee EJ, Poindexter HBW, West MS, Pivarnik JM, Risser JMH, Hickson JF (Univ of Texas, Houston; Rice Univ; Univ of Houston–Univ Park)
Med Sci Sports Exerc 20:116–121, April 1988   15–3

The prevalence of iron deficiency with and without anemia and prevalence changes during competitive seasons have been studied in endurance athletes, especially runners. The prevalence of iron deficiency in female intercollegiate athletes in a variety of sports, the effect on iron status of treating deficient athletes with iron during competitive seasons, and the impact of iron deficiency and its treatment on the athletes' and coaches' assessment of performance were determined in 100 athletes and 66 nonathletes.

Thirty-one athletes initially had iron deficiency, compared with 30 controls. Iron-deficient athletes did not have more symptoms of iron deficiency or differences in mood state when compared with normal athletes, but they considered their performance to be poorer. Total iron intakes were similar, as were menstrual blood losses. At reassessment, 15.6% of initially normal athletes were iron deficient and 63.6% of iron-deficient athletes had normal iron levels. Athletes taking an iron supplement and their coaches did not perceive greater improvement in performance or mood compared with athletes taking placebo.

Female varsity college athletes in this series had a high prevalence of iron deficiency, but the findings did not differ among athletes in different sports or between athletes and nonathletes.

▶ This study found that iron deficiency was not significantly different among female runners, other female athletes, and women who were not athletes. It appears that iron deficiency is a common problem for female college students and is not primarily an athlete's problem. We can conclude that mild iron deficiency has little effect on the performance of elite athletes. However, this study did show that most female athletes increased their iron stores when given one 325-mg ferrous sulfate capsule (65 mg of iron) daily for a 3-month period.—Col. J.L. Anderson, PE.D.

Iron Deficiency in Adolescent Female Dancers
Mahlamäki E, Mahlamäki S (Univ of Kuopio, Finland)
Br J Sports Med 22:55–56, June 1988   15–4

Iron deficiency affects 10% to 20% of women of fertile age in western countries. Physically active children during growth are also prone to iron deficiency. A comparative study was made of the occurrence of iron deficiency in 25 adolescent female dancers and 23 age-matched controls. Concentrations of fasting blood hemoglobin, serum iron, serum transferrin, and serum ferritin were determined. Iron supplementation was begun if body iron stores were low. Blood samples were obtained again after 10 weeks.

Low hemoglobin concentrations were more prevalent among the dancers than among controls (Fig 15–1). Decreased iron stores and completely absent iron stores were equally common in both groups. Iron supplementation decreased the number of anemic girls from 16 to 4. The highly significant difference in hemoglobin levels between the treated and untreated groups disappeared. However, 10 weeks of iron therapy were not sufficient to increase iron stores.

That low hemoglobin concentrations were more prevalent among adolescent female dancers than among age-matched controls may be explained partly by the fact that endurance training increases plasma volume and thus causes dilution anemia. A closer look at the diets of adolescent female dancers is warranted.

▶ Some investigators have made an entire career out of the diagnosis of anemia in various types of athletes. There are many possible reasons why hemoglobin levels might be low in athletes, including a low iron intake as a result of diet fads or an excessive proportion of fat in the diet, iron losses in sweat, a decreased rate of red blood cell formation, an increased rate of red blood cell breakdown because of mechanical trauma, and hemorrhage from such sites as

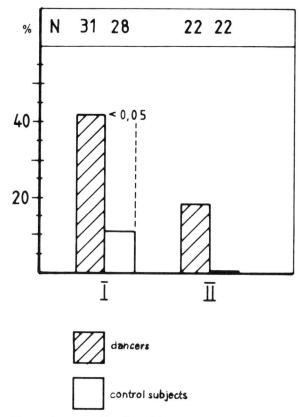

Fig 15–1.—The prevalence (%) of low hemoglobin concentrations (<125 gm/L) in adolescent female dancers and their controls before (I) and after (II) iron supplementation for 10 weeks. (Courtesy of Mahlamäki E, Mahlamäki S: *Br J Sports Med* 22:55–56, June 1988.)

the bladder. However, the most common explanation is undoubtedly pseudoanemia, associated with expansion of plasma volume. In this situation the body's total hemoglobin content is normal, although the hemoglobin is dispersed in a larger total plasma volume (1).

If the athlete's condition is indeed a pseudoanemia, one would anticipate finding normal iron saturation and no evidence of immature red blood cells or increase of iron-carrying protein transferrin in the circulation. Female ballet dancers are likely to consume an inadequate diet, because of current stereotypes of the ideal body build for a ballerina; given also a demanding daily physical schedule, they are particularly prone to true anemia. Mahlamäki and Mahlamäki found that 15% of the dancers, but none of the controls, had telltale evidence of a low serum iron level and increased transferrin concentration in association with low hemoglobin levels. Even more conclusively, iron supplementation increased the hemoglobin concentrations to an acceptable figure in 75% of those who were initially abnormal. Plainly, it is desirable to encourage dancers to eat more; if they refuse to do this, a careful watch should be kept for signs of anorexia nervosa, with iron and protein supplementation of their diet in the interim.—R.J. Shephard, M.D. Ph.D.

Reference

1. Hallberg L, Magnusson B: *Acta Med Scand* 216:145–148, 1984.

Foot Impact Force and Intravascular Hemolysis During Distance Running
Miller BJ, Pate RR, Burgess W (Univ of South Carolina, Columbia)
Int J Sports Med 9:56–60, February 1988   15–5

Iron depletion, a suboptimal hemoglobin (Hb) concentration, and anemia have been found in endurance athletes. Distance runners may be particularly prone to these conditions. Several researchers have suggested that intravascular hemolysis may be an important factor contributing to the depressed iron status in runners. The causes of hemolysis occurring with prolonged bouts of running are not known. The relationship between foot impact force and the magnitude of changes in markers of intravascular hemolysis during distance running was investigated.

Fourteen male distance runners completed 2 treadmill runs and a resting procedure. The treadmill tests involved running at 215 m per minute^{-1} for 10,000 footstrikes at elevations of $+5\%$ or -6%. The mean foot impact force was 11% greater on downhill running. The hemoglobin, plasma free hemoglobin, and haptoglobin concentrations and hematocrit were assayed in blood samples drawn 15 minutes and immediately before exercise and immediately, 1 hour, and 2 hours after exercise.

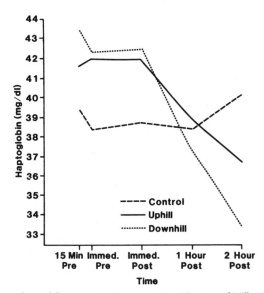

Fig 15–2.—Serum haptoglobin concentrations across time. (Courtesy of Miller BJ, Pate RR, Burgess W: *Int J Sports Med* 9:56–60, February 1988.)

Analysis of variance demonstrated that haptoglobin was significantly decreased and plasma-free hemoglobin was significantly increased after treadmill running (Fig 15−2). These changes were significantly greater with downhill running than with uphill running.

The findings support the theory that mechanical trauma to red blood cells occurring at footstrike is a major cause of hemolysis during running. The hematologic effects of chronic participation in distance running with various levels of foot impact force are unknown and warrant investigation.

▶ The idea that the mechanical trauma of running contributes to anemia in athletes has been current for a number of years. However, the concept of exploiting the difference in impact forces between uphill and downhill running is a neat way of putting the trauma hypothesis to an experimental test. Given the increase of free hemoglobin in the plasma and the decrease of serum haptoglobins, it seems fairly conclusive that trauma occurs in an experiment of 10,000 paces (equivalent to running a substantial distance, perhaps 10 miles, or 16 km). It is worth stressing that the average runner would not normally go downhill continuously for a distance of 16 km, and the running surface might also be less hard than a treadmill; the data reported thus indicate a maximum likely effect. Although measurable, the increase of free hemoglobin observed (5 mg/dl) is small relative to total hemoglobin (around 15 gm/dl), so that the contribution of hemolysis to anemia is probably quite small; using a procedure suggested by Noyes and Garby (1), the authors set the loss of red blood cells at 0.85 ml, hardly the major hemolysis that they claim.—R.J. Shephard, M.D. Ph.D.

Reference

1. Noyes W, Garby L: *Scand J Lab Clin Invest* 20:33−38, 1967.

Serum Erythropoietin in Cross-Country Skiers
Berglund B, Birgegård G, Hemmingsson P (Karolinska Hosp, Stockholm; Akademiska Hosp, Uppsala; Skogshälsan, Östersund, Sweden)
Med Sci Sports Exerc 20:208−209, April 1988   15−6

Previous studies in cross-country skiers who have undergone "blood doping" or autologous reinfusion of blood show that the serum concentration of erythropoietin (s-Epo) before reinfusion significantly higher than in healthy normal persons. Whether this is the result of earlier venesection or whether values are generally higher in elite athletes is unknown. To examine the concentrations of s-Epo and hemoglobin in cross-country skiers 41 male and 31 female elite cross-country skiers were studied during the winter season. All lived and trained at low altitude. The results were compared with those of 12 male and 13 female normal, sedentary, low-altitude residents.

As expected, the hemoglobin concentration was significantly higher in male than in female skiers. However, the s-Epo concentration did not differ significantly between male and female skiers. No significant difference in the concentrations of s-Epo and hemoglobin from baseline was detected in 18 skiers from whom a second blood sample was drawn after an average of 2.3 months of training. Similarly, the s-Epo concentration did not differ significantly between elite cross-country skiers and the sedentary controls.

The serum concentration of s-Epo in cross-country skiers who live and train at low altitudes is similar to that of normal nonathletic persons and appears to be unaltered during the winter season.

▶ Considerable disquiet was caused by the disclosure that several competitors in the Los Angeles Olympic competition had engaged in autologous "blood doping." Although early attempts to improve performance by this technique were rather unsuccessful because of deterioration of the stored blood, there is good evidence that with modern methods, "blood doping" can enhance physical performance. Advances of transfusion technology now allow a dishonest endurance competitor to withdraw a substantial sample of blood some weeks before competition, await regeneration of the body's hemoglobin stores, and then boost the baseline hemoglobin concentration by reinfusion of the stored blood.

The challenge plainly is to find an adequate method of detecting this abuse. An earlier report from Berglund and associates (1) raised the hope that venesection might give rise to a telltale increase in s-Epo levels. Unfortunately, this sign probably depends on the duration of blood storage. If the blood is kept at a temperature of 4 C, storage is kept to a ceiling of about 4 weeks because of the build-up of cellular aggregates and the progressive loss of erythrocytes. Increments of s-Epo may be detectable at this stage. However, if blood is kept in the frozen state, a longer period of storage is possible, and once the baseline hemoglobin level has been restored, it seems unlikely that there would be a detectable increase in the s-Epo concentration. Further search for a detection technique is thus urgently required.— R.J. Shephard, M.D. Ph.D.

Reference

1. Berglund B, et al: *Int J Sports Med* 8:66–70, 1987.

Mechanism of the Haematological Changes Induced by Hyperventilation
Stäubli M, Bigger K, Kammer P, Rohner F, Straub PW (Neumünster Hosp, Zollikerberg, Switzerland; Univ of Bern, Switzerland)
Eur J Appl Physiol 58:233–238, December 1988   15–7

Voluntary hyperventilation in healthy men results in increases in lymphocyte and platelet counts. After hyperventilation, lymphocyte and platelet counts were at or near initial levels; neutrophil counts nearly doubled, although they did not change during hyperventilation. These phenomena were investigated in 11 normal, 9 splenectomized, and 12 β blocked men to investigate the pathophysiology of hyperventilation-induced blood cell alterations. Hyperventilation consisted of deep, synchronized breathing at 20 breaths per minutes for 20 minutes. Blood was sampled from supine persons immediately before hyperventilation, 15 minutes into the hyperventilation period, and 75 minutes after hyperventilation.

All of the men had mean decreases in carbon dioxide pressure of 19 torr, and identical changes in pH and red blood cell counts. Neutrophil counts increased only slightly and marginally significantly during hyperventilation but nearly doubled afterward in all groups. Lymphocyte counts during hyperventilation were similar among the groups. Thrombocyte counts during hyperventilation increased in the normal and β-blocked men but not in the splenectomized men.

These data suggest that neutrophil mobilization after hyperventilation is not affected by β-blockade or splenectomy. This implies that β-adrenergic mechanisms are not involved, although because epinephrine and norepinephrine levels increase during hyperventilation, α-adrenergic mechanisms may be active. Because splenectomy had no effect on increases in lymphocyte counts during hyperventilation or on neutrophil count increases after hyperventilation, these cells must be rapidly mobilized from extralienal pools such as the lymphatics or lungs. Increases in thrombocytes during hyperventilation seem entirely related to mobilization from the spleen.

▶ In a series of thought-provoking experiments, these investigators have shown that merely lying quietly and hyperventilating for 20 minutes evokes many, if not all, of the "acute hematologic changes of strenuous exercise": hemoconcentration, thrombocytosis, lymphyocytosis, and leukocytosis.—E.R. Eichner, M.D.

Plasma Volume During Heat Stress and Exercise in Women
Stephenson LA, Kolka MA (US Army Research Inst of Environmental Medicine, Natick, Mass)
Eur J Appl Physiol 57:373–381, March 1988   15–8

There are conflicting data on the plasma volume response to heat stress and exercise in women, even when menstrual phase is controlled for. To learn how the cycle affects dynamic fluid exchange, 5 healthy women, none using oral contraceptives, were passively heated to a dry bulb temperature of 50.4 degrees in the follicular and luteal phases of the cycle. In other studies they exercised at about 80% of peak oxygen uptake in both cycle phases.

Plasma volume decreased by a mean of 156 ml during passive heating in the follicular phase of the cycle and by 300 ml in the luteal phase. During exercise, the plasma volume decreased by 463 ml in the follicular phase and by 381 ml in the luteal phase of the cycle.

The menstrual cycle influences plasma volume dynamics during passive heating; more fluid leaves the vasculature in the luteal phase. During marked exercise there is greater fluid loss in the follicular phase of the cycle, but final plasma volume values do not differ significantly in the 2 phases.

▶ The observations from this study that women hemoconcentrate less during passive heating in the follicular phase than in the luteal phase is new, and there is no complete explanation for this phenomenon.— Col. J.L. Anderson, PE.D.

Polycythemia and Hydration: Effects on Thermoregulation and Blood Volume During Exercise-Heat Stress

Sawka MN, Gonzalez RR, Young AJ, Muza SR, Pandolf KB, Latzka WA, Dennis RC, Valeri CR (US Army Research Inst of Environmental Medicine, Natick, Mass; Boston Univ)
Am J Physiol 255:R456–R463, September 1988   15–9

Acute polycythemia reportedly tends to reduce body heat storage during exercise in a hot environment in euhydrated but nonheat-acclimated humans. Several questions were raised about the effect of acute polycythemia on thermoregulation during exercise in the heat. The effects of autologous erythrocyte infusion on thermoregulation and blood volume during exercise in the heat were studied to determine whether heat-acclimated persons and hypohydrated persons would have a thermoregulatory advantage from acute polycythemia.

Five heat-acclimated men attempted 4 heat stress tests (HST), 2 before infusion and 2 after infusion. Autologous erythrocyte infusion was accomplished with 500 ml of a sodium chloride-glucose-phosphate solution of about 60% hematocrit. One HST, both before and after infusion, was performed while the men were euhydrated and 1 was performed while they were hypohydrated. The HST consisted of a 120-minute exposure in a hot environment.

Polycythemia increased the sweating rate and reduced core temperature during exercise-heat stress in both euhydrated and hypohydrated men. Erythrocyte infusion increased plasma and blood volumes. The increased plasma volume was associated with an elevated total circulating protein mass. The increased total circulating protein mass tended to maintain plasma volume better when hypohydrated. Heat acclimation appeared to increase the extravascular protein mass (Fig 15–3).

Erythrocyte infusion appears to provide a thermoregulatory advantage during exercise in the heat for acclimated persons during both euhydration and hypohydration.

▶ Polycythemia may present as an independent disease process, as a response to congenital cardiac lesions or high-altitude exposure, and as a consequence of "blood doping." The quantity of blood reinfused in the present experiment (500 ml at 60% hematocrit) is comparable with the infusions that are believed to have occurred in many instances of "blood doping." One might speculate that the increased viscosity of the blood would reduce the maximum

A

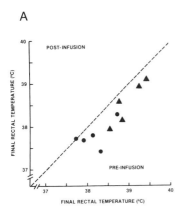

B

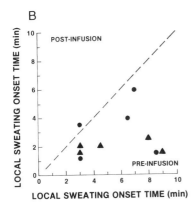

C

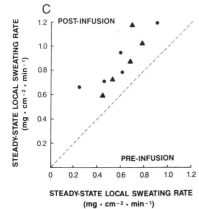

Fig 15–3.—Individual data for final exercise rectal temperature (**A**), local sweating onset time (**B**), and steady-state local sweating responses (**C**) to pre- and postinfusion heat stress tests. *Circles,* euhydration experiments; *triangles,* hypohydration experiments. (Courtesy of Sawka MN, Gonzalez RR, Young AJ, et al: *Am J Physiol* 255:R456–R463, September 1988.)

cardiac output and thus reduce the thermoregulatory ability after blood transfusion. This may be true in extreme cases of polycythemia, but at the levels evaluated by Sawka et al., the effects of plasma volume expansion (resulting in part from the added mass of plasma proteins) seem dominant. Thus, after transfusion, the subjects were able to produce sweat at a greater rate and with a shorter latency, whether initially euhydrated or hypohydrated. Certainly, the present experiments give no cause for concern about thermoregulation during exercise in patients with moderate polycythemia.—R.J. Shephard, M.D. Ph.D.

Changes in Blood Platelet Function, Coagulation, and Fibrinolytic Activity in Response to Moderate, Exhaustive, and Prolonged Exercise

Drygas WK (Med Academy, Lodz, Poland)
Int J Sports Med 9:67–72, February 1988   15–10

Reports on exercise-induced hemostatic changes have yielded conflicting results. Some authors have concluded that there are beneficial hemostatic effects from exercise in coronary heart disease (CHD) prevention because of enhanced fibrinolytic activity, whereas others call for caution. To investigate these discrepancies the effects on coagulation, blood platelet function, and fibrinolytic activity were studied in 47 healthy men aged 25–55 years who underwent moderate, exhaustive, and prolonged exercise.

Static exertion of short duration and moderate intensity did not produce significant changes in any of the indices analyzed. Prolonged exercise on a cycle ergometer in aerobic conditions resulted in strong activation of the fibrinolytic system and a slight increase in platelet count but did not cause significant changes in platelet factor 4 or platelet aggregate ratio, recalcification, and prothrombin time. Repeated bouts of maximum exercise resulting in considerable acidosis produced a significant rise in blood platelet count and an increase in platelet factor 4 release. These alterations were accompanied by strong intensification in fibrinolytic activity (table). Unfavorable hemostatic changes were noted after intensive exercise in some individuals.

The mode of exercise and its intensity and duration are important factors affecting blood platelet function and fibrinolytic activity. More attention should be directed to the problem of verifying the hemostatic changes associated with preventive and rehabilitative training programs.

▶ There is increasing evidence that exercise has a biphasic impact on blood clotting, enhancing platelet counts, and increasing thrombin activity while at the same time encouraging the lysis of clots post exercise. The precise response observed in any given experiment thus varies with the time of sampling and other conditions of the experiment. In general, intensive exercise seems required to activate clotting; possible mechanisms include endothelial damage induced by an increased sheer-stress on blood vessels, mobilization of newly formed platelets from the pulmonary circulation, an increase of plasma cate-

Changes in Blood Platelet Function, Coagulation, and Fibrinolytic Activity With Various Models of Exercise

	Isometric exercise with 50% of max. power (n=12)			Submaximal 18 min bicycle ergometer test (n=25)			Prolonged submaximal bicycle ergometer test (n=26)			Maximum stepwise bicycle ergometer test (n=7)		
	Before	After	P	Before	After	P	Before	After	P	Before	After	P
RT sec	116 ±25	123 ±33		117 ±16	121 ±16		118 ±15	119 ±17		122 ±15	112 ±16	*
PT %	95 ±10	93 ±8		96 ±7	96 ±8		93 ±9	93 ±15		96 ±5	82 ±19	
PC 10^9/l	205 ±53	211 ±28		185 ±56	194 ±50	**	193 ±57	213 ±51	**	174 ±37	195 ±35	*
PF4 Uml^{-1}	0.06 ±0.03	0.06 ±0.03		0.06 ±0.02	0.08 ±0.04	***	0.06 ±0.02	0.07 ±0.02		0.06 ±0.03	0.10 ±0.04	
CPA %	0.92 ±0.04	0.94 ±0.03		0.90 ±0.04	0.87 ±0.07		0.91 ±0.04	0.90 ±0.05		0.93 ±0.04	0.91 ±0.06	
FG mgdl^{-1}	236 ±37	230 ±54		239 ±40	224 ±47		236 ±37	224 ±46		253 ±66	233 ±73	
ELT min	217 ±33	213 ±27		205 ±49	154 ±64	***	208 ±31	88 ±46	***	202 ±54	75 ±39	*

Values are means ± SD. RT, recalcification time; PT, prothrombin time; PC, platelet count corrected for hemoconcentration; PF4, platelet factor 4; CPA, circulating platelet aggregates; FG, fibrinogen corrected for hemoconcentration; ELT, euglobulin lysis time; P, statistical level of significance; $*P < .05$; $**P < .1$; and $***P < .001$.
(Courtesy of Drygas WK: Int J Sports Med 9:67–72, February 1988.)

cholamines, increases in factor VIII, increased core temperature, lactate acidosis, and hemoconcentration. In healthy individuals, fibrinolysis is also stimulated by a release of plasminogen activator from the walls of blood vessels and increased production of prostacyclin and antithrombin III. An optimal exercise prescription considers potential adverse effects of very vigorous exercise on the blood coagulation system and adjusts the dose of exercise to avoid such effects, which could give rise to exercise fatalities.—R.J. Shephard, M.D. Ph.D.

Effects of Exercise on Plasma Atrial Natriuretic Factor and Cardiac Function in Men and Women
Donckier JE, de Coster PM, Buysschaert M, Levecque P, Cauwe FM, Brichant CM, Berbinschi AC, Ketelslegers J-M (Catholic Univ of Louvain; Univ Clinics of Mont-Godinne; Faculté de Médecine, Brussels)
Eur J Clin Invest 18:415–419, August 1988   15–11

Atrial natriuretic factor (ANF), a peptide with potent diuretic and natriuretic activity, is normally released in response to volume loading; however, it is also released in certain pathologic conditions and is reported to increase in plasma after exercise. The relationship between changes in ANF and cardiac volumes was studied in 7 men and 6 women who had normal histories and normal findings on physical examination, resting electrocardiography, chest films, and maximal exercise stress tests. All 13 were hospitalized and given a 4-day constant sodium diet of 150 mmol/day. A light breakfast containing 0.8 gm of protein, 5 gm of lipids, 20 gm of carbohydrates, and 45 mg of sodium was served 1 hour before exercise testing. Cardiac function and ventricular volumes were assessed by multigated radionuclide angiography during 3 levels of graded exercise and 2 recovery periods of 5 minutes and 30 minutes.

At the second and third levels of exercise and after 5-minute recovery, the mean ANF levels increased in all subjects (Fig 15–4). After a 30-minute recovery the subjects had normal values. Mean ANF levels were higher in women, but not significantly so. In both sexes there were significant decreases in ventricular volumes and increases in ejection fraction and rate-pressure product during exercise. Compared with the increase in rate-pressure product, the kinetics of plasma ANF concentrations were characterized by a delayed rise and persistent elevation in recovery.

The study demonstrated that ANF is released during exercise, but the relevance remains to be explained. The persistent elevation in recovery, which was also present in the changes in ventricular volume, suggests that other factors such as catecholamines may still be influential after termination of exercise.

▶ This study failed to find a relationship between cardiac volume assessed by radionuclide angiography and ANF. This is not surprising as ventricular, not

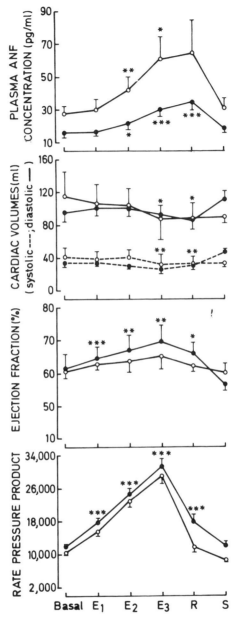

Fig 15–4.—Changes in plasma concentrations of ANF, systolic *(dashed lines)* and diastolic *(solid lines)* ventricular volumes, ejection fractions, and rate-pressure- products during 3 graded exercise levels (E1, E2, E3, corresponding to 20%, 40%, and 60% of maximal workload) after 5-minute recovery (R) and 30-minute supine rest (S). Readings are compared with basal readings for concentrations of ANF separately in women *(open circles)* and men *(solid circles)*; for other parameters sexes are considered together. Data are expressed as means ± SEM. *P < .05; **P < .01; ***P < .005. (Courtesy of Donckier JE, de Coster PM, Buysschaert M, et al: *Eur J Clin Invest* 18:415–419, August 1988.)

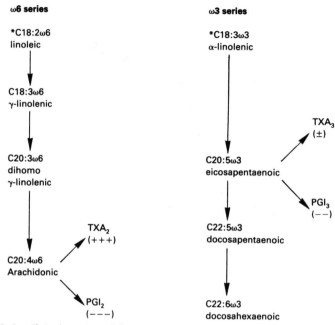

Fig 15-5.—Chain elongation and desaturation of polyunsaturated fatty acids and their relationship to prostaglandins affecting platelet function. *PGI*, prostacycline; *TX*, thromboxane; *plus sign*, promotes platelet aggregation and blood vessel vasoconstriction; *minus sign*, inhibits platelet aggregation and promotes blood vessel vasodilation; *asterisk*, the number after the C refers to the number of carbon atoms, that after the colon to the number of double bonds, and ω3 or ω6 indicates that the first double bond counting from the methyl end is in the 3-position or 6 position, respectively. (Courtesy of Haigh JR, Fruin CA, Pinn R, et al: *Br J Sports Med* 22:66–70, June 1988.)

atrial, volumes were measured, and if any relationship would make physiologic sense, it would be ANF secretion with atrial volume or pressures.—J.R. Sutton, M.D.

Lipids and Platelet Function in Runners
Haigh JR, Fruin CA, Pinn R, Lea E JA (Univ of East Anglia, Norwich; Norfolk and Norwich Hosp, Norwich, England)
Br J Sports Med 22:66–70, June 1988   15–12

Exercise has become a symbol of protection against heart disease. The role of lipids and lipoproteins in coronary heart disease is controversial (Fig 15–5). The effect of distance running on the fatty acid composition of platelet and erythrocyte membranes was studied. Platelet aggregation and levels of high-density lipoprotein cholesterol (HDL-c), low-density lipoprotein cholesterol (LDL-c), total cholesterol, and triglycerides were also investigated.

Eleven runners and 12 healthy, age-matched, nonrunners were studied. Platelet aggregation and fatty acid composition of membrane lipids in both platelets and erythrocytes were similar in both groups, with some exceptions: In platelets, docosahexaenoic acid was significantly higher in runners; in erythrocytes, the fatty acids C20:3ω6/C22:1ω9 and C22:5ω3 were significantly higher in runners. No significant differences were found between levels of HDL-c, LDL-c, and total cholesterol in runners and controls. Triglycerides were significantly lower in the runners.

These findings suggest that if altered serum lipid and lipoprotein concentrations are related to the development of cardiovascular disease, this may not result from a direct effect of lipids and lipoproteins on platelets.

▶ One interesting finding in this paper is that runners who were covering as much as 30–50 miles (50–80 km) per week did not have an increase of HDL-c relative to controls. A possible factor is that many of the previous studies of exercise and lipid profiles have been conducted in the United States, where the baseline total cholesterol is higher than in Great Britain; even in the controls, Haigh and associates noted a total cholesterol level of only 170 mg/100 ml (4.6 mM/L). The significance of the higher docosahexaenoic acid levels in the platelets of runners is unclear. The compound is a side product of the reaction that forms prostaglandin-3 (an inhibitor of platelet aggregation); however, platelet aggregation is itself unchanged relative to controls; given a Student's t ratio of 2.3, with 11 comparisons of different fatty acids in the plasma cell membrane, it may be no more than a chance finding.—R.J. Shephard, M.D. Ph.D.

16 Doping

Effect of L-Tryptophan Supplementation on Exercise Performance
Segura R, Ventura JL (Univ of Barcelona)
Int J Sports Med 9:301–305, October 1988   16–1

Strenuous exercise is associated with a degree of pain and fatigue; training increases tolerance to both. Increased plasma levels of β-endorphins play an important role in the regulation of pain perception. Because 5-hydroxytryptamine (5-HT) affects nociception through its effects on the enkephalin-endorphin system, supplementation with L-tryptophan, the immediate precursor of 5-HT, might improve endurance and the perception of effort.

Twelve healthy athletes underwent 2 trials of treadmill testing to 80% of maximum oxygen uptake until exhaustion. The athletes received either placebo or L-tryptophan the night before the test and at breakfast, lunch, and 1 hour before the test. Patients who received placebo at the first trial had L-tryptophan at the second and vice versa.

In all but 2 athletes, total exercise time to exhaustion was increased when they took L-tryptophan. The mean increase was 49.4%. Two individuals had a decrease of 15.5% in exercise time with L-tryptophan therapy. When these were excluded, exercise time for the other 10 increased by 62.6% with L-tryptophan treatment (table). Athletes taking L-tryptophan also perceived less exertion, although their workloads were increased. There were no differences in other variables between the groups. Moderate doses of L-tryptophan may increase pain tolerance and thus permit longer exercise time and greater workload.

▶ There have been various reports that administration of essential amino acids can improve physical performance, although generally the implication has been that such substances provide no more than a convenient metabolic substrate for energy production. This paper makes the interesting suggestion that L-tryptophan might increase pain tolerance by altering the brain levels of 5-hydroxytryptamine and thus the output of endorphins. The gain in treadmill running time (49%) is quite striking. Although the duration (6–8 minutes of effort) is not in the range in which endorphins normally have a major role, previous experiments have suggested that L-tryptophan can modify the pain threshold of animals (1). Moreover, although the normal diet contains some L-tryptophan, the authors of the present paper argue that the enzyme tryptophan hydroxylase is never fully saturated, and increased tryptophan levels can thus increase brain serotonin levels. The double-blind experiment seems well conducted, and although the subjects could possibly have distinguished

Running Time (s) During the Placebo and Tryptophan Trials

Subjects	1	2	3	4	5	6	7	8	9	10	11	12	Mean
Placebo	270	150	450	150	300	210	360	390	570	390	540	240	335 ± 140
L-tryptophan	300	240	510	390	1080	270	300	570	480	480	600	270	457 ± 233
Increased (decreased) percentage	11%	60%	13%	160%	260%	28%	(16%)	46%	(15%)	23%	11%	12%	49.4% ± 80.8%

(Courtesy of Segura R, Ventura JL: *Int J Sports Med* 9:301–305, October 1988.)

the nature of the lactose placebo by biting into the capsule, these observations seem to merit further investigation.— R.J. Shephard, M.D. Ph.D.

Reference

1. Telner J, et al: *Pharmacol Biochem Behav* 10:657–661, 1979.

Caffeine in Sport: Urinary Excretion of Caffeine in Healthy Volunteers After Intake of Common Caffeine-Containing Beverages
van der Merwe PJ, Müller FR, Müller FO (Univ of the Orange Free State, Bloemfontein, South Africa)
S Afr Med J 74:163–164, 1988   16–2

According to the International Olympic Committee (IOC), a caffeine concentration of 15 μg/ml or more in athletes is a disqualifying factor. Because caffeine-containing beverages such as coffee, tea, and Coca-Cola are consumed socially, a study was done to determine how much of these beverages has to be taken to approach or exceed the IOCs permissible level of caffeine. For a period of at least 3 days, 9 healthy volunteers participated in this randomized trial. Within a 15-minute period they drank various beverages containing caffeine in amounts ranging from 1.52 mg/kg to 17.53 mg/kg. The latter dose is equivalent to 8 cups of percolated coffee.

There was a significant correlation between the amount of caffeine taken and the maximum concentration measured in urine, which was 14.02 μg/ml. Despite the high dose, this is less than the IOC limit of 15 μg/ml. Apparently, the nature of the caffeine-containing beverage does not influence the absorption of caffeine.

Participants in competitive sports will not attain the IOC limit of 15 μg of caffeine per ml of urine merely by the social intake of caffeine-containing beverages. If the IOC limit is exceeded, it may be assumed that caffeine ingestion was done on purpose.

▶ Even hardened coffee addicts would flinch at the thought of drinking 8 cups of coffee in the course of 15 minutes; given that this yielded peak urinary concentrations of 5.3–14.0 μg/ml, the permitted IOC ceiling of 15.0 μg/ml seems inherently reasonable in allowing for social consumption of tea and coffee. The implication is that those who are disqualified have, on average, drunk the equivalent of 11 or more cups of coffee within 15 minutes; what this does to motor coordination is hard to imagine!— R.J. Shephard, M.D. Ph.D.

Drug Abuse In Athletes: Anabolic Steroids and Human Growth Hormone
Council on Scientific Affairs (American Medical Association, Chicago)
JAMA 259:1703–1705, March 18, 1988   16–3

The Council on Scientific Affairs examined the abuse of anabolic hormones—steroids and growth hormone (GH)—by athletes. Anabolic steroids are synthetic androgens with greater anabolic activity relative to androgenic activity than testosterone. The probable benefits of steroids in athletic performance include increased body weight, which may include an increase in lean mass, increased muscular strength when coupled with a high-protein diet, and increased aggressiveness. Because small, difficult-to-measure increments in muscular performance or psychological benefit may constitute the difference between winning and losing, these changes may be perceived as critical by the athlete, particularly during professional or world-class competitions. However, adverse effects are clear and include oligospermia and temporary infertility, gynecomastia, abnormal liver effects, development of an atherogenic blood lipid profile, and an increase in acne formation, irritability, and aggressiveness. Masculinizing effects are common in women, and accelerated pubertal changes in children.

Anabolic steroids are widely used at all levels of athletic activity, and steroid abuse is common, particularly among athletes in sports requiring great strength. They are easily obtained illegally through gymnasiums or mail-order sources, and some athletes even claim being given a prescription for the drugs.

The abuse of human GH (hGH) is a recent phenomenon of undetermined extent. Human GH is indicated in GH deficiency and other legitimate investigational uses, but it also has great potential for misuse. Human HG is favored by athletes because of anticipated body growth and increased strength potential, and because it is not detectable in drug testing procedures. Its use is limited by its great expense, however. Adverse effects have not been documented but can be predicted on the basis of the known effects of endogenous hypersecretion. Two recombinant DNA-derived hGH products are available, but bogus GH preparations, animal GH preparations, and foreign products should also be considered. The source of illicit supply is questionable.

Federal efforts to curtail the illegal distribution of these drugs should be endorsed, as should educational activities, with emphasis on the adverse effects and limited benefits on the use of these drugs.

▶ The Seoul Olympic Games, the disqualification of sprinter Ben Johnson, and the subsequent Dubbin Inquiry in Canada have focused attention on the abuse of anabolic steroids and the host of drugs used in attempts to enhance athletic performance. The extent of drug abuse appears much greater than most had appreciated, and the widespread use of steroids and hGH among high school athletes is very worrying.

This report by the American Medical Association in *JAMA* adds clout to the position previously taken by the American College of Sports Medicine and the Canadian Academy of Sports Medicine.

The issue is a simple one of ethics, and no amount of education regarding the lack of effect of these substances will work. (They *are* effective, and such statements are responsible for professional organizations losing credibility.) By the same token, overemphasis on the deleterious side effects, including hepatoma and severe liver malfunction, decreased libido, and impaired testicular function will also not deter the determined steroid abuser. The arguments can only logically be on ethical grounds.—J.R. Sutton, M.D.

Body Composition Response to Exogenous GH During Training in Highly Conditioned Adults

Crist DM, Peake GT, Egan PA, Waters DL (Univ of New Mexico)
J Appl Physiol 65:579–584, August 1988   16–4

Reportedly, physiologic growth hormone (GH) replacement therapy in sedentary older women with impaired endogenous GH secretion significantly increases the fat-free weight (FFW) and decreases the fat weight (FW) compartments. A double-blind, placebo-controlled study was carried out to assess the effects of chronic alternate-day treatment with supraphysiologic doses of biosynthetic methionyl-human GH (met-hGH) on FFW, percent body fat (%fat), FFW-FW, endogenous secretion of GH, and secretion of insulin-like growth factor I in exercising young adults aged 22–33 years whose body composition response to exercise was presumably attenuated by extensive training.

The 5 men and 3 women were all well trained in progressive resistance exercise. Each person was randomly assigned to 6 weeks of treatment with either placebo or met-hGH and then was assigned to the other treatment for the next 6 weeks. All 8 trained with progressive resistance exercise throughout and were maintained on a high-protein diet monitored by extensive compositional analyses of daily dietary intake records.

Treatment with met-hGH resulted in significant decreases in %fat and significant increases in FFW and FFW-FW (table). The magnitude of change in body composition correlated directly with the relative dose of met-hGH. There were no apparent relationships between the hormone-induced percent change in FFW-FW and either the endogenous GH response to stimulation with L-dopa-arginine or the levels of insulin-like growth factor I obtained after treatment with placebo. There were no differences between treatments in the dietary intakes of total kilocalories, protein, carbohydrates, and fat. However, mean levels of insulin-like growth factor I were increased after treatment with

Fat-Free Weight, Percent of Body Fat, Ratio of Fat-Free Weight to Fat Weight in 8 Adults Studied Before and After Treatment With met-hGH

Body Composition	Placebo		met-hGH	
	Pre	Post	Pre	Post
FFW, kg	60.8±4.5	61.8±4.0	61.8±4.0	64.5±3.9*
%Fat	13.4±1.6	13.0±0.9	12.8±1.0	11.3±1.2*
FFW/FW	7.8±1.9	6.9±0.6	7.3±0.7	9.1±1.7*

*Significant difference between pretest and posttest means ($P < .05$).
(Courtesy of Crist DM, Peake GT, Egan PA, et al: *J Appl Physiol* 65:579–584, August 1988.)

met-hGH, when compared with postplacebo levels. Five of 7 individuals had a suppressed GH response to stimulation from either L-dopa-arginine or submaximal exercise after treatment with met-hGH.

These findings indicate that treatment with supraphysiologic doses of met-hGH significantly alter body composition in highly conditioned adults in a relative dose-dependent manner. However, such treatment may impair the stimulated release of endogenous GH in some individuals.

▶ The Ben Johnson scandal should finally have convinced athletes and their advisers that sports pharmacologists can detect the abuse of androgens by those who seek an unfair advantage over other competitors. However, there are disturbing reports that the more sophisticated of such cheats are now turning to hGH as a less readily detectable method of achieving similar results. Surprisingly, Crist and associates make no mention of this potential application of their findings, although they were using as subjects the most likely candidates for GH abuse—athletes who had engaged in progressive resistance exercise for a number of years. In 5 of 7 subjects there was evidence of a depressed release of endogenous GH in response to standard stimuli, and in the remaining 2 the lack of suppression may have reflected low levels of exogenous hormone [as in most experiments on doping, it was necessary to use somewhat marginal doses of exogenous hormone relative to those used in "doping"). If suppression of endogenous hGH secretion is confirmed, this may offer a possible avenue for detection of abuse. In addition to ethical considerations relating to fair competition, GH can, of course, lead to premature closure of epiphyses in adolescents, whereas in adults large doses of hGH can cause hyperglycemia and overgrowth of soft tissue.—R.J. Shephard, M.D. Ph.D.

Self-Reported Use of Anabolic-Androgenic Steroids by Elite Power Lifters
Yesalis CE III, Herrick RT, Buckley WE, Friedl KE, Brannon D, Wright JE (Pennsylvania State Univ, University Park; US Powerlifting Federation; Madigan Army Med Ctr, Fort Lewis, Wash; US Army Fitness School, Fort Harrison, Ind)
Phys Sportsmed 16:91–100, December 1988   16–5

Although steroid use by athletes is thought to be widespread, there is disagreement as to whether the level of use is increasing or decreasing. Given the concern about the potential health effects of these drugs, it is important to estimate the size and characteristics of the population at risk. Sixty-one athletes who competed in the 1987 National Championship of the United States Powerlifting Federation were surveyed to ascertain attitudes toward anabolic-androgenic steroids, patterns of use, and health effects. A subsample of 20 athletes was also interviewed by telephone.

Fifteen of 45 athletes who responded to the survey acknowledged having used steroids as did 11 of 20 athletes telephoned. Improved athletic performance was most often cited as the reason. Other reasons cited were treatment of injury, prevention of illness or injury, and appearance or other personal reasons. Overall, 73% of the athletes obtained steroids on

Survey Results in 15 Steroid Users	No.	%
Median length of cycle (week)		
<6	4	27
6–9	5	33
10–12	6	40
>12	0	0
Primary source of steroids		
Black market*	11	73
Physician or pharmacist	3	20
Mail order	1	7
Main reason for use†		
Improved athletic performance	10	67
Treatment of injury	4	27
Prevention of illness/injury	3	20
Appearance or other personal reasons	2	13
Mean longest cycle of use	12 weeks	
Mean age at first use of steroids	21.5 years	
Mean number of cycle of use	7.9	

*Other athletes, gym owners/managers.
†Respondents could select up to 2 reasons.
(Courtesy of Yesalis CE III, Herrick RT, Buckley WE, et al: *Phys Sportsmed* 16:91–100, December 1988.)

the black market, 20% obtained them from physicians or pharmacists, and 7% obtained them by mail order (table). Heightened libido, acne, and increased body hair were the most common side effects. Of the users, 60% favored stopping steroid use in sports. Most athletes thought that for drug testing to be effective, it would have to be conducted on a random, unannounced basis throughout the year, not just as competition time.

The small number of admitted users suggests that athletes underreported their steroid use. The reported level of use probably represents the lower boundary of steroid use among power lifters. Future studies should create alternative methods to deal with the problem of underreporting.

▶ The hearings of the Dubbin Commission in Canada have highlighted the extensive use of steroids, not only by power-lifters but by many other categories of athlete, including top members of national track teams. The paper by Yesalis et al. notes the substantial proportion of competitors who were supplied with steroids by physicians or licensed pharmacists, and a disturbing feature of the Dubbin inquiry has also been the apparent complicity not only of physicians but also of senior members of national sports associations. Sometimes, it appears, athletes have had foreknowledge of supposedly random drug testing, and a witness suggested that an eastern European nation brought an elaborate gas chromatograph system to the Montreal games to make sure that "doped" athletes had become free of steroids on the day that they were scheduled to compete. Given the prevalence of such cheating, and the development of forms of doping such as human growth hormone treatment (for which there is no basis of control), one may well wonder whether we can return to international sport for the joy of competing rather than for the dubious satisfaction of winning at all costs.—R.J. Shephard, M.D. Ph.D.

Estimated Prevalence of Anabolic Steroid Use Among Male High School Seniors
Buckley WE, Yesalis CE III, Friedl KE, Anderson WA, Streit AL, Wright JE (Pennsylvania State Univ, University Park; Madigan Army Med Ctr, Fort Lewis, Wash; Michigan State Univ; US Army Physical Fitness School, Fort Harrison, Ind)
JAMA 260:3441–3445, Dec 16, 1988   16–6

The use of anabolic-androgenic steroids (AS) is perceived by the public to have grown to epidemic proportions. However, the incidence and prevalence of AS use among elite, amateur, and recreational athletes are not well documented. A study was conducted to identify AS use patterns among 3,403 senior boys in 46 private and public high schools across the United States who completed a questionnaire eliciting current or previous use of AS and user and nonuser characteristics.

The overall participation rate on a schoolwide basis was 68.7%, and 50.3% on an individual basis. Of 12th grade boys, 6.6% use or have used AS, and more than two thirds of users began the practice when they were aged 16 years or younger. About 21% of users reported that a health professional was their primary source of AS.

This was the first study to establish the prevalence of anabolic AS use among male high school students. It is probable that there was some underreporting. Educational intervention strategies should begin as early as junior high school and should not be directed only toward those who participate in school-based athletics.

▶ The reported use of AS by 6.64% of high school seniors suggests that, at a minimum, between 250,000 and 500,000 adolescents in the United States have tried or are currently using these drugs. It appears that the authors are correct in their suspicion that their data are on the low side because of underreporting. Equally disturbing is the fact that a health professional was identified as the primary source of AS by 21% of the users.—J.S. Torg, M.D.

Assessment of Laboratory Quality in Urine Drug Testing: A Proficiency Testing Pilot Study
Davis KH, Hawks RL, Blanke RV (Research Triangle Inst, Research Triangle Park, NC; Natl Inst on Drug Abuse, Rockville, Md; Virginia Commonwealth Univ)
JAMA 260:1749–1754, Sept 23/30, 1988   16–7

Concerns about the proliferation of urine testing laboratories in the United States that do not operate under any particular professional or governmental guidelines prompted the federal government in 1986 to establish standards for accreditation of these laboratories. Urine drug testing must be performed under controls that will stand up to judicial challenge for the handling of evidence and meeting high standards of accuracy.

A pilot study, which consisted of an open proficiency testing phase and a blind testing phase, was carried out in 50 civilian commercial laboratories, all of which participated voluntarily. Drug-free urine specimens were obtained from paid volunteers. The urine was pooled and samples were tested by 2 reference laboratories to insure that the urine samples were free of interfering concentrations of prescription and over-the-counter drugs. The samples were fortified with commonly abused drugs at concentrations comparable to casual use or were left as unfortified blanks.

During the open phase of the study, 12 laboratories reported 16 false positive results (1.6%) in a total of 1,000 control specimens submitted, and 50 laboratories reported 100 false negative results (17%) in 600 positive drug challenges submitted. During the blind phase 4 laboratories reported 5 false positive results (1.3%) in 389 control specimens submitted and 109 false negatives (31%) among 350 positive challenges submitted. Most false positive errors in the blind phase resulted from misidentifications within drug classes.

The substance most often missed in false negative results in the blind phase was phencyclidine, which was detected only 49% of the time, followed by morphine (missed 47% of the time), cocaine (missed 38% of the time), and methamphetamines (missed 28% of the time).

The overall rankings of laboratory performance in the open and blind phases of this pilot study showed that 25 laboratories confirmed more than 92% of challenges correctly in the open phase and 9 laboratories confirmed more than 88% correctly in the blind phase.

▶ There is an ever-increasing demand for urine testing, both in terms of random spot-checks on athletes and as a means of controlling drug abuse in the North American labor force. In international competition the accused athlete may make a perfunctory attempt to protest innocence, but the standards of control for both the collection of specimens and subsequent analysis of urine specimens are currently so rigorous that there is little possibility an athlete can be falsely accused of drug abuse.

However, there is much more concern about the standards of drug testing currently accepted in industry, and if the testing of athletes becomes more commonplace, similar problems of poor-quality work may well arise. It is particularly interesting that many of the laboratories that are presently undertaking industrial testing are able to provide only qualitative results. The National Institute of Drug Abuse is currently seeking methods of accrediting testing laboratories, but there is little chance either of improving the accuracy of analyses or of correcting the disturbing total of 1.6% false positive results until all laboratories are able to report quantitative results for specimens distributed by a standardizing laboratory.—R.J. Shephard, M.D. Ph.D.

Blood Doping as an Ergogenic Aid

American College of Sports Medicine
Physician Sportsmed 16:131–134, January 1988   16–8

The American College of Sports Medicine has defined its position on the use of blood doping as an ergogenic aid for athletic performance:

Blood doping, or reinfusion of autologous or homologous red blood cells (RBC), is used to induce normovolemic erythrocythemia. The resultant hemoconcentration enhances oxygen delivery to skeletal muscles and improves maximal oxygen uptake and endurance capacity. Blood doping has been used in experimental procedures to examine the effect of hemoglobin on oxygen transport during dynamic exercise under both normoxic and hypoxic conditions. These studies support the ergogenic properties of RBC transfusion, but documentation of these effects in actual competitive conditions is lacking.

The ergogenic effectiveness of blood doping depends on several factors. Postreinfusion hemoconcentration occurs only when normocythemia is restored before reinfusion. In addition, improvements in maximum aerobic capacity are achieved only when athletes receive 2,000 ml of homologous blood or 900–1,800 ml of freeze-preserved autologous blood. Blood is preserved either by refrigeration at 4 C or by a glycerol freezing technique. The latter is preferable because it is possible to delay reinfusion until normocythemia has been reestablished in the donor. In contrast, with refrigeration there is a progressive loss of erythrocytes, and the recommended 3-week maximum storage period is not enough to restore the pre-phlebotomy hemoglobin level. Blood doping is not a procedure without risk. Hyperviscosity syndrome may develop, as well as known side effects from homologous and autologous transfusions, such as transfusion reactions, delayed reactions, and viral infections.

Autologous RBC transfusion is considered to be a scientifically valid and acceptable laboratory procedure to induce erythrocythemia for legitimate scientific inquiry under clinically controlled conditions. However, it is the position of the American College of Sports Medicine that the use of blood doping as an ergogenic aid during athletic competition is unethical and unjustifiable.

▶ This position statement could well be linked to all aspects of ergogenic aids. I would prefer the College simply to condemn all such practices on ethical grounds alone. Thus it would circumvent the need to issue a new position statement every time a new ergogenic aid hits the athletic world.—J.R. Sutton, M.D.

Use of Smokeless Tobacco in Major-League Baseball

Connolly GN, Orleans CT, Kogan M (Massachusetts Dept of Health, Boston; Fox Chase Cancer Ctr, Philadelphia)
N Engl J Med 318:1281–1285, May 12, 1988   16–9

Two types of smokeless tobacco—moist snuff and chewing tobacco—are popular among baseball players today. The patterns and consequences of the use of smokeless tobacco were assessed among professional baseball players by means of an anonymous self-report questionnaire given to members of 7 major league baseball teams during the 1987 spring training season.

In all, 265 men (mean age, 27 years) completed the questionnaire. They had been playing professional baseball for an average of 8 years. Thirty-four percent reported current use of smokeless tobacco, 17% reported past use, and 49% reported never having used it. Among current users, 63% used snuff only, 30% used both snuff and chewing tobacco, and 8% used only chewing tobacco. Use was higher during the baseball season than during the off-season. Fifteen percent of current users also smoked cigarettes. The brand of snuff most commonly used was Copenhagen, which provides a higher level of nicotine bioavailability than other brands. Most current users reported that they used smokeless tobacco "for something to do," because it is a habit, or because it helps them relax. Thirty-eight percent of current users reported that they had noticed sores, white patches, or gum problems where they held the tobacco in their mouths. Two thirds of the current users said they would be interested in a players' guide to help them quit using smokeless tobacco.

The expected relationships were found between self-reported use of smokeless tobacco and addiction. Interventions for users of smokeless tobacco should include providing information about the serious adverse effects of smokeless tobacco on health and should emphasize the improvements in health, well-being, and athletic performance that result from quitting. Influential peers who have quit may be powerful role models.

▶ This is an interesting historical, if not anecdotal, review of the use of moist "snuff" and "chewing tobacco" since organized baseball was established in 1845. Related are such pearls as this: ". . . Babe Ruth, who was a heavy snuff 'dipper', tobacco chewer, and cigar smoker . . . apparently used snuff internasally and was advised by his physician to discontinue the practice because of impacted nasal passages." Although the report relies on the conclusions of the Surgeon General's report on the health consequences of smokeless tobacco use and the Consensus Conference Report on smokeless tobacco of the National Institutes of Health, no actual data substantiating the deleterious effects of these practices are given. Rather, it is simply stated: "Both reports concluded that the use of smokeless tobacco was causally related to oral cancer and gum recession, that it can lead to dependence on nicotine, and that it is not a safe alternative to smoking." It is further pointed out that Babe Ruth died of an oropharyngeal tumor at age 52 that was believed to be related to heavy tobacco consumption, whereas Honus Wagner, an outspoken critic of tobacco, outlived Ruth, dying at the age of 81. This paper can be best described as an interesting but anecdotal account of a perceived problem.—J.S. Torg, M.D.

17 Diet and Body Composition

Resting Metabolic Requirements of Men and Women
Owen OE (Temple Univ)
Mayo Clin Proc 63:503–510, May 1988   17–1

The measured resting metabolic rates (RMR) in normal persons are less than their predicted rates based on the formulas and tables from the largest, most authoritative reports published in the first half of this century. A systematic study was thus conducted to reappraise the caloric requirements of lean and obese women and men.

Forty-four lean and obese women, 8 of whom were trained athletes, and 60 lean and obese men had RMRs measured by indirect calorimetry. The women were aged 18–82 years and weighed 43–171 kg; all were mentally and physically active. Body composition was calculated by densitometry and skinfold thickness. Body compositional variables reflecting active protoplasmic tissue were all highly interrelated. Body weight alone had prediction values for RMR similar to those of other variables of active protoplasmic tissue mass. The influence of age on RMR in this group was minimal, and the regional distribution of fat had no effect on RMR.

Metabolic efficiency is not necessarily or exclusively related to obesity. The caloric requirements of human beings, based on body weight or active protoplasmic tissue mass, may vary by twofold.

▶ This is an interesting and very valuable report explaining how the author developed new regression equations for predicting RMRs for healthy and obese men and women. He found that the old equation from the first half of this century overestimated the RMRs of men and women today. Some interesting information that he also reported showed that, although the human brain constitutes about 2% of the body weight, it consumes about 20% of the RMR. Similarly, the liver constitutes about 2% of the body weight and consumes about 20% of the RMR. Much of the energy consumption by the liver is used to synthesize glucose and ketone bodies as fuels for the brain. Muscle comprises 35% to 40% of the body weight and consumes about 20% of the RMR. Adipose tissue is normally about 20% of the body weight but consumes only about 2% to 5% of the RMR.—Col. J.L. Anderson, PE.D.

Carbohydrate Ingestion and Muscle Glycogen Depletion During Marathon and Ultramarathon Racing

Noakes TD, Lambert EV, Lambert MI, McArthur PS, Myburgh KH, Benade AJS
(Univ of Cape Town; MRC Research Inst for Nutritional Diseases, Tygerberg, South Africa)

Eur J Appl Physiol 57:482–489, March 1988   17–2

Previous studies have suggested that ingestion of carbohydrate during prolonged exercise prevents the development of hypoglycemia and increases the overall rate of carbohydrate utilization. Two studies were undertaken to characterize the effects of carbohydrate ingestion on exercise performance, the blood fuel-hormone response to exercise, and the utilization of muscle glycogen during prolonged competitive exercise.

In the first study 18 male runners in 3 subgroups matched for maximum oxygen consumption and blood lactate turnpoint underwent a 3-day carbohydrate depletion phase followed by 3 days of carbohydrate loading (500–600 gm/day). During a 42.2-km standard marathon race the runners drank a solution containing 2% glucose, 8% glucose polymer, or 8% fructose. In the second study the 18 runners, placed in 2 matched subgroups, drank a solution containing either 4% glucose or 10% glucose polymer during a 56-km ultramarathon race.

Race performance was not different between groups in either race. The

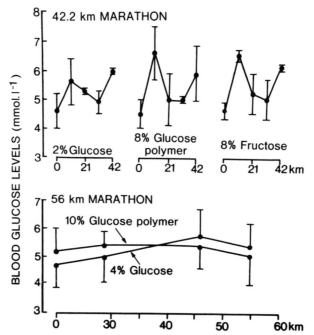

Fig 17–1.—Level of blood glucose before and during 42.2-km marathon *(top)* and 56-km ultramarathon *(bottom)* in groups of numbers ingesting various carbohydrate solutions. (Courtesy of Noakes TD, Lambert EV, Lambert MI, et al: *Eur J Appl Physiol* 57:482–489, March 1988.)

blood glucose level, serum level of free fatty acids, and insulin concentrations did not differ significantly between groups during the 2 races (Fig 17–1). Neither the nature nor amount of carbohydrate ingested influenced the rate of utilization of muscle glycogen in these runners.

The data show that hypoglycemia is uncommon in athletes during prolonged competitive exercises provided they are carbohydrate loaded before the race and ingest a minimum of 10 gm of carbohydrate per hour during competition. The type and amount of carbohydrate CHO do not affect performance in a race or the extent of muscle glycogen depletion during prolonged exercise. It appears that ingestion of carbohydrate enhances performance by preventing hypoglycemia and by providing oxidizable substrate when liver and muscle glycogen stores are depleted.

▶ The extent of muscle glycogen depletion over long-distance athletic events remains a matter of some controversy. There have been papers describing serum glucose concentrations so low that immediate transfusion of glucose/saline was required. On the other hand, in our studies of postcoronary marathon runners, blood samples obtained a few minutes after the runners passed the finish line actually showed supranormal blood glucose readings despite 4–5 hours of jogging. Presumably, much depends not only on preloading of the muscle glycogen reserves but also on the intensity of activity, particularly the extent of anaerobic exercise during an event; if the speed is held below the anaerobic threshold, then much of the required energy may be derived from fat rather than from carbohydrate. The intensity of effort was around 75% of maximum oxygen intake in the present 42-km event and 65% of maximum oxygen intake in the 56-km run, both values being well below the anaerobic threshold for this sample of well-trained individuals.

In theory, glucose polymer and fructose can be ingested at higher concentrations than glucose, because they have a lower osmotic pressure and are thus less liable to delay gastric emptying. In the present experiments, ingestion of "glucose equivalents" was 40 gm/hour for the glucose polymer and fructose vs. 10 gm/hour for the glucose solution. No difference of muscle glycogen levels was found among the 3 mixtures, and it is worth stressing that over 3 hours of running, the total ingestion of carbohydrate (30 gm or 120 gm) made only a marginal contribution to the energy requirements of a race. Such amounts are also small relative to the combined muscle and liver glycogen stores of almost 1,000 gm in a runner who has systematically preloaded with carbohydrate. Previous studies in which major benefit was claimed for carbohydrate ingestion were often unrealistic in that subjects were tested in the postabsorptive state, rather than when preloaded with glycogen, which is the norm for the present generation of distance runners; moreover, in the present experiments, all of the solutions tasted sweet, thus avoiding any psychologically induced deterioration of performance under conditions in which water alone was provided.

Plainly, the value of the carbohydrate component of fluid increases with the length of the event, and this should be the guiding factor in recommending beverages to athletes. Over a 24-hour race, the glycogen reserves are still no more than 1 kg, but ingested glucose polymer is then able to provide a very useful additional 1 kg of fuel.—R.J. Shephard, M.D., Ph.D.

Attitudes Toward Eating and Body Weight in Different Groups of Female Adolescent Athletes

Brooks-Gunn J, Burrow C, Warren MP (Univ of Pennsylvania; Columbia Univ; St. Luke's-Roosevelt Hosp, New York)
Int J Eating Disord 7:749–757, November 1988   17–3

Female athletes frequently have low weight and delayed menarche. However, sports differ in their requirements for body shape and size. It was hypothesized that dancers and figure skaters, who are required to have low weights, would have more negative attitudes about eating, lower weights, and later menarche than swimmers, who are not required to maintain low weights.

A survey was made that included regional and national athletes aged 14–18 years. There were 25 figure skaters, 64 ballet dancers, and 72 swimmers. Nonathletic adolescents served as a control group. Height, weight, menarchal age, and attitudes toward eating were elicited. Dancers and skaters were lighter and leaner than swimmers and nonathletes, and they also were more likely to have delayed menarche. Dancers and skaters also had higher dieting, bulimia, and oral control scores than the swimmers and nonathletes. Dancers scored higher on dieting and lower on oral control than skaters.

Dancers and skaters had more negative eating attitudes. Dancers showed more restraint eating than skaters, which suggested that low weights might be difficult to maintain given the relatively low energy demands required for dancing.

▶ Coaches and trainers must carefully monitor their female athletes to insure they are getting sufficient nutrients and are not bulimic. Any athletes, men or women, who are practicing weight control to improve athletic performance need to be properly counseled concerning nutrition. Unfortunately, many coaches push for the weight loss and are not worried about what the possible long-term consequences may be. Of course, at this time we cannot identify any long-term consequences if the poor nutritional intake is only short term.—Col. J.L. Anderson, PE.D.

Body Image and Eating Disturbance in Obligatory Runners, Obligatory Weightlifers, and Sedentary Individuals

Pasman L, Thompson JK (Univ of South Florida, Tampa)
Int J Eating Disorders 7:759–769, November 1988   17–4

Some individuals addicted to exercise have come to be called obligatory exercisers. To examine the concept of obligatory exercise and its possible connection with eating disturbance, body image and eating dis-

Group Comparisons for All Dependent Variables

Group*

	Male			Female		
	R	W	C	R	W	C
SELF-EST†						
Global	13 (13)	3 (24)	9 (11)	21 (24)	3 (13)	15 (8)
Waist	13 (16)	4 (23)	10 (13)	25 (25)	3 (13)	20 (12)
Hips	18 (12)	8 (25)	15 (14)	26 (31)	7 (17)	13 (9)
Thighs	7 (14)	−5 (28)	2 (17)	12 (21)	1 (20)	13 (20)
MAN-EST†						
Global	10 (17)	3 (23)	12 (11)	14 (18)	3 (13)	1 (20)
Waist	18 (19)	12 (25)	17 (12)	20 (23)	9 (14)	3 (25)
Hips	16 (21)	6 (24)	14 (15)	12 (15)	8 (14)	2 (16)
Thighs	−5 (15)	−9 (24)	4 (12)	10 (21)	−7 (19)	−1 (26)
QUEST‡ §						
EDI-DT	5.20 (5.18)	3.80 (5.12)	0.40 (0.91)	10.13 (5.25)	7.73 (6.10)	2.40 (2.47)
EDI-B	0.53 (0.74)	0.80 (1.26)	0.40 (0.74)	1.33 (1.99)	0.87 (1.41)	0.47 (0.91)
EDI-BD ‖	3.13 (4.75)	7.33 (5.14)	4.47 (6.46)	12.60 (7.43)	7.27 (4.95)	10.33 (10.38)
BSRQ-PAE	3.77 (0.49)	3.55 (0.53)	3.45 (0.67)	3.08 (0.65)	3.68 (0.51)	3.42 (0.91)

*R, runners; W, weight lifters; C, controls.
†SELF-EST, Size Estimation of Self; MAN-EST, Size Estimation of Mannequin (in terms of percentage overestimation or underestimation).
‡QUEST, Questionnaire: EDI-DT, Eating Disorders Inventory, Drive for Thinness Subscale; EDI-B, Eating Disorders Inventory, Bulimia Subscale; EDI-BD, Eating Disorders Inventory, Body Dissatisfaction Subscale; BSRQ-PAE, Body Self-Relations Questionnaire, Physical Appearance Evaluation Subscale.
§Numbers in parentheses are standard deviations. Lower numbers indicate more dissatisfaction.
(Courtesy of Pasman L, Thompson JK: *Int J Eating Disorders* 7:759–769, November 1988.)

turbance were studied in obligatory runners, obligatory weight lifters, and sedentary controls.

There were 15 men and 15 women in each of the 3 groups. They were asked to estimate the size of their waists, hips, and thighs using an adjustable light-beam apparatus. Estimations were repeated on a mannequin. A Gneupal anthropometer was used to measure the actual size of body sites. The groups also were evaluated for eating disorders and body satisfaction using subscales of the Eating Disorders Inventory and the Body Self Relations Questionnaire (table).

Weight lifters were significantly more accurate in estimating body size than were runners or controls; there was no difference between runners and controls. All persons overestimated waist and hip sizes to a greater degree than they did thigh sizes, whether on their own bodies or on the mannequin. More women than men were dissatisfied with their bodies except for male weight lifters who were as dissatisfied as female weight lifters. Both runners and weight lifters had more eating disturbances than controls, and women had greater eating psychopathy than men had.

Athletes who engage in certain types of physical activity may have superior ability to estimate body size. The type of physical activity and gender may also be related to body satisfaction and incidence of eating disorders.

▶ Given that anorexia is often accompanied by obsessional exercise, there has been much discussion for several years as to whether addiction to a physical activity such as long-distance jogging is another expression of the same basic clinical disorder. The present paper supports the current consensus: Although there is some evidence of eating disturbance in both weight lifters and runners, relative to controls, the anorectic tendencies are much milder than in true anorectic patients, perceptions of body size are more realistic, and there is never evidence of an associated bulimia.—R.J. Shephard, M.D., Ph.D.

Dissimilarities in Eating Attitudes, Body Image Distortion, Depression, and Self-Esteem Between High-Intensity Male Runners and Women With Bulimia Nervosa
Nudelman S, Rosen JC, Leitenberg H (Univ of Vermont)
Int J Eating Disorders 7:625–634, September 1988   17–5

It has been suggested that the habit of intense running in men bears some resemblance to the features of eating disorders in women and that such a habit in men could be associated with the same characteristics of negative body image, lower self-esteem, fears of weight gain, anxiety, depression, and other traits that are assumed to underlie eating disorders in women.

Twenty high-intensity exercising men (mean age, 25.3 years) were compared with 20 sedentary, moderately exercising men (mean age, 25.3 years) and with 20 women (mean age, 26.1 years) who had bulimia nervosa. The 3 groups did not differ in education or deviation from average weight. The 2 groups of men completed the Obligatory Running Questionnaire, which measures compulsive exercising tendencies. All 3 groups completed the Eating Attitudes Test (EAT) and the Eating Disorders Inventory (EDI). In addition, all were asked to estimate their body dimensions, which were then verified by actual measurement.

Interpretation of the test scores revealed that the high-intensity exercising men did not resemble women with eating disorders (table). They were not anxious about eating or overly preoccupied with food, did not engage in excessive binge eating or purging, were not negatively preoccupied with their weight or intent on losing weight, did not have the personality traits presumed to underlie eating disorders, and were not depressed or low in self-esteem. The high-intensity exercisers were actu-

Differences Between Groups in Symptoms of Eating Disorders, Size of Distortion, Behavioral Traits, Depression, and Self-Esteem

	Male runners		Male controls		Female bulimics		
	M $\dagger$	SD	M $\dagger$	SD	M $\dagger$	SD	Statistic
Eating disorder symptoms							
EAT							
Total	13.0^a	8.3	9.4^a	5.5	47.2^b	17.4	$F = 64.65^{***}$
Dieting	3.4^a	4.0	2.3^a	2.4	18.3^b	8.6	$F = 49.19^{***}$
Bulimia	0.4^a	1.3	1.2^a	2.9	11.7^b	3.9	$F = 92.47^{***}$
Oral control	1.9^{ab}	1.6	1.3^a	1.3	3.7^b	4.7	$F = 3.33^*$
EDI-symptom scales							
Drive to thinness	0.9^a	2.3	1.5^a	2.1	14.2^b	4.9	$F = 97.76^{***}$
Bulimia	0.8^a	1.6	0.8^a	2.5	10.8^b	3.9	$F = 81.96^{***}$
Body Dissatis.	1.5^a	2.1	3.7^a	4.7	13.6^b	8.3	$F = 26.36^{***}$
Size estimation	12.3^{ab}	13.3	6.1^a	12.2	17.8^b	13.1	$F = 3.79^*$
Psych. adjustment							
EDI-trait scales							
Ineffectiveness	0.8^a	1.6	1.0^a	1.8	10.9^b	6.8	$F = 40.74^{***}$
Perfectionism	5.4	3.8	5.9	4.5	7.8	4.8	$F = 1.63$
Interpersonal Distrust	2.4^a	3.8	2.8^a	3.4	5.8^b	4.0	$F = 4.72^*$
Interoceptive Awareness	0.5^a	0.9	1.5^a	2.5	11.1^b	6.8	$F = 38.64^{***}$
Maturity Fears	1.2^a	1.7	2.6^a	3.5	5.3^b	5.1	$F = 6.29^{**}$
Depression	3.5^a	4.4	5.3^a	4.7	19.9^b	7.8	$F = 47.62^{***}$
Self-esteem	35.1^a	4.5	34.2^a	3.7	23.5^b	5.2	$F = 41.07^{***}$
Social self-esteem	136.4^a	25.9	138.5^a	19.4	117.1^b	30.1	$F = 4.23^*$

$^*P < .05.^{**}P < .01^{***}P < .001.$
$\dagger$Means with different superscripts are significantly different at $P < .05$.
(Courtesy of Nudelman S, Rosen JC, Leitenberg H: *Int J Eating Disorders* 7:625–634, September 1988.)

ally significantly better adjusted than women with eating disorders and were nearly identical on any measure to controls. High-intensity exercising in men does not appear to be analogous to eating disorders among women.

▶ Some bulimia and anorexia nervosa patients engage in compulsive exercising as a further method of producing a pathologically low body mass, and there have been fears that the person who chooses to run (say) 50 miles per week may have the same type of psychological disorder. The report by Nudelman and colleagues provides a fairly categoric disproof of such a hypothesis. Although a form of addiction to prolonged exercise can undoubtedly develop, perhaps as a consequence of the associated secretion of endorphins, the body image and personality of the distance runner seem very normal. It would be interesting to repeat this type of study with other classes of athlete; a distortion of body image seems more likely in those who engage compulsively in body-building programs.—R.J. Shephard, M.D., Ph.D.

The Role of Selectivity in the Pathogenesis of Eating Problems in Ballet Dancers

Hamilton LH, Brooks-Gunn J, Warren MP, Hamilton WG (Adelphi Univ, Garden City, NY)
Med Sci Sports Exerc 20:560–565, December 1988   17–6

Ballet dancers must meet rigid requirements with regard to body weight and shape. The high incidence of anorexia nervosa and bulimia in ballet dancers suggests that chronic dieting behavior may be involved in the pathogenesis of eating disorders.

Thirty-two dancers from 3 American ballet companies and 17 dancers from the national ballet company of the People's Republic of China were surveyed (table). The Chinese company and 1 American company choose their dancers exclusively from ballet schools, where the dancers are enrolled at an early age and where they must maintain rigid standards with regard to body weight and shape. The other 2 American companies choose their dancers from general auditions. Dancers were questioned about familial obesity, eating problems, and menstrual history. Dancers also completed an eating problems scale.

American dancers from the less selective companies reported significantly more eating problems, anorexic behavior, and familial obesity than did either Americans chosen from the company school or the Chinese dancers. All groups had delayed menarche and body weight approximately 14% below the ideal for height.

Dancers who survive a stringent process of early selection may be more naturally inclined toward the thin body image required for ballet and

Mean Differences in Anthropometric Measures and Eating Behavior in Highly Selected (HS) and Less Selected (LS) Dancers

	HS Chinese		HS Americans		LS Americans	
	$\bar{X}$	SD	$\bar{X}$	SD	$\bar{X}$	SD
Height (cm)	163.09*	3.89	168.45*	4.39	166.67	4.60
Weight (kg)	45.57*	3.38	51.92*	2.96	50.24	4.53
Ideal weight	−15.31	4.03	−12.00	3.54	−13.08	5.39
Menarche	14.40	1.18	14.62	1.88	14.77	1.88
% Menarche ≥14	59%		63%		69%	
% Irregularity	57%		39%		77%	
% Anorexia	00%		5%		23%	
% Bulimia	24%		5%		23%	
% Purge	00%		00%		15%	
EAT-26	2.45	0.49	2.37	0.74	2.93	1.18
Anorexic sum	1.47	0.87	1.11 †	1.76	2.77 †	2.05

*HS Chinese vs. HS Americans.

†HS Americans vs. LS Americans; X values in the same row with similar superscripts are significantly different from each other at $P < .05$; 17 HS Chinese, 19 HS Americans, 13 LS Americans.

(Courtesy of Hamilton LH, Brooks-Gunn J, Warren MP, et al: Med Sci Sports Exerc 20:560–565, December 1988.)

may be at less risk for the development of eating problems. Delayed menarche is typical in these dancers and is probably related to both genetic and environmental factors.

▶ This paper once again illustrates the unrealistic body build required of ballet dancers. Competition for places in top companies is such that it is possible to select performers who are 6% to 12% below the actuarial ideal body mass, and among those who join the ballet companies later in life, as many as 23% have a tendency to become bulimic to meet this requirement. Plainly, there is a need to make more realistic demands on the shape and appearance of female participants.—R.J. Shephard, M.D., Ph.D.

Physical Activity, Diet, and Risk of Colon Cancer in Utah
Slattery ML, Schumacher MC, Smith KR, West DW, Abd-Elghany N (Univ of Utah; Utah Cancer Registry, Salt Lake City)
Am J Epidemiol 128:989–999, November 1988   17–7

Individuals who are more physically active usually consume more calories and have lower cardiovascular death rates; however, although physical activity also appears to reduce the risk of colon cancer, a higher caloric intake has been associated with an increased risk of this disease developing. To assess these factors, combined effects of physical activity and diet on colon cancer risk were studied using a population-based, case-control method.

Data were obtained for a reference period of 2 years before interview for the control group (204 women and 180 men) and 2 years before diagnosis for patients (119 women and 110 men). Leisure-time and occupational activities were categorized by level of intensity and were converted to calories expended per week. Dietary data were obtained from a quantitative food-frequency questionnaire. Physical activity and dietary data were divided into quartiles based on the distribution in the study population.

When high and low quartiles of physical activity were compared, total physical activity protected against the development of colon cancer in both men and women. Intense physical activity offered the greatest protection for both sexes, but more so for men. The relationship between physical activity and risk of colon cancer was not altered by dietary intake of calories, protein, or fat; a higher caloric intake did increase the risk of colon cancer. Adding total activity to the model did not alter the relationship between dietary calories and colon cancer.

High levels of physical activity appear to reduce the risk of colon cancer associated with high levels of dietary intake, especially of fat. Physical activity may stimulate colon peristalsis, thus decreasing the time that potential carcinogens remain in the colon.

▶ This is one of an increasing number of well-designed epidemiologic studies that show a reduced risk of cancer of the colon in highly active individuals. The major additional contribution of this study was the ability of the authors to assess the potentially confounding variables of caloric intake, which itself is positively related to the rate of colonic cancer. Intriguing though this study is, epidemiologic studies per se are rarely able to establish definitively a mechanistic relationship, although they can establish causality.—J.R. Sutton, M.D.

Body Composition: Practical Considerations for Coaches and Athletes
Bishop PA, Smith JF (Univ of Alabama, Tuscaloosa)
Natl Strength Conditioning Assoc J 10:27–32, June–July 1988   17–8

Estimating body composition is probably one of the most popular of all modern technical procedures of exercise science. Most methods for estimating fatness are fairly simple, but there are many ways to err greatly in assessing measurements, computing, and interpreting body composition estimates. Correct use of assessment techniques allows coaches and athletes to monitor body composition changes and thus optimize training techniques and performance.

Appropriate tested techniques and prediction equations must first be selected (table). Indiscriminate use of skinfold equations results in errors in most groups of athletes. Established methods must be followed carefully with attention to detail. Residual volume should be determined if

---

Estimated Body Fat Percentage From Jackson & Pollock * and Jackson, Pollock, and Ward Equations†

Age Skinfold Sum ‡ §	20 M	20 F	25 M	25 F	30 M	30 F	35 M	35 F
16-20	4.2	--	4.7	--	5.3	--	5.8	--
21-25	5.8	--	6.3	--	6.9	--	7.4	--
26-30	7.3	12.3	7.9	12.6	8.4	12.9	9.0	13.2
31-35	8.9	14.2	9.4	14.5	10.0	14.8	10.5	15.1
36-40	10.4	16.0	11.0	16.3	11.5	16.6	12.1	16.9
41-45	11.9	17.7	12.5	18.1	13.0	18.4	13.6	18.7
46-50	13.4	19.5	13.9	19.8	14.5	20.1	15.1	20.4
51-55	14.8	21.2	15.4	21.5	16.0	21.8	16.5	22.1
56-60	16.2	22.8	16.8	23.2	17.4	23.5	18.0	23.8
61-65	17.6	24.5	18.2	24.8	18.8	25.1	19.4	25.4
66-70	19.0	26.0	19.6	26.4	20.2	26.7	20.7	27.0
71-75	20.3	27.6	20.9	27.9	21.5	28.2	22.1	28.5
76-80	21.7	29.1	22.2	29.4	22.8	29.7	23.4	30.0
81-85	22.9	30.5	23.5	30.8	24.1	31.2	24.7	31.5
86-90	24.1	31.9	24.8	32.2	25.4	32.6	26.0	32.9
91-95	25.4	33.3	26.0	33.6	26.6	33.9	27.2	34.3

*Jackson AS, Pollock ML: *Br J Nutr* 40:497–504, 1980.
†Jackson AS, Pollock ML, Ward A: *Med Sci Sports Exerc* 12:175–182, 1978.
Male equation is $1.10938 - .008267 (SM3) + .0000016 (SM3^2) - .0002574 (AGE)$.
‡Male skinfolds (SM3) used are sum of chest, abdomen, and thigh;
Female equation is $1.0994921 - .0009929 (SF3) + .0000023 (SF3^2) - .000139 (AGE)$.
§Female skinfolds (SF3) used are sum of triceps, thigh, and suprailium.
(Courtesy of Bishop PA, Smith JF: *Natl Strength Conditioning Assoc J* 10:27–32, June–July 1988.)

underwater weighing is performing. Skinfold sites should be carefully identified in accordance with the directions of the equation used. The limitations on the accuracy of the procedure should be understood; individual errors can be large in all methods. Results should be interpreted and applied cautiously, being careful not to overinterpret small differences in body composition.

Because of the likelihood of substantial error in body composition evaluation, coaches and athletes should be concerned about the use of estimators in athletes. These numbers are best used for monitoring the progress of an individual, not for making comparisons among individuals or against arbitrary standards. Body composition estimation can be a useful measurement for evaluating athletes if done correctly.

▶ The authors have warned us, and we should heed their warnings, regarding the limitations and accuracy of these procedures. They offer very good advice when warning that these numbers are best used for monitoring the progress of an individual, not for making comparisons among individuals or against arbitrary standards.—F.J. George, ATC, PT

Changes in Plasma Lipids and Lipoproteins in Overweight Men During Weight Loss Through Dieting as Compared With Exercise
Wood PD, Stefanick ML, Dreon DM, Frey-Hewitt B, Garay SC, Williams PT, Superko HR, Fortmann SP, Albers JJ, Vranizan KM, Ellsworth NM, Terry RB, Haskell WL (Stanford Univ; Univ of Washington)
N Engl J Med 319:1173–1179, Nov 3, 1988   17–9

Obese individuals have a greater risk of coronary heart disease developing. This may partially be the result of the low concentration of high-density lipoprotein (HDL)-cholesterol that is characteristic of obesity. Weight loss elevates the concentration of HDL-cholesterol as does exercise, but an increase in HDL has not been shown to be independent of the loss of body fat.

The loss of body fat through dieting was compared with loss of fat from exercise without dieting to determine the relative effect on levels of plasma lipids and lipoproteins.

Forty-two dieters, 47 exercisers, and 42 controls were studied. Food intake for dieters was designed to reduce baseline total body fat by one third in a 9-month period. Exercisers followed a supervised exercise program to accomplish the same goal without dieting. Controls maintained their usual diet and exercise regimens throughout the 1 year trial.

As compared with controls, dieters had significant loss of total body weight, both fat weight and lean weight. Exercisers had significant loss of total body weight and fat weight but not lean weight. Fat weight loss was similar in dieters and exercisers. Both study groups had significant increases in plasma concentrations of HDL-cholesterol and significant decreases in levels of triglycerides. Levels of low-density lipoproteins remained constant in controls and did not differ significantly between the 2 study groups.

Fat loss either through dieting or exercise has a comparable favorable effect on plasma concentrations of lipoproteins. Dieting without exercise, however, also produces loss of lean body weight.

▶ This meticulous study has demonstrated the value of exercise compared with diet to reduce weight in overweight males. If you wish to lose fat rather than lean body mass, exercise will do it, but diet alone will not. Both approaches led to comparable increases in the HDL-cholesterol content. Although the study did not attempt to examine whether there was a further advantage in adding a diet to an exercise program, this implication should not escape the reader.—J.R. Sutton, M.D.

Body Compositions of Eumenorrheic, Oligomenorrheic, and Amenorrheic Runners
De Souza MJ, Maresh CM, Abraham A, Camaione DN (Univ of Connecticut, Storrs)
J Appl Sport Sci Res 2:13–15, February–March 1988   17–10

Body composition was measured of 27 female runners aged 18–33 years who had run at least 25 miles a week for a year or longer. Nine persons were eumenorrheic and 9 were oligomenorrheic. Nine others— with cycles at intervals of 90 days or longer—were categorized as amenorrheic. Only 1 had primary amenorrhea. The underwater weighing method was used.

Both the amenorrheic and oligomenorrheic runners weighed significantly less than the eumenorrheic individuals. Those who were amenorrheic ran more miles a week than the eumenorrheic runners did. Underwater weighing and skinfold thickness measurements indicated a significantly lower body fat percentage in amenorrheic and oligomenorrheic women than in those who were eumenorrheic. Fat weight was less in the former groups, but lean body weights were similar in all groups.

The Jackson, Pollock, and Ward generalized regression equation can provide accurate estimates of body composition in female athletes. These estimates can be helpful in monitoring training responses and nutritional interventions. Further studies are needed to learn how the interaction of body composition and menstrual status relates to successful sports performance.

▶ Because there is considerable inconsistency among the various indirect methods of estimating body fat percentage in both eumenorrheic and amenorrheic athletes, the authors decided to do what they believe to be the first study to compare body fat percentages derived from a generalized regression equation to values obtained by hydrostatic weighing. Their subjects were eumenorrheic, oligomenorrheic, and amenorrheic runners. Because the latter 2 groups were very similar in body composition measures, they collapsed those 2 groups. Their finding that the Jackson, Pollock, Ward regression equation gives a reasonably accurate estimate of percent body fat in women runners should be helpful to general practitioners who are monitoring the body composition of their patients who are runners.— Col. J.L. Anderson, PE.D.

Body Composition Analysis by Bioelectrical Impedance: Effect of Skin Temperature
Caton JR, Molé PA, Adams WC, Heustis DS (Univ of California, Davis)
Med Sci Sports Exerc 20:489–491, November 1988   17–11

Bioelectrical impedance analysis (BIA) systems have been used to determine body water and body composition. The validity and reliability of the BIA method need to be evaluated, especially with regard to factors that introduce variation in whole-body resistance. The effect of changes in ambient and skin temperatures on measurement of resistance and estimation of body composition using BIA was studied in 8 men.

Electrodes were placed on prepared sites on the right hand and foot. Using the prediction equations supplied with the instrumentation, body composition and body water were estimated. After completing the BIA measurements, body composition was determined by hydrodensitometry.

The dry bulb temperature of the chamber ranged from 14.4 C in the cool condition to 35.0 C in the warm condition, with relative humidity at 45.4% and 35.9%, respectively. Hand and foot skin temperatures were significantly different in the 2 conditions, ranging from 24.1 C in the cool condition to 33.4 C in the warm condition. Resistance was significantly greater in the cool condition as compared with the warm condition. Estimated body water was significantly lower in the cool condition than in the warm condition. Also, fat mass and percent fat predicted by BIA were significantly greater in the cool than in the warm condition. Using BIA without considering the ambient temperature thus does not yield reliable results and should be avoided.

To determine whether the demonstrated effect of temperature on resistance results from redistribution of blood flow and body water between compartments, further studies are needed in which body water distribution and skin flow are manipulated without any change in ambient temperature.

▶ There has been considerable commercial pressure in the past few years to adopt BIA as a convenient standard clinical method of estimating the percentage of body fat. In essence, a high-frequency electrical signal applied to 2 extremity electrodes is used to measure the impedance between 2 more proximal electrodes. The main determinant of impedance is the average cross-section of the cylinder of fluid interposed between the proximal electrodes, so that assumptions about body geometry are an inherent part of the error of the impedance method and discrepancies in fat predictions occur between tall and shorter individuals. However, the skin also contributes a substantial and highly variable impedance, and this is likely to be modified by sweating in a warm environment.

I had some personal experience with the bioimpedance method many years ago when I was interested in the measurement of forearm blood flow (another possible application of the impedance technique); at that time I abandoned the method, largely because of the influence of changes in skin impedance with sweating. High-input impedance detectors are now supposed to overcome this problem; the present authors are thus inclined to attribute the disturbing effects of heat to an increase in the superficial blood volume, and thus an altered geometry for the electrical signal. Irrespective of mechanisms, the conclusion seems inescapable that bioimpedance techniques give only a very rough indication of body fat content. Greater information (including an indication of the critical patterning of body fat) can be obtained more cheaply and more simply by the use of skinfold calipers.—R.J. Shephard, M.D., Ph.D.

Body Building and Myoglobinuria: Report of Three Cases
Doriguzzi C, Palmucci L, Mongini T, Arnaudo E, Bet L, Bresolin N (Univ degli Studi di Torino, Italy; Univ degli Studi di Milan, Italy)
Br Med J 296:826–827, March 19, 1988   17–12

Body building has not been mentioned among the various kinds of exercise that can cause myoglobinuria. Myoglobinuria occurred in 3 healthy young adults after a first session of body building. All 3 regularly engaged in sports activities.

After their first session of body building aimed at strengthening pectoral and abdominal muscles, the 3 men complained of muscle pain and weakness and of passing dark urine. Determination of serum creatine kinase activity several days later showed increases of 5-fold to 180-fold over normal. Results of all other laboratory tests were normal. Results of electromyography, forearm ischemic exercise test, biochemical and histochemical analysis of biopsy samples of the quadriceps muscle, and all other laboratory findings, including serum creatine kinase activity, were normal 1–4 months later.

Thus in the first training session, the myoglobinuria resulted from unaccustomed effort. Body building, in contrast to other types of physical activity, uses muscles usually less trained, such as the pectorals, trapezii, and abdominal muscles.

▶ These cases demonstrate that muscle damage is common whenever we engage in new or unusual physical activity. The classic type of exercise to induce such damage is the so-called eccentric or lengthening contraction, e.g., when we go downhill. Usually the pain and soreness are delayed for 24–48 hours and the maximum rise in creatine phosphokinase activity occurs within 2–5 days. Myoglobin, by contrast, often appears in the urine earlier. It is possible to avoid such an alarming clinical course by beginning a new activity quietly and building up slowly. Even such activities as stepping down from a height, which invariably causes muscle damage, can be trained. The problem in most patients, as in those described in this report, can be adequately diagnosed by history alone and the clinical response to a graduated training program. In the vast majority of patients a common sense clinical appraisal obviates the need for more extensive and invasive investigations.—J.R. Sutton, M.D.

The Effects of Strength Training in Patients With Selected Neuromuscular Disorders
McCartney N, Moroz D, Garner SH, McComas AJ (McMaster Univ, Hamilton, Ont)
Med Sci Sports Exerc 20:362–367, October 1988   17–13

Progressive resistance strength training increases muscle size, strength, and endurance capacity in healthy individuals, but the effects of this training have not been well documented in patients with neuromuscular disorders. The effects of progressive resistance strength training on muscle strength, size, and structure were investigated in 5 patients with limb-girdle or facioscapulohumeral muscular dystrophy or spinal muscular dystrophy.

Maximum isometric, dynamic, and isokinetic strength was measured in single-arm curl and double-leg press exercises before and after training. The contractile properties of the elbow flexors were also measured and computed tomography (CT) scans of the upper arms and thighs. Three persons underwent muscle biopsy of the biceps brachialis muscle of each arm. All 5 participated in dynamic weight training 3 times a week for 9 weeks. In arm exercises 1 arm was trained while the other acted as a control.

Strength in the trained arm increased from 19% to 34%. In the control arm strength went from −14% to +25%. Leg strength increased from 11% to 50%. Patients were able to lift the pretraining maximum load at least 3 times and up to 48 times after arm training. With the untrained arm they were able to lift the load from 1 to 13 times before fatigue. Training had no influence on the contractile properties of the elbow flexors, but before training 3 individuals had incomplete motor unit activation. Biopsy specimens and CT studies were inadequate to derive findings, but there was no evidence of additional structural damage to muscles.

Strength training may result in substantial increases in the strength and endurance capacities of individuals with slowly progressive neuromuscular disorders. Most gains in strength apparently result from neural adaptation rather than from muscle hypertrophy.

▶ Although we have the techniques readily available to quantify effects of a training program on muscle morphology, ultrastructure, biochemistry, and neurophysiology, little has been learned about patients with neuromuscular disorders. This is partly because of the anecdotal reports that a training program may be injurious to patients with various dystrophies. Albeit with few numbers, the present study was well designed with graduated exercise and did not demonstrate any adverse effect.

Furthermore, the improvement in strength and endurance achieved could have a substantial effect on the quality of life of such patients. Studies of this type are to be encouraged; in addition, more longitudinal studies are required.—J.R. Sutton, M.D.

Metabolic Effects of Repeated Weight Loss and Regain in Adolescent Wrestlers
Steen SN, Oppliger RA, Brownell KD (Univ of Pennsylvania; Univ of Iowa)
JAMA 260:47–50, July 1, 1988   17–14

Weight "cutting" by wrestlers can lead to adverse body composition changes, renal dysfunction, disordered thermal regulation, abnormal testosterone levels, and impaired strength. The effects on energy requirements of cyclic weight loss and regain were studied in 27 high school wrestlers, 14 of whom were classified as cyclic losers. The resting metabolic rate was measured by indirect calorimetry.

The resting metabolic rate was 14% less in cyclers than in noncyclers, who required 1,071 J less energy expenditure than the noncyclers under resting conditions. Oxygen consumption—but not respiratory quotient—differed significantly in the 2 groups. There were no important differences in pulse, blood pressure, or oral temperature.

It is possible that a low metabolic rate precedes weight cycling or even makes it necessary. As wrestlers lose and regain weight, fat may be lost and then regained in different areas of the body.

▶ It is increasingly recognized that reduction in the intake of food energy does not necessarily lead to a corresponding reduction of body mass. Although various factors contribute to this anomaly, one important influence is a reduction of the metabolic rate; resting metabolism is reduced, eating induces a smaller increase in metabolism, and there is a smaller elevation of the metabolic rate in the period after vigorous exercise. These findings have now been well documented in studies of patients with chronic obesity who are dieting, and also in malnourished individuals from developing countries, but it is interesting to note that the same type of metabolic response can be induced by the cyclic loss of body weight practiced by some wrestlers.

Some contribution to decreased metabolism might be anticipated from loss of lean tissue, but in the present report the lean mass was similar in those with and those without a cyclic pattern of weight loss. It is unfortunately not possible to infer a direct cause-and-effect relationship, because the study was cross-sectional in type. The authors advance the ingenious possibility that initial obesity gave the "cyclers" a low basal metabolic rate, and the resultant difficulty in reducing body mass led them to adopt the more dramatic and undesirable techniques common among the "cyclers."—R.J. Shephard, M.D., Ph.D.

Differences in Basal and Postexercise Osteocalcin Levels in Athletic and Nonathletic Humans

Nishiyama S, Tomoeda S, Ohta T, Higuchi A, Matsuda I (Kumamoto Univ Med School, Japan)
Calcif Tissue Int 43:150–154, 1988   17–15

In 9 athletic and 10 nonathletic male students, osteocalcin levels were monitored together with calcium metabolic hormones in relation to exercise. The ages ranged from 20 to 24 years. Nine practiced volleyball for 2 hours 5 days a week; the other 10 engaged in no comparable physical activity. Concentrations of osteocalcin, parathyroid hormone (PTH), calcitonin, and alkaline phosphatase, in addition to other serum concentrations, were monitored in these 2 groups before, immediately after, and 60 minutes after 30 minutes of exercise on a running ergometer. An adequate amount of drinking water was given to prevent hemoconcentration.

Similar changes in all concentration levels occurred in both groups. Immediately after exercise the serum PTH, phosphorus, and free fatty acid concentrations increased, and the serum ionized and total calcium concentrations decreased, in both groups. Before exercise, serum osteocalcin levels were significantly higher in the athletic students. The response to exercise differed between the 2 groups. Serum osteocalcin levels in the athletic group were unchanged immediately after exercise and increased 60 minutes later. In the nonathletic group the levels increased immediately after exercise and reverted to the preexercise level 60 minutes later.

The serum osteocalcin level in combination with the serum calcium and PTH levels were monitored because previous studies have indicated that osteocalcin reflects osteoblastic activity or bone formation and may be a sensitive index of component bone turnover. In these 19 students short-term, moderate-intensity exercise induced a significant elevation of osteocalcin levels immediately after exercise in nonathletes and 60 minutes after exercise in athletes, even when the circadian rhythm was considered. The serum osteocalcin concentration may be an indicator of the rate of bone turnover in physically active persons.

▶ Human plasma normally contains about 10.5 mg of calcium per dl. About a half of this total is loosely combined with the protein osteocalcin and thus cannot readily diffuse from the plasma. An excess of free calcium in the plasma would have adverse consequences for neuromuscular function, and it might thus be anticipated that increased calcium turnover in bone would be compensated by an increase of carrier protein. As in other tissues, an increased turnover is probably a prelude to a strengthening of bone, and the high preexercise osteocalcin levels in athletes may thus be considered a positive adaptation.—R.J. Shephard, M.D., Ph.D.

Premenopausal Bone Mass Is Related to Physical Activity
Aloia JF, Vaswani AN, Yeh JK, Cohn SH (Winthrop–Univ Hosp, Mineola, NY; Brookhaven Natl Lab, Upton, NY; State Univ of New York, Stony Brook)
Arch Intern Med 148:121–123, January 1988   17–16

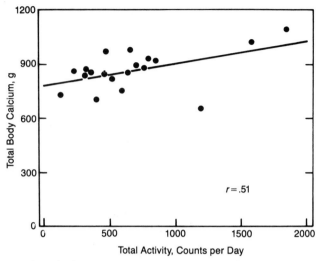

Fig 17–2.—Relationship between activity counts and total body calcium levels. (Courtesy of Aloia JF, Vaswani AN, Yeh JK, et al: *Arch Intern Med* 148:121–123, January 1988.)

Learning the effect of exercise on bone mass in the general population has been hindered by the inability to estimate habitual physical activity reliably in sedentary persons. Motion sensors—mechanical devices that measure body movement—are now available. The large-scale integrated (LSI) motion sensor provides measurements that correlate with other

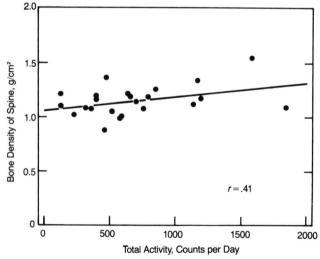

Fig 17–3.—Relationship between activity counts and bone density of spine. (Courtesy of Aloia JF, Vaswani AN, Yeh JK, et al: *Arch Intern Med* 148:121–123, January 1988.)

physiologic measures of the level of physical activity, has a low variability among units, and successfully distinguishes between population groups.

To determine the relationship between physical activity, as measured by the LSI and bone mass, 24 healthy, white, premenopausal, sedentary women were studied. Bone mineral levels were measured by single- and dual-photon absorptiometry and neutron activation analysis.

Total physical activity levels were related to both bone mineral density of the spine and total body calcium levels. No significant relationship was found between the bone density of the distal part of the radius and activity (Figs 17–2 and 17–3). Negative correlations were found between cigarette smoking and bone density of the spine and radius.

Physical activity is a major determinant of bone mass in white premenopausal women.

▶ Using the new activity monitoring device, large-scale integrated motion sensor, these authors have determined that there is a positive correlation between physical activity and bone mass in white premenopausal women. They point out that increasing activity to moderate levels in premenopausal women should result in the development of a higher peak bone mass. Being cautious, however, they believe that the findings from this cross-sectional study should be interpreted cautiously until clinical trials can be done to establish that the association observed between physical activity and bone mass is in fact causal.—Col. J.L. Anderson, PE.D.

Weight-Bearing Exercise Training and Lumbar Bone Mineral Content in Postmenopausal Women
Dalsky GP, Stocke KS, Ehsani AA, Slatopolsky E, Lee WC, Birge SJ Jr (Washington Univ)
Ann Intern Med 108:824–828, 1988   17–17

To evaluate weight-bearing exercise training and subsequent detraining on lumbar bone mineral content, 35 healthy, sedentary, postmenopausal women aged 55–70 years were assessed. Nineteen women exercised and 16 served as controls. Short-term and long-term weight-bearing exercise lasting for 9 months and 22 months, respectively, was undertaken, followed by 13 months of reduced training. All women were given 1,500 mg of calcium daily. The exercise group did weight-bearing exercise—walking, jogging, and stair climbing at 70% to 90% of maximal oxygen uptake capacity for 50–60 minutes 3 times a week.

Bone mineral content increased by 5.2% above baseline in participants in short-term training (Fig 17–4); there was no change in the control group. After 22 months of exercise, bone mineral content in training participants was 6.1% above baseline. After 13 months of decreased activity, the bone mass had decreased to 1.1% above baseline.

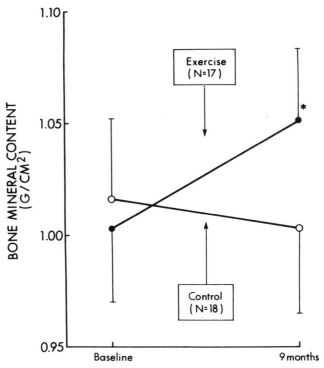

Fig 17–4.—Effect of weight-bearing exercise training on lumbar bone mineral content (gm/cm²). Values are mean ± SE. (*Closed circles* represent exercise group; *open circles,* control group.) *Significantly higher than 0 month of exercise (P = .0054). (Courtesy of Dalsky GP, Stocke KS, Ehsani AA, et al: *Ann Intern Med* 108:824–828, June 1988.)

Weight-bearing exercise apparently leads to significant increases in bone mineral content that are maintained with continued training in older, postmenopausal women. With reduced weight-bearing exercise, bone mass reverted to baseline values. Further studies should determine the threshold exercise prescription that will produce significant increases in bone mass.

▶ The results of this study showed that weight-bearing exercise training of the frequency, intensity, and duration used in this study can significantly increase the lumbar bone mineral content above baseline levels in postmenopausal women who have an adequate calcium intake. Although the exercise program used produced a significant increase in $\dot{V}O_{2max}$, there was no correlation between improved aerobic power and bone mineral content, which suggests that the stimulus for increasing bone mineral content may not be the same as needed to improve aerobic power. It appears likely that the critical element in the adaptation of bone to weight-bearing exercise is the stress or intensity applied to the skeleton, which would be a function for body weight and type and duration of exercise.—Col. J.L. Anderson, PE.D.

Hormone and Bone Mineral Status in Endurance-Trained and Sedentary Postmenopausal Women

Nelson ME, Meredith CN, Dawson-Hughes B, Evans WJ (Tufts Univ)
J Clin Endocrinol Metab 66:927–933, May 1988   17–18

If exercise is associated with lower weight and body fat, and lower weight is a risk factor for osteoporosis, exercise itself must alter calcium metabolism to enhance bone mineral density (BMD). The mechanisms by which exercise affects BMD are not known. The relationships between bone density at sites most often fractured in the elderly, endocrine status, and body composition were studied in 15 endurance-trained and 18 sedentary postmenopausal women (mean age, 62 years).

Endurance-trained women had lower body weight, lower body fat, and higher aerobic capacity. No differences in current calcium intake were noted between the 2 groups, but carbohydrate intake was higher in the endurance-trained women. Bone mineral density of the spine, proximal femur, and radius did not differ between groups; however, when normalized for body weight, the BMDs of the spine and radius in the endurance-trained group were higher than in the sedentary group (Fig 17–5). Serum esterone and parathyroid hormone levels were lower and 1,25-dihydroxyvitamin D and somatomedin-C levels higher in the endurance-trained women. Serum growth hormone levels tended to be higher in the endurance-trained group, and a postexercise increase in the

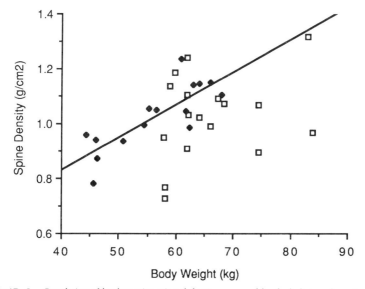

Fig 17–5.—Correlation of lumbar spine mineral density measured by dual-photon absorptiometry, and body weight in endurance-trained *(filled circles)* and sedentary *(open circles)* postmenopausal women(endurance-trained women: $r = .81$; $P = .0002$; sedentary women: $r = .31$; $P = .22$). Only the regression line for the endurance-trained women is shown ($y = .01188x + .3562$). (Courtesy of Nelson ME, Meredith CN, Dawson-Hughes B, et al: *J Clin Endocrinol Metab* 66:927–933, 1988.)

serum level of growth hormone was noted in the endurance-trained, but not the sedentary, women.

The major effect of regular exercise in this series was on body weight and hormone status. Although leanness and low serum esterone levels are risk factors for osteoporosis, these were not associated with lower BMD in this group of endurance-trained women. Improved calcium absorption in endurance-trained women may be the result of a higher carbohydrate intake and higher serum 1,25-dihydroxyvitamin D levels.

▶ And the search goes on! We are still trying to understand the relationship between a number of variables and osteoporosis. This study suggests that altered nutrient intake, to include elevated amounts of carbohydrates, and altered endocrine status enabled the endurance-trained postmenopausal women to maintain the same bone mineral status as the heavier sedentary postmenopausal women who had higher serum estrone levels.—Col. J.L. Anderson, PE.D.

Suitability of Cyproterone Acetate in the Treatment of Osteoporosis Associated With Athletic Amenorrhea
De Crée C, Lewin R, Ostyn M (Catholic Univ of Leuven, Belgium; Univ of Copenhagen)
Int J Sports Med 9:187–192, June 1988   17–19

A sharply reduced spine mineral content is associated with long-distance running in women. The link between menstrual irregularity and osteoporosis in athletes appears obvious, but no satisfactory explanations have been offered.

The efficacy of the antiandrogenic agent cyproterone actetate (CA) in its contraceptive form was evaluated in the treatment of osteoporosis associated with athletic amenorrhea in 7 high-performance athletes and 4 women with similar characteristics who served as controls. The mean age was 22 years. Training began at a mean age of 14 years, and mean training intensity expressed as kilometers run per week was 35.

Mineral density was primarily affected by the hypoestrogenic status of the athletes. All participants had low serum progesterone and luteinizing hormone profiles during the midluteal phase. Cyproterone acetate was given for 8 months to treat the increased bone loss in the 7 athletes. Vertebral density appeared to be elevated; cortical base mineral content measured at the radius was not changed significantly.

Cyproterone acetate, given in combination with estrogens, is suitable for the treatment of osteoporosis caused by a hypoestrogenic status. This treatment could replace other contraceptive agents. Women with the most severe estrogen deficiency had a more pronounced reaction to this therapy.

▶ It has become generally accepted that prolonged exercise-induced amenorrhea and anovulation in women who are long-distance runners may result in a sharply decreased spine mineral content. As yet, there are no satisfactory explanations to explain this link between exercise-induced amenorrhea and osteoporosis. This study appears to show that estrogen replacement, complemented with cyproterone acetate as an alternative gestagen, is a suitable approach to treatment of osteoporosis associated with athletic amenorrhea. This is the same treatment that was previously found effective in treating postmenopausal osteoporosis.—Col. J.L. Anderson, PE.D.

Menstrual Status in Female Athletes: Correlation With Reproductive Hormones and Bone Density
Baker E, Demers L (Richland Mem Hosp/Univ of South Carolina, Columbia; Pennsylvania State Univ, Hershey)
Obstet Gynecol 72:683–687, November 1988   17–20

Previous studies have reported that amenorrheic athletes appear to have reduced bone density and a higher risk of stress fractures. To determine the effects of strenuous exercise on reproductive function and skeletal integrity, serum hormone concentrations, bone mass, and dietary practices were studied in college athletes and sedentary controls.

Ten eumenorrheic and 6 oligomenorrheic athletes and 12 control women matched for age, height, and weight were studied. The eumenorrheic women began sports training earlier than the oligomenorrheic women. Oligomenorrheic women had significantly lower serum estradiol concentrations during cycle weeks 2 and 3, but had an increase in this hormone concentration during cycle week 4. Significant differences in serum gonadotropin concentrations during week 4 were noted in the oligomenorrheic women. There was no significant difference in spinal mineral density values in the 3 groups.

In these collegiate athletes, minimal but significant changes in serum hormonal and gonadotropin concentrations may result in menstrual dysfunction, but bone density appears to be unaffected.

▶ This study is included because it does not totally agree with other previous studies that have reported bone density among amenorrheic athletes. The difference may be explained because of the difference in the study groups. These authors examined collegiate athletes, whereas other authors have usually reported on elite athletes. We can assume that elite athletes train at a higher level of intensity than collegiate athletes do.— Col. J.L. Anderson, PE.D.

18 Environmental Factors

Sleep Patterns

Submaximal Exercise Effects on Sleep Patterns in Young Women Before and After an Aerobic Training Programme
Driver HS, Meintjes AF, Rogers GG, Shapiro CM (Univ of the Witwatersrand Med School, Johannesburg; Univ of Edinburgh)
Acta Physiol Scand 133:8–13, 1988   18–1

Most studies can be interpreted as supporting the hypothesis that sleep serves a restorative function, but some studies have not found a significant effect of exercise on slow-wave sleep. The interaction of the state of fitness and performance of an exercise task in persons acting as their own controls has not been studied. The effects of submaximal exercise on the sleep patterns of young women, untrained and after training, were examined in an attempt to disentangle life-style and fitness effects, establishing the impact of exercise on sleep.

Nine untrained women underwent a 12-week fitness program. Baseline sleep patterns and sleep patterns after 1 hour of submaximal exercise performed in the evening were compared at 0 and 12 weeks. Sleep was divided into rapid eye movement (REM) and non-REM (NREM) sleep, with NREM sleep being subdivided into slow-wave sleep (stages 3 and 4) and stages 1 and 2. The submaximal exercise involved cycling for 1 hour at 70% of maximal oxygen consumption. A significant improvement in cardiorespiratory fitness did not produce any changes in baseline sleep parameters. The response to the submaximal exercise was an increase in stage 2 NREM sleep and a reduction in slow-wave sleep, stages 3 and 4, which may indicate a stress effect. Compared with the untrained state, slow-wave sleep in the trained state was significantly higher after an exercise load.

These data demonstrated that although improvement in cardiorespiratory fitness did not change baseline sleep parameters, the response to the exercise load did change; slow-wave sleep levels were higher when the women were trained than when untrained. Training and submaximal exercise tended to shorten sleep-onset latency and lengthen the latency to REM sleep, although this result was not significant.

▶ If sleep is to serve its intended restorative function, it is important that it contain an adequate component of deep (slow EEG wave) sleep. Although the present bout of exercise (70% of maximum oxygen intake for 1 hour) was performed quite early in the evening (between 4:00 PM and 7:00 PM), it nevertheless caused some decrease of slow-wave sleep in the unfit women. Twelve weeks of training, inducing an increase of about 10% in maximal oxygen intake, were apparently sufficient to correct this problem. The findings suggest that a training program may help patients who complain of unsatisfying sleep.—R.J. Shephard, M.D., Ph.D.

Epidemiology of Exercise Effects on Sleep

Vuori I, Urponen H, Hasan J, Partinen M (Central Hosp, Hämeenlinna, Finland; Univ of Helsinki)
Acta Physiol Scand 133:3–7, 1988   18–2

Quality of sleep, a major element of quality of life, is affected by many factors. It is generally thought that leisure-time exercise is a sleep-enhancing activity. This belief is partly supported and partly challenged by experimental evidence. A survey was designed to study the characteristics of sleep and perceived factors promoting and disturbing sleep.

Several living habits, including exercise, and sleep characteristics were studied independently of each other by a pretested questionnaire and a sleep diary mailed to a stratified random sample of 200 men and women in each of 4 age groups: 36, 41, 46, and 50 years. The total sample was 1,600, and the response rate was 75%.

Every third respondent believed that exercise (e.g., jogging) had a positive impact on the quality of sleep. The most frequently perceived positive effects of exercise were ease of falling asleep, depth of sleep, a sense of well-being, and greater alertness in the morning. Negative perceived effects of exercise were uncommon. The balance of positive and negative perceived exercise effects was more favorable when the activity was performed early in the evening compared with late at night. When both intensity and timing of exercise were considered, light and moderate exercise, particularly in the early evening, had mainly positive effects on sleep. The frequency of negative influences increased when the exercise was performed vigorously late at night. However, a considerable proportion of vigorous late-night exercisers reported mostly positive effects (table).

These data suggest that light and moderate exercise early in the evening should be emphasized in health education as a way to enhance and improve the quality of sleep. Epidemiologic data on exercise and sleep require further investigation and verification using objective methods and controlled interventions.

▶ Lack of adequate or satisfying sleep is a common complaint in the office of the general practitioner, and it is widely held that moderate exercise may be helpful in alleviating sleep problems. The positive effects reported here can be explained in terms of mental or physical relaxation and possibly by a slight elevation of body temperature. However, vigorous exercise is also recognized as

Perceived Effects of Exercise, Alcohol, and Mental Work on Sleep*

	Exercise	Alcohol		Mental work
	early %	little %	much %	%
Easier to fall asleep	70	63	71	32
Deeper sleep	66	36	42	14
Difficult to fall asleep	7	16	26	71
Restless sleep	6	23	54	55
Early awakening	5	18	42	34
Better feeling in the morning	65	13	12	11
More tired in the morning	2	28	80	40

*Proportions (%) of those who evaluated the habit as having some or a clear influence on sleep.
(Courtesy of Vuori I, Urponen H, Hasan J, et al: *Acta Physiol Scand* 133:3–7, 1988.)

an arousing stimulus; an increased blood level of catecholamines, a greater rise in body temperature, and increased nerve traffic through the reticular formation of the brain wake the patient up. For instance, the expressway driver who is starting to feel sleepy on a night drive is commonly advised to take a brief walk around a rest area. It is thus not surprising that exercise can cause sleep problems if it is undertaken too late at night. Timing is all important. This is particularly true in a hot part of the world, where it may be necessary to wait until after supper before the outdoor temperature is cool enough to permit many forms of activity.—R.J. Shephard, M.D., Ph.D.

Circadian Variation in Blood Pressure Responses to Muscular Exercise
Cabri J, De Witte B, Clarys JP, Reilly T, Strass D (Free Univ of Brussels; Liverpool Polytechnic, England; Univ of Freiburg, West Germany)
Ergonomics 31:1559–1565, November 1988   18–3

Metabolic responses to steady-state exercise vary with the time of day. To assess the impact of circadian rhythms on safety in recreational exercise, 12 men performed short-term intense exercise 6 times daily at 2:00 AM, 6:00 AM, 10:00 AM, 2:00 PM, 6:00 PM, and 10 PM. Body weight, rectal temperature, muscle function, and blood pressure were examined for circadian rhythmicity.

Blood Pressure (mm Hg) Post Exercise in 12 Individuals at 6 Different Times of Day

Test	02:00	06:00	10:00	14:00	18:00	22:00
Rest						
Systolic	129±9	125±7	126±10	127±8	129±11	134±14
Diastolic	86±7	83±6	83±9	81±6	83±8	82±10
Slow isokinetic movement						
Systolic	141±7	137±11	142±13	142±10	144±12	147±13
Diastolic *	88±10	82±8	79±10	82±10	82±7	83±11
Fast isokinetic movement						
Systolic	142±8	137±10	141±12	140±10	140±12	145±15
Diastolic	90±10	84±8	83±10	84±7	85±10	84±10
Isometric test						
Systolic	145±12	139±13	143±16	146±15	142±16	151±16
Diastolic *	87±11	83±8	77±9	78±7	82±9	83±11
Fatigue test						
Systolic	152±14	147±15	150±13	151±20	153±12	154±17
Diastolic *	87±12	85±8	78±10	75±10	82±11	83±12

*Includes significant rhythm.
(Courtesy of Cabri J, De Witte B, Clarys JP, et al: *Ergonomics* 31:1559–1565, November 1988.)

Rectal temperature had a significant circadian rhythm, peaking at 6:18 PM. Body weight did not vary significantly during the day. Blood pressure variation with time of day was not significant at rest. Postexercise systolic pressures did not have significant rhythms, but diastolic pressures had significant circadian rhythms after slow isokinetic movements, after the 20-second maximum isometric test, and after the 60-second fatigue test (table). The peak time varied between 00:37 AM and 02:05 AM.

Blood pressure is most disturbed by acute exercise at night and in the early morning. Exercisers should be cautioned about performing brief bouts of intense exercise at these times.

▶ Many body functions vary over the 24-hour cycle, and there has been much discussion of methods to optimize such "circadian" rhythms, particularly when athletes are crossing several time zones to participate in international competitions. Probably the most significant shift from the competitive point of view is the disturbance of vigilance. Physiologic changes are relatively small, although the 8–10 mm Hg variation of exercise diastolic pressure could be significant in an older individual with somewhat marginal coronary circulation.—R.J. Shephard, M.D., Ph.D.

Air Pollutants

Physical Training and Fasting Erythrocyte Activities of Free Radical Scavenging Enzyme Systems in Sedentary Men

Ohno H, Yahata T, Sato Y, Yamamura K, Taniguchi N (Asahikawa Med College; Nagoya Univ; Osaka Univ, Japan)
Eur J Appl Physiol 57:173–176, February 1988   18–4

Several hematologic changes may be induced by long-distance running. Reportedly, brief submaximal physical exercise increases total glutathione reductase (GR) activity in human erythrocytes. The effects of endurance training on the free radical scavenging enzyme systems in human erythrocytes were assessed in 7 sedentary healthy males aged 18–19 years who underwent 10 weeks of physical training that included running more than 5 km 6 times a week.

Maximum oxygen uptake and the 12-minute walk-run performance increased significantly after training. Of the antioxidant enzyme systems studied in the erythrocytes, both catalase activity and concentration and total GR activity were significantly higher after the training period (table). The erythrocyte GR activity coefficient also increased significantly.

Chronic aerobic exercise increases riboflavin requirements and has positive effects on antioxidative processes. However, the exact mechanisms that cause these changes are unknown.

▶ One of the potentially adverse effects of vigorous exercise is the accumulation of an increased concentration of "free radicals," intermediate products in

Effects of 10-Week Running on Free Radical Scavenging Enzyme Systems in Human Erythrocytes

Biochemical parameter	Before	After	Probability
GSH, mg·gHb^{-1}	2.36±0.10	2.44±0.11	N. S.
G-6-PD, IU·gHb^{-1}	12.1±0.9	12.3±1.3	N. S.
6-PGD, IU·gHb^{-1}	8.80±0.33	9.17±0.35	N. S.
GSH-Px, IU·gHb^{-1}	31.6±1.9	31.5±1.8	N. S.
GR, IU·gHb^{-1}			
Total (with FAD)	10.4±0.5	13.3±0.7	$P<0.02$
Active (without FAD)	7.38±0.39	8.20±0.45	N. S.
CAT			
Activity, ×10^4 IU·gHb^{-1}	15.2±1.1	17.1±11.3	$P<0.05$
Concentration, mg·gHb^{-1}	1.77±0.06	1.90±0.08	$P<0.05$
SOD			
Activity, ×10^3 unit·gHb^{-1}	9.66±0.58	10.4±0.7	N. S.
Concentration, mg·gHb^{-1}	0.610±0.018	0.647±0.013	N. S.
Hb, g·100 ml^{-1} of whole blood	15.1±0.3	14.8±0.5	N. S.
Hct, %	44.6±1.0	44.4±1.2	N. S.
ΔCV†, %		2.14±1.86	

*Values are means ±SEM.
†Red blood cell volume change.
(Courtesy of Ohno H, Yahata T, Sato Y, et al: Eur J Appl Physiol 57:173–176, February 1988.)

the oxidation of hydrogen ions to water (1). Among other undesirable actions, free radicals can lead to errors of DNA replication (accelerating the process of aging at the cellular level) and can destroy cellular membranes. Leakage of cellular contents is a well-recognized consequence of very prolonged exercise, and could reflect oxidant damage. Likewise, red blood cells show altered mechanical properties suggestive of metabolic changes in their membranes after a

100-km run (2). Taken alone, such findings might destroy a physician's enthusiasm for exercise! However, the positive side of the equation is that regular training also increases the concentrations of various enzymes that break down free radicals. Jenkins et al. (3) previously demonstrated this for skeletal muscle, and the present paper demonstrates a parallel change in erythrocytes.—R.J. Shephard, M.D., Ph.D.

References

1. Shephard RJ: *Biochemistry of Exercise.* Springfield, Ill, Charles C Thomas, 1983.
2. Reinhart WH, et al: *J Appl Physiol* 54:827–830, 1984.
3. Jenkins RP, et al: *Int J Sports Med* 5:11–14, 1984.

Effects of Ambient Ozone on Respiratory Function in Healthy Adults Exercising Outdoors
Spektor DM, Lippmann M, Thurston GD, Lioy PJ, Stecko J, O'Connor G, Garshick E, Speizer FE, Hayes C (New York Univ, Tuxedo, NY; Brigham and Women's Hosp, Boston; Harvard Med School; US Environmental Protection Agency, Research Triangle Park, NC)
Am Rev Respir Dis 138:821–828, October 1988   18–5

Previous studies of the effects of ambient air pollution on the respiratory function in children have shown consistent associations between decrements in spirometric indexes and concentrations of ozone (O_3). The extent to which O_3 and other air pollutants affect the respiratory function during outdoor exercise was examined in 30 healthy adult nonsmokers. The exercises were performed in a largely wooded area in upstate New York. Before each exercise period the participants completed an acute symptoms questionnaire and performed at least 3 acceptable spirometric maneuvers. After exercising on the same course at the same level each day, they took their own pulses. Spirometric maneuvers were performed post exercise. A mobile laboratory monitored pollutant and environmental data.

Ozone concentrations ranged from 21 to 124 parts per billion. During only 4 of 448 exposures did the O_3 concentration exceed the current national ambient air quality standards. All measured functional indexes showed significant O_3 associated mean decrements (table). Mean decrements were smaller in 10 persons with minute ventilations of more than 100 L than in 10 others with minute ventilations between 60 L and 100 L or in 10 with minute ventilations of less than 60 L. In 10 individuals with minute ventilations similar to those used in controlled 1-hour and 2-hour exposures to O_3 in purified air in chambers, the effects were almost twice as large as those found in the chamber studies.

Ambient cofactors can potentiate responses to O_3. Results of studies in

Mean Regression Slopes (±SE) for Changes in Respiratory Function Indexes After Outdoor Exercise vs. Ambient Ozone Concentrations

Data Set	FVC (ml/ppb O_3)	FEV_1 (ml/ppb)	PEFR (ml/s/ppb)	FEF_{25-75} (ml/s/ppb)	FEV_1/FVC (%/ppb)
Full, n = 30	-2.08 ± 0.46†	-1.35 ± 0.35†	-9.21 ± 1.69†	-6.00 ± 1.04†	-0.0376 ± 0.0084†
Male, n = 20	-2.45 ± 0.65†	-1.86 ± 0.73*	-12.07 ± 2.14†	-6.28 ± 1.49†	-0.0410 ± 0.0122†
Female, n = 10	-1.35 ± 0.41†	-1.31 ± 0.44*	-3.47 ± 1.72*	-5.44 ± 1.01†	-0.0309 ± 0.0068†
< 60 L§, n = 10	-1.91 ± 0.71*	-1.75 ± 0.59*	-4.89 ± 2.36*‡	-6.74 ± 1.32†	-0.0418 ± 0.0132*
60 to 100 L§, n = 10	-2.30 ± 0.95*	-1.74 ± 0.71*	-14.26 ± 2.61†	-8.64 ± 1.93†	-0.0437 ± 0.181*
> 100 L§, n = 10	-2.03 ± 0.78*	-0.55 ± 0.45‡	-8.50 ± 3.20‡	-2.63 ± 1.72‡	-0.0273 ± 0.0125*
< 80 ppb, n = 29	-1.42 ± 0.63*	-1.30 ± 0.62*	-6.60 ± 2.40*	-5.51 ± 1.38*	-0.0359 ± 0.0097†

*Significantly different from zero slope at $P < .05$.
†Significantly different from zero slope at $P < .01$.
‡Significantly different from slope of middle range at $P < .05$ by analysis of variance.
§Estimated minute volume during exercise in liters based on individually determined pulse rate–ventilation rate calibrations.
(Courtesy of Spektor DM, Lippmann M, Thurston GD, et al: Am Rev Respir Dis 138:821–828, October 1988.)

chambers may substantially underestimate O_3-associated responses in individuals engaged in outdoor recreation.

▶ Previous chamber studies have suggested that the threshold concentration of O_3 exposure affecting respiratory function is about 0.75 ppm at rest, dropping to 0.35 ppm in moderate exercise, and possibly as low as 0.1 ppm in all-out effort. Such levels are encountered only in major conurbations on very polluted days. The present report illustrates the danger of relying simply on-controlled chamber experiments, because it suggests that under normal ambient conditions (which may include exposure to other pollutants, or to cold and dry air), the threshold is substantially lower than in the laboratory.

From the viewpoint of the team physician, the important lesson is that O_3 is produced by sunlight. Pollutant levels are thus dramatically lower in the early morning than in mid-afternoon, and exposure can be controlled rather readily by adjustment in the times of practice and competition.—R.J. Shephard, M.D., Ph.D.

High Altitude

Operation Everest II: Oxygen Transport During Exercise at Extreme Simulated Altitude
Sutton JR, Reeves JT, Wagner PD, Groves BM, Cymerman A, Malconian MK, Rock PB, Young PM, Walter SD, Houston CS (McMaster Univ, Hamilton, Ont; Univ of Colorado; Univ of California, San Diego, La Jolla; US Army Research Inst of Environmental Medicine, Natick, Mass; Univ of Vermont)
J Appl Physiol 64:1309–1321, 1988   18–6

Operation Everest II is a project in which a series of studies examine the physiologic effects of high altitude. Direct circulatory measurements were made of cardiac output and gas exchange using arterial and Swan-Ganz catheterization during exercise in a decompression chamber.

Eight healthy young men took part in the study. Most were active athletes, but only 2 had climbing experience at high altitudes. Six completed all of the altitude tests. The decompression chamber was at sea level. In a 40-day period the barometric pressure was lowered to achieve the effect of an ascent of Everest. Measurements obtained included electrocardiogram, arterial O_2 saturation, expired ventilation, mixed expired O_2 (FE_{O_2}) and CO_2 (FE_{CO_2}), blood lactate, arterial and mixed venous blood gases, cardiac output, and hemoglobin and hematocrit.

At all barometric pressures, an increase of work brought about an increase in $\dot{V}O_2$ and $\dot{V}CO_2$. As PI_{O_2} decreased, there was a decrease in maximal O_2 uptake from a mean of 3.98 L/minute at sea level to 1.17 L/minute at PI_{O_2} 43 torr. At this point, profound hypoxemia and hypocapnia occurred.

For a given $\dot{V}O_2$, $PI_{O_2}-PA_{O_2}$ during maximal exercise at altitude is far less than at an identical $\dot{V}O_2$ at sea level. The most important factors involved in transport of O_2 from the atmosphere to the tissues were adaptations in ventilation and maximal extraction of oxygen at the tissue. Altitude did not change diffusion from alveolus to end-capillary blood. Except at PI_{O_2} 43 torr, mass circulatory transport of O_2 to tissue capillaries remained unaffected by altitude.

The work capacity seen in these 8 men suggests that they would have been unable to climb to the summit of Everest without supplementary oxygen. Increased ventilation and a reduction of $P\bar{v}_{O_2}$ maintains O_2 transport. Oxygen was moved from the atmosphere to the alveolus and diffused from the capillary to the tissue mitochondria. The results, although not in a natural setting, demonstrate that humans can work at barometric pressures and O_2 pressure considered to be at the limits of survival.

▶ This is a key paper in the series "Operation Everest II (OEII)," a decompression chamber study simulating a climb of Mt. Everest. Inspired oxygen pressure was simulated, but none of the other variables of the mountain environment such as varying temperature, dehydration, or lack of access to food was present. Of the 8 men who began the study, 6 made it to the "summit" and had the first direct blood measurements made of key variables.

Various exercise studies were performed in OEII including (1) a traditional $\dot{V}O_2$ max test, (2) a progressive test to exhaustion in which blood and muscle biopsy samples were taken, (3) an isolated test of the tibialis anterior muscle with and without electrical stimulation, and (4) the test described in this paper, involving steady-state exercise on a cycle ergometer at several exercise intensities, infusion of inert gases to quantify V/Q, and sampling of blood from indwelling arterial and pulmonary artery catheters. The usual cardiorespiratory variables were also measured.

The most dramatic findings were a reduction in $\dot{V}O_2$ max from 50 ml/kg/minute to 15 ml/kg/minute and a fourfold increase in alveolar ventilation. Blood gases showed a progressive decrease in P_{CO_2} as $P_{I_{O_2}}$ fell. Whereas $(A-a)D_{O_2}$ and cardiac output did not vary at altitude, O_2 extraction was maximal. A further point of interest is confirmation of Edwards' earlier work that, with acclimatization, the blood lactate concentration decreases at altitude despite decreasing $P_{I_{O_2}}$ and $P_{A_{O_2}}$, which might be expected to increase it. Clearly, such an invasive study would not be possible at extreme altitudes on the mountain, but its success has given us a wealth of new and rather unique physiologic information to help explain how such feats are possible. However we interpret the physiology, it is obvious that even superhumans such as Messner and Habeler, the first to reach the summit of Everest without using supplementary oxygen, were on the very limits of human survival.—J.R. Sutton, M.D.

Operation Everest II: Pulmonary Gas Exchange During a Simulated Ascent of Mt Everest
Wagner PD, Sutton JR, Reeves JT, Cymerman A, Groves BM, Malconian MK (Univ of California, San Diego, La Jolla; US Army Research Inst of Environmental Medicine, Natick, Mass)
J Appl Physiol 63:2348–2359, December 1987   18–7

Eight normal individuals of varying athletic ability were subjected to decompression at a barometric pressure of 240 torr for 40 days, simulating an ascent to the summit of Mt. Everest. In 6 who completed the experiment, ventilation-perfusion relationships were evaluated by the multiple inert gas elimination technique evaluated both at rest and while performing exercise (up to 80% to 90% of maximal oxygen uptake).

Dispersion of the blood flow distribution increased by 64% from rest to a workload of 215 W, both at sea level and at a barometric pressure of 428 torr. At 347 torr the increase was 79% (exercise to 159 W), and at 282 torr it was 112% (exercise to 108 W). At 240 torr an increase of 9% occurred (exercise to 60 W). The dispersion did not correlate with cardiac output, ventilation, or pulmonary wedge pressure but did so with mean pulmonary artery pressure.

Variable but increasing ventilation-perfusion mismatching is associated with long-term exposure to both altitude and exercise. Alveolar interstitial edema is the likely primary cause of inequality. The predominant pulmonary abnormalities associated with exposure to extreme altitude probably result from pulmonary interstitial fluid accumulation.

▶ This is also one of the series of papers entitled "Operation Everest II" in which subjects simulated a climb of Mt. Everest and had a variety of investigations performed. In spite of a fourfold increase in alveolar ventilation at the "summit of Everest," which is one of the most important adaptations to altitude, gas exchange function of the lung showed some degree of impairment. The authors speculate that interstitial edema was a possible cause.—J.R. Sutton, M.D.

Effects of Altered CSF [H⁺] on Ventilatory Responses to Exercise in the Awake Goat

Smith CA, Jameson LC, Dempsey JA (Univ of Wisconsin)
J Appl Physiol 65:921–927, August 1988   18–8

An experiment was designed to reveal how medullary chemoreception might interact with ventilatory stimuli brought about by exercise and increases in metabolic rate. Five adult female goats were trained to exercise on a treadmill and wear a tight-fitting respiratory mask at intervals.

Cerebrospinal fluid (CSF) was altered until a new steady condition of alveolar hypo- or hyperventilation was reached. The goats completed 2 levels of steady-state treadmill exercise. The animals usually hyperventilated somewhat from rest through exercise when the CSF had a normal acid-base state. Changing CSF[H⁺] during exercise did not normally alter the regulation of partial pressure of CO_2 in arterial blood (Pa_{CO_2}).

As far as alteration in the gain of exercise ventilatory response, the alteration did not need a chronic shift in the resting level. Even when resting levels are markedly changed, the alteration occurs with equal precision in the regulation of exercise Pa_{CO_2}.

In the steady state the primary controller(s) of exercise hyperpnea can function independently from the central or peripheral chemoreceptors. By using unanesthetized animals it was possible to study physiologic states with unmodified receptor sites, neural pathways, and response gains.

▶ This is a particularly elegant study in which the authors were able to examine independently the effect of the peripheral chemoreceptor by using carotid body-denervated goats in which the acid-base medium of the central chemoreceptors was altered by perfusing mock CSF into the cisternum with H^+ concentrations varying from 21 to 95 nEq/L. In spite of these major perturbations, ventilation was dependent primarily on metabolic rate, i.e., $\dot{V}CO_2$, although as expected, the set point varied enormously. The study again emphasizes how well matched ventilation is to metabolic demands.—J.R. Sutton, M.D.

The Lung at High Altitude: Bronchoalveolar Lavage in Acute Mountain Sickness and Pulmonary Edema
Schoene RB, Swenson ER, Pizzo CJ, Hackett PH, Roach RC, Mills WJ Jr, Henderson WR Jr, Martin TR (Univ of Washington; Seattle VA Med Ctr; St Anthony's Hosp, Denver; Univ of Alaska, Anchorage)
J Appl Physiol 64:2605–2613, June 1988   18–9

High altitude can bring about a number of medical problems including high-altitude pulmonary edema (HAPE) and acute mountain sickness (AMS). High-altitude pulmonary edema, a noncardiogenic edema, is a severe illness associated with high concentrations of proteins and cells in lavage fluids. Acute mountain sickness is characterized by impaired gas exchange and is less serious than HAPE. In this study the cellular and biochemical content of fluid obtained by bronchoalveolar lavage was compared in 7 climbers with AMS or HAPE and in a normal healthy person. Studies were performed at an altitude of 4,400 m (barometric pressure of 440 torr). Cell counts and differentials were performed at the research site, and the remainder of the fluids were frozen for later analysis.

The healthy control had an arterial O_2 saturation of 83%. Climbers with HAPE had a mean O_2 saturation of 55%, and those with AMS, 70%. The patients with HAPE had the highest leukocyte count. They also tended to have higher percentages of neutrophils. Those with severe HAPE had notable increases in the total protein concentration in lavage fluid and corresponding increases in levels of albumin and IgG. Patients with AMS had protein concentrations in lavage fluid similar to those in normal individuals. Other measurements showed equivalent results in AMS and normal persons.

Although gas exchange was impaired with AMS, concentrations of proteins and cells in the air space were not altered. Acute mountain sickness was not proven to be an earlier stage of HAPE. Remarkably, HAPE resolved rapidly with movement to a lower altitude, even after protein concentrations in the alveolar fluid were higher than those found in acute respiratory distress syndrome. Climbers with both HAPE and AMS recovered, and 6 were able to resume their ascent.

▶ This important study helps to shed light on the possible mechanisms of the high-altitude medical problems of AMS and HAPE. In a tent at an altitude of 4,400 m on Mt. McKinley, these investigators performed bronchoalveolar lavage on normal climbers and a number of "patients" with AMS or HAPE. The major mechanistic controversy regarding the pathogenesis of HAPE is whether the edema is caused by increased "permeability" or by increased transudation.

Another popular hypothesis was that both AMS and HAPE were of a similar etiology, with HAPE being simply a more severe form of AMS. Although the numbers of subjects and patients were small, there seemed to be a very clear-cut distinction, those with HAPE and severe hypoxemia having markedly increased proteins in the alveolar lavage fluid. In addition, some of the mediators such as C5a and thromboxane B2 were markedly increased in the HAPE victims.

It is important that this study be repeated and the findings confirmed by other workers as it seems seminal in high-altitude medicine.—J.R. Sutton, M.D.

Effect of Carbon Dioxide in Acute Mountain Sickness: A Rediscovery
Harvey TC, Winterborn MH, Lassen NA, Raichle ME, Jensen J, Richardson NV, Bradwell AR (Univ of Birmingham, England; Washington Univ; Bispebjerg Hosp, Copenhagen; Univ of Liverpool, England)
Lancet 2:639–641, Sept 17, 1988   18–10

To study the effect of CO_2 in acute mountain sickness 6 patients with moderate acute mountain sickness were studied at altitudes between 3,400 m and 5,400 m. As they became ill with clinical symptoms (headache, vomiting, nausea, ataxia), each patient was placed on a mattress and breathed air for several minutes via a nonreturn valve until a steady state was reached. A 3% CO_2 air mixture was then inhaled for between 12 and 25 minutes. Earlobe capillary blood samples were obtained and blood and gas samples analyzed.

A striking increase in PaO_2 and SaO_2, a small decline in pH, and a rise in $PaCO_2$ as a consequence of increased ventilation were noted during inhalation of CO_2. Considerable improvement in oxygenation with corresponding clinical benefit was achieved. The patients noted prompt relief of headache and other features such as nausea, ataxia, drowsiness, and weakness. In 3 patients cerebral blood flow was increased by 17% to 39%, suggesting that oxygen delivery to the brain was improved. It was feared that the predicted increase in cerebral blood flow induced by the breathing of CO_2 might precipitate acute cerebral edema and exacerbated headache; however, despite an increase in cerebral blood flow, relief of neurologic symptoms occurred within minutes. The rapid response suggests that the cerebral symptoms of acute mountain sickness result from hypoxic nervous tissue rather than from edema. The beneficial effects of CO_2 inhalation at high altitudes were confirmed.

▶ Those interested in mountaineering and aviation medicine have recognized for many years that acute exposure to high altitude leads to an uneasy compromise between hyperventilation, which increases alveolar and thus arterial oxygen pressure, and the dangers of a resultant hypocapnia (with such adverse consequences as intermittent breathing and a reduction of cerebral blood flow). As early as 1898 the Italian physiologist Mosso was using carbon dioxide mixtures to relieve the symptoms of men in a hypobaric chamber. If carbon dioxide is available, this can be added to the inspirate in sufficient quantities to relieve hypocapnia, without greatly reducing the inspired oxygen pressure; by restoring the chemoreceptor drive, ventilation may even be improved, with an increase in arterial oxygen pressure, as in the present experiments.

The early research on the therapeutic value of carbon dioxide was largely forgotten with the advent of drugs such as Diamox (acetazolamide). However, the increase of cerebral blood flow found by Harvey and associates is impressive, given that some physiologists have argued for a maximum change in cerebral flow of 10%. A 39% augmentation of cerebral flow would make an enormous difference to brain function under conditions of marginal oxygenation.

In recent years there has been growing concern about the cerebral component of acute mountain sickness, and it is instructive to find confirmation of the early observations of Yandell Henderson (1) that the headache and other acute symptoms of high-altitude exposure are relieved rather than worsened by carbon dioxide. On a long mountaineering expedition, Diamox tablets are likely to prove more popular than heavy carbon dioxide cylinders, but nevertheless the breathing of carbon dioxide may have some role in the treatment of acute mountain sickness, particularly in a hospital environment.—R.J. Shephard, M.D., Ph.D.

Reference

1. Henderson Y: *Adventures in Respiration.* London, Baillière, Tindall and Cox, 1938.

Incidence of Acute Mountain Sickness at Intermediate Altitude
Montgomery AB, Mills J, Luce JM (San Francisco Gen Hosp; Univ of California, San Francisco)
JAMA 261:732–734, Feb 3, 1989   18–11

Acute mountain sickness (AMS) may occur in persons who ascend quickly to high altitudes. To examine the incidence of AMS at intermediate altitudes, a questionnaire was given to 454 persons who attended week-long continuing medical education seminars in the Rocky Mountains at base elevations of approximately 2,000 m. A control group of 96 persons attending seminars at sea level completed similar questionnaires. To be classified as having AMS, respondents had to have experienced at least a moderate degree of 3 or more of these symptoms: headache, dyspnea, insomnia, anorexia, or fatigue.

Twenty-five percent of respondents in the Rocky Mountain survey reported acute AMS-like symptoms as compared with only 5% of persons at sea level. Those who had come from lower altitudes were most at risk for AMS. Medication was used by half of those with symptoms. Ninety percent of symptoms occurred in the first 72 hours and their duration was short.

Further studies of preventive or therapeutic measures for AMS are needed.

Effects of Dexamethasone on the Incidence of Acute Mountain Sickness at Two Intermediate Altitudes
Montgomery AB, Luce JM, Michael P, Mills J (San Francisco Gen Hosp; Univ of California, San Francisco)
JAMA 261:734–736, Feb 3, 1989   18–12

Dexamethasone acetate reportedly can ameliorate symptoms of acute mountain sickness (AMS) in patients at high altitudes. It also is effective prophylaxis in climbers rapidly ascending to these altitudes. To determine the effects of dexamethasone in individuals at intermediate altitudes, 70 health professionals attending a seminar at an elevation of 2,700 m were examined. Of these, 35 were given dexamethasone acetate and 35 took placebo every 6 hours for 6 doses beginning at the time of exposure. In a similar experiment at another location at 2,050 m, 24 persons were given dexamethasone and 25 placebo. To be classified as having AMS, study participants had to report at least moderate severity of 3 or more of these symptoms: insomnia, headache, anorexia, dyspnea, or fatigue.

The mean AMS score decreased by 50% in the dexamethasone-treated group compared with the placebo-treated group at 2,700 m. The incidence of AMS was only 20% of that of controls at this altitude. At 2,050 m, however, there was no difference between the treatment and placebo groups in either the mean AMS symptom score or incidence of AMS.

The routine use of dexamethasone is not recommended for individuals ascending to higher altitudes because side effects can be considerable. The drug should be reserved for individuals at high risk or for those in whom symptoms are unusually severe.

▶ These 2 papers document the occurrence of a complex of symptoms that the authors identify with the syndrome of AMS. However, the role that dexamethasone plays in prevention is unclear. This may well be because the participants in this study started their medication after arrival at altitude, thus differing from previous prophylactic studies of AMS in which medication was given before ascent.—J.S. Torg, M.D.

Acetazolamide and Dexamethasone in the Prevention of Acute Mountain Sickness
Zell SC, Goodman PH (Univ of Nevada)
West J Med 148:541–545, May 1988   18–13

Thirty-two healthy backpackers were randomly assigned to receive either placebo, or 250 mg of acetazolamide twice daily, or 4 mg of dexamethasone acetate 4 times daily, or both medications together in conjunction with a climb to 12,000–13,300 ft. The group drove to a base camp at 7,000 ft the evening before ascent and were taken to 9,000 ft before climbing the rest of the way.

The incidence of sickness was less in actively treated persons than in those given placebo. Combined drug treatment was superior to either drug alone, and dexamethasone alone did not significantly reduce the rate of acute mountain sickness (AMS). Several climbers reported marked depression after discontinuing the use of dexamethasone.

Routine prophylaxis is not necessary in view of the mild nature of AMS. Acetazolamide may be appropriate for those with a history of illness, or if a rapid ascent to high altitude is planned. Dexamethasone should not be used alone, and combined treatment should be reserved for persons who are resistant to prophylaxis with acetazolamide.

A Randomized Trial of Dexamethasone and Acetazolamide for Acute Mountain Sickness Prophylaxis
Ellsworth AJ, Larson EB, Strickland D (Univ of Washington)
Am J Med 83:1024–1030, December 1987   18–14

The efficacy of dexamethasone as prophylaxis for acute mountain sickness (AMS) was compared with that of acetazolamide, the accepted prophylactic drug regimen at altitude, in a double-blind, randomized trial. Forty-seven climbers received dexamethasone (4 mg), acetazolamide (250 mg), or placebo every 8 hours as prophylaxis during rapid, active ascent of Mount Rainier (elevation, 4,392 m). A combined, abbreviated version of the Environmental Symptoms Questionnaire and the General High-Altitude Questionnaire was used to evaluate symptoms of AMS.

Forty-two climbers (89.4%) reached the summit in an average of 34.5 hours after leaving sea level. At the high point, climbers taking dexamethasone reported significantly less headache, fatigue, nausea, dizziness, and clumsiness, and a greater sense of feeling refreshed, than climbers taking placebo or acetazolamide. In addition, climbers taking dexamethasone reported fewer problems of runny nose and chills, symptoms that were unrelated to AMS. At low elevations, climbers taking acetazolamide reported more feelings of nausea, fatigue, and sleepiness, and less feeling of being refreshed. Because these drug side effects probably obscured the previously established prophylactic effects of acetazolamide at higher elevations, a separate analysis of the acetazolamide subgroup was undertaken. Those who did not experience side effects at low elevations demonstrated a prophylactic effect of acetazolamide similar in magnitude to the dexamethasone effect but lacking that drug's euphoric effects.

Dexamethasone is as effective as acetazolamide as a prophylactic agent for AMS and apparently causes fewer side effects. Acetazolamide is still the drug of choice for prophylaxis, but in view of the side effects obscuring its prophylactic effects at low elevations, the substitution of dexamethasone may be effective during rapid ascent to a high altitude.

▶ The studies reviewed in Abstracts 18–13 and 18–14 indicate that dexamethasone is as good as acetazolamide in the prevention of AMS. Neither attempts to determine how the drug acts to prevent mountain sickness. In view of the ever-increasing numbers of people traveling to altitude for recreation, the absolute number of those experiencing AMS will continue to increase. Both articles agree that acetazolamide is the drug of choice, particularly if inadvertent long-term use occurs and adrenal suppression with dexamethasone results. Of even greater importance, it must be emphasized that a slow ascent to altitude, allowing for acclimatization, makes the most sense. Furthermore, taking either dexamethasone or acetazolamide will not guarantee immunity from AMS or the more severe forms of altitude illness, e.g., high altitude pulmonary or cerebral edema. In fact, taking drugs may give a false sense of security and lessen the desire for sensible and adequate acclimatization.—J.R. Sutton, M.D.

Underwater Exploration

Drowning Mortality in Los Angeles County, 1976 to 1984
O'Carroll PW, Alkon E, Weiss B (Los Angeles County Dept of Health Services; Univ of California, Los Angeles)
JAMA 260:380–383, July 15, 1988   18–15

Drowning is the fourth leading cause of accidental death in Los Angeles County. Data collected by the Los Angeles County Coroner's Office on drownings occurring from 1976 to 1984 were analyzed.

In this 9-year period, 1,587 drownings occurred. The victims included 1,130 males and 457 females. This yields an annual rate of 2.36 drownings per 100,000 persons. The largest proportion of drownings—44.5%—occurred in private swimming pools. Children aged 2–3 years had the highest swimming pool drowning rate. Elderly persons also experienced high drowning rates, mostly in swimming pools and bathtubs. Drowning site profiles varied dramatically by age and sex.

Los Angeles County should address the problem of drownings among infants and toddlers in private swimming pools and explore the failure of regulations requiring fencing of swimming pools to prevent these deaths. There are several potential opportunities for preventive intervention by physicians; health care professionals cannot rely on national drowning site profiles for developing local drowning prevention strategies.

Drowning and Near-Drowning on Australian Beaches Patrolled By Life-Savers: A 10-Year Study, 1973–1983
Manolios N, Mackie I (Prince of Wales Hosp, Randwick, NSW, Australia)
Med J Aust 148:165–171 1988   18–16

Expired-air resuscitation and cardiopulmonary resuscitation are standard practice for lifeguards in Australia. Resuscitation report forms of the Surf Life-Saving Association of Australia for 1973–1983 were analyzed. During the study period there were 262 immersion victims at patrolled beaches. Sixty-one victims received expired-air resuscitation and 29 underwent cardiopulmonary resuscitation.

One hundred victims died; there were no deaths in children aged younger than 5 years. Vomiting and regurgitation were the major problems associated with attempts at resuscitation. Twenty-six patients who survived were apneic and without a pulse at initial assessment. Three victims sustained cardiopulmonary arrest after apparently successful resuscitation. Most of the victims who drowned were either unfamiliar with the area, were swimming during unpatrolled hours, or were swimming outside the patrolled area. Eleven victims who died had predisposing medical conditions.

The major factors contributing to drowning are preventable. These include an inability to swim, swimming outside patrolled areas, unfamiliarity with the beaches, previous medical conditions, and consumption of alcohol. Resuscitation techniques are effective in most near-drownings. Regurgitation is the major problem during resuscitation.

▶ These 2 articles (Abstracts 18–15 and 18–16) vividly demonstrate the variation in local drowning site patterns. Specifically, in the Los Angeles County study the major drowning problem occurs among infants and toddlers in private swimming pools. On the other hand, in the Australian study there were no deaths in the surf involving children under 5 years of age. Both studies recognize drowning as a major problem necessitating appropriate preventive measures. Also, both studies identify males in the second and third decades as being at greatest risk.—J.S. Torg, M.D.

Gastric Rupture by Diving Accident: Review of Two Cases and the Relevant Literature

Hassen-Khodja R, Batt M, Legoff D, Gagliardi JM, Valici A, Wolkiewicz J, Le Bas P (Ctr Hosp Univ, Nice; Hôpital Pasteur, Nice, France)
J Chir (Paris) 125:170–173, March 1988   18–17

Gastric rupture as a consequence of scuba diving is rare; only 5 patients have been described in the literature. This type of accident may occur when a large amount of oxygen suddenly enters the stomach and increases the intraluminal pressure until it becomes high enough to cause the gastric wall to rupture. Although these accidents are similar to those reported in association with resuscitation procedures, they differ in physiopathology and clinical presentation.

Case 1.—Woman, 31, experienced scuba diver, descended to 42 m. Just before diving she had taken 2 tablets of effervescent aspirin. While submerged, she discovered that her equipment was faulty and she swallowed sea water. When reascending, she experienced abdominal pain, which became intolerable after resurfacing. At arrival in the hospital, her abdomen was distended and tympanic. Radiography confirmed a large pneumoperitoneum without pneumothorax. After a session in the hyperbaric chamber, the pneumoperitoneum was evacuated under pressure, and a 3-cm wound on the vertical portion of the small curvature was sutured. Her postoperative course was uneventful. Examination of her diving equipment confirmed that it was defective.

Case 2.—Man, 54, experienced diver, descended to 40 m. During reascent he experienced severe abdominal pain and was taken to the hospital in a state of extreme anxiety. The patient's abdomen was distended from a large radiographically confirmed pneumoperitoneum. The pneumoperitoneum was compressed and evacuated, and a 3-cm linear wound on the upper third of the small gastic curve was sutured. His postoperative course was uneventful.

Gastric rupture caused by a scuba diving accident should be treated by urgent operation with radiographic confirmation of a large pneumoperitoneum.

▶ Rupture of the stomach is a rare complication of diving, but it is worth remembering that the stomach is a relatively thin-walled organ. Rupture has been observed during mouth-to-mouth resuscitation with application of excess pressure of 100–150 mm Hg (1), a pressure that can easily be reached if diving equipment is defective, the diver swallows effervescent substances, or air is gulped into the stomach. Normally, the body is protected by burping or expulsion of gas into the intestines, but the circumstances of underwater exploration may discourage use of both of these mechanisms of pressure relief.—R.J. Shephard, M.D., Ph.D.

Reference

1. Cassenbaum WH, et al: *J Trauma* 14:811–814, 1974.

---

⁹⁹TCᵐ-HMPAO Single Photon Emission Tomography in the Diagnosis of Cerebral Barotrauma
Macleod MA, Adkisson GH, Fox MJ, Pearson RR (Inst of Naval Medicine, Gosport, Hampshire, England)
Br J Radiol 61:1106–1109, December 1988   18–18

There is mounting clinical and psychological evidence that pathologic changes occur in the central nervous system (CNS) when a person experiences decompression pulmonary barotrauma, but a cerebral or spinal cord lesion has not been demonstrated in vivo after a decompression incident. Two divers sustained decompression accidents during submarine escape training. Cerebral arterial gas embolism was diagnosed in both. A third patient, a recreational diver, experienced type II decompression sickness.

All 3 patients had normal neurologic findings after recompression. They were admitted to the hospital within 5 hours to several days after their accidents. Single-photon emission computed tomography (SPECT) was performed after injection with 555 MBq ⁹⁹ᵐTc-labeled hexamethyl propyleneamine oxime (⁹⁹ᵐTc-HMPAO). One patient underwent a second SPECT study 1 week later. The SPECT examinations showed well-defined cerebral ischemic lesions in all 3 patients. In the patient having 2 SPECT studies, a hypoperfused area was seen in 2 transaxial slices in the left frontoparietal region on the first examination (Fig 18–1); the

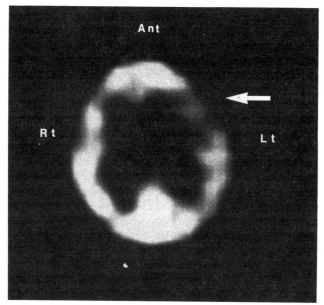

Fig 18-1.—Transaxial view showing an ischemic lesion in the left frontoparietal region *(arrow)*. (Courtesy of Macleod MA, Adkisson GH, Fox MJ, et al: *Br J Radiol* 61:1106–1109, December 1988.)

second SPECT test showed improvement in perfusion in the initial lesion but also a new ischemic area in the left posterior parietal region.

Imaging with ^{99m}Tc-HMPAO provides a significant advance in locating and demonstrating cerebral ischemic lesions after barotrauma. These studies will advance understanding of the pathologic processes involved.

▶ The sensitivity of techniques to investigate cerebral barotrauma appears to have increased markedly with the introduction of positive emission tomography (PET). Despite previous clinical findings indicating definite impairment, results of electroencephalography and high-resolution computed axial scanning have usually been normal. Although it is unrealistic to expect PET scanners to be readily available (they also require a cyclotron nearby to make the necessary isotopes), their value as an investigative tool is very broad indeed, as this study indicates.—J.R. Sutton, M.D.

Thermoregulation

Precedence of Head Homoeothermia Over Trunk Homoeothermia in De-hydrated Men
Caputa M, Cabanac M (Univ Claude Bernard, Oullins, France)
Eur J Appl Physiol 57:611–615, Spring 1988   18–19

When the human body becomes dehydrated, sweat decreases and body temperature increases. It has been suggested that, in a dehydrated state, the body might give precedence to head cooling for the heat-susceptible brain, rather than attempt evaporative cooling of the entire body. Under these conditions it would be expected that facial sweating would be less inhibited than sweating on the trunk. An attempt was made to identify the partitional effects of dehydration on facial and trunk sweating in 3 men.

The men participated in 4 experimental sessions: 2 control sessions and 2 sessions in a dehydrated state. Dehydration was accomplished by abstinence from liquids for 24–36 hours and by sweating during 20-minute exercise periods on a bicycle ergometer. Tympanic and esophageal temperatures were recorded and sweat rates on the back and forehead were measured.

The forehead sweat rate was unchanged after dehydration, but sweat was significantly reduced on the back, resulting in an increase in esophageal temperature. Tympanic temperature was decreased by dehydration (Fig 18–2). The men were allowed to drink water 20 minutes after the

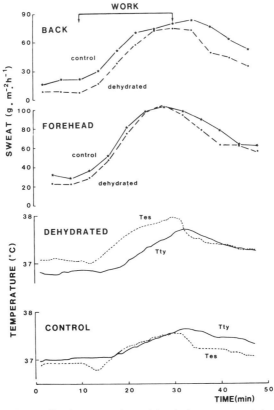

Fig 18–2.—Evolution of local sweat secretion and deep body temperatures before, during, and after 20 minutes of work on a cycle ergometer. Each curve is the mean of 6 sessions (3 subjects taken twice each). *Back, forehead:* locus where sweating was measured. *Control, dehydrated:* data obtained during experiments on control or dehydrated subjects. (Courtesy of Caputa M, Cabanac M: *Eur J Appl Physiol* 57:611–615, Spring 1988.)

end of the exercise session. Compared with findings in the control period, a potohidrotic response was seen on the backs of the men only in the dehydrated state.

Dehydration inhibits sweating on the body. The forehead, however, continues to sweat to provide evaporation for selective cooling of the brain.

▶ A cool brain seems to be a high priority when we exercise in a dehydrated state. Rowell suggested previously that perfusion of vital organs such as the brain takes precedence over whole-body thermoregulation (1). This study suggests that within the body's thermoregulatory control, another hierarchy exists that favors facial sweating to cool the brain when the body is dehydrated. It makes good sense, and the study also indicates the importance of quantifying regional differences in both sweat rates and measurements of "core" temperature.—J.R. Sutton, M.D.

Reference

1. Rowell LB, et al: *J Appl Physiol* 31:864–869, 1971.

Physical Assessment of Heat Insulation Rescue Foils
Ennemoser O, Ambach W, Flora G (Univ of Innsbruck, Austria)
Int J Sports Med 9:179–182, April 1988   18–20

Different materials used to warm hypothermic individuals have different insulating capabilities. The efficiency of aluminum-coated foils as both rescue blankets and rescue suits was assessed. A cylindrical, warm-water-filled, dull-black vessel was used as a phantom and foil blankets or suits were applied. The change of temperature of the phantom was recorded; results were transferred to reactions of hypothermic individuals. One assumption used was a definition of hypothermia as a core temperature of 32 C.

Both a rescue foil and woolen blanket are necessary for thermal stabilization if the hypothermic individual is not well dressed (Fig 18–3). In this case the blanket alone performed better than the foil alone, but if the individual is warmly dressed, either alone suffices. The use of "Hibler packing" also was evaluated. This is a tight wrapping of 3 layers of blankets over a hot water-soaked sheet on the chest. This method gave good results over both wet and dry clothing but was improved if a rescue foil also was applied.

These model experiments on a water-filled vessel provide evidence that aluminum-coated foils are useful in thermal stabilization of the hypothermic patient. In combination with a woolen blanket or "Hibler packing," excellent results are obtained, even with an inadequately dressed individual.

▶ Aluminum foil has had widespread empiric use for prevention of hypothermia under cold conditions; however, the physical environment in most real-life

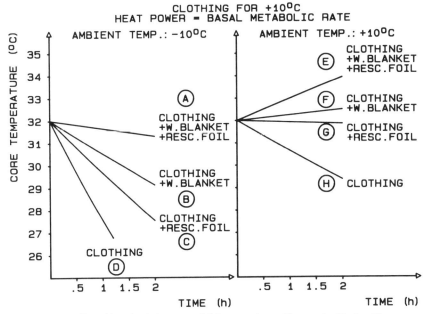

Fig 18–3.—Effect of heat insulation rescue foil in comparison with a woolen blanket. Heat power equals the basal metabolic rate. **Left panel:** ambient temperature −10 C, adequate clothing. *A,* woolen blanket and foil together; thermal stabilization. *B,* woolen blanket alone, further cooling off. *C,* rescue foil alone: stronger cooling off than with woolen blanket alone. *D,* inadequate clothing: strong cooling off. **Right panel:** ambient temperature + 10 C, adequate clothing. *E,* woolen blanket and foil together: reheating. *F,* woolen blanket alone: thermal stabilization. *G,* foil alone: thermal stabilization. *H,* adequate clothing: cooling off. (Courtesy of Ennemoser O, Ambach W, Flora G: *Int J Sports Med* 9:179–182, April 1988.)

emergencies is so varied that it is difficult to obtain more than the strong opinions of rescue parties for or against such treatment. It is thus helpful to have laboratory data supporting the use of aluminum foil. The present results suggest that a blanket can be as effective or more effective than foil, and it is important to use whatever protection is to hand to increase the insulation of a person who has lost the ability to sustain core temperature.—R.J. Shephard, M.D., Ph.D.

Rewarming Techniques for Hypothermia
Nelson MS (Stanford Univ Hosp)
Top Emerg Med 10:23–29, April 1988   18–21

Hypothermia—a core body temperature of less than 35 C—is a common problem in emergency medicine and may occur at any time of year. The signs and symptoms of hypothermia may be overlooked or mistaken for alcohol intoxication, head injury, or drug overdose.

Special hypothermia thermometers should be used in treating patients with initial temperatures of less than 35 C. Victims of mild hypothermia, with temperatures of 32.2 C or higher, may experience alterations in consciousness and often complain of being cold. Shivering is a common indication of hypothermia but is not always present. Patients with severe hypothermia are usually confused and may have slurred speech, a staggering gait, decreased mental skills, and little or no shivering.

Patients with mild hypothermia usually respond well to active external rewarming. Problems occurring during rewarming may reflect the presence of various other illnesses, such as sepsis, endocrinopathy, drug overdose, head trauma, or acute myocardial infarction. Patients with severe hypothermia or cardiovascular instability should be hospitalized immediately and given warm, humidified air or oxygen and warm fluids intravenously. Under some circumstances, peritoneal dialysis or partial cardiopulmonary bypass should be initiated. No patient should be pronounced dead until he or she has been rewarmed and still cannot be revived. In general, patients with mild hypothermia usually respond well to active internal rewarming methods, whereas those with severe hypothermia require both internal and external techniques for rewarming.

▶ Any treatment of hypothermia is more effective if there is early diagnosis; too frequently, the condition is overlooked until the victim is losing consciousness and has difficulty in standing or walking. The lesson that hypothermia can develop in the summer as well as in the winter is important and should be impressed not only on physicians but also on all those who supervise outdoor activities. In hill and mountain walking, common problems are inadequate clothing (deprived teenagers with little warm clothing are often sent to summer camps by well-meaning philanthropists), drenching rain and mist, and a lack of fitness in either the victim or other members of the party (so that the pace of climbing slows to a speed inadequate to maintain body temperature). Poor initial muscle glycogen stores and inadequate reserves of food to cover the possibilities of getting lost or injured can add to the patient's problems by causing a cessation of shivering and ketotic confusion. Occasionally (particularly in snowmobiling parties), there is also a history of alcohol intake, with resultant cutaneous vasodilatation and exacerbation of the confusion caused by cold and ketosis.

Boating accidents and whitewater canoeing are further causes of hypothermia, particularly in the early part of the summer, when rivers are running rapidly at temperatures close to freezing. Because water has much greater thermal conductivity than air, chilling is much more rapid in the water, and a person can quickly reach the severe stage of hypothermia at which they experience a paradoxical sensation of warmth and want to peel off their clothes. When found by a rescuer, it is important to distinguish such cases of paradoxical hypothermia from rape; occasionally, attempts to leave the victim undisturbed for inspection by the police have contributed to death.—R.J. Shephard, M.D., Ph.D.

The Use of Extracorporeal Rewarming in a Child Submerged for 66 Minutes
Bolte RG, Black PG, Bowers RS, Thorne JK, Corneli HM (Primary Children's Med Ctr, Salt Lake City)
JAMA 260:377–379, July 15, 1988   18–22

Submersion injury is a significant cause of morbidity and mortality in children and young adults. A young child who had been submerged in cold water for at least 66 minutes had a good neurologic outcome.

Child, 2½ years, fell into a creek near Salt Lake City. After 66 minutes rescue workers finally located her under water. She had been wedged against the upstream side of a rock; there was no evidence of an air pocket. She was cyanotic, apneic, and flaccid, with fixed and dilated pupils and no palpable pulse. Her rectal temperature was 22.4 C. Core rewarming with mist/oxygen at 40 C through an endotracheal tube, warmed isotonic intravenous fluids, and continuous 40 C gastric lavage was begun, but active external rewarming techniques wee withheld. About 3 hours after the accident, extracorporeal rewarming (ECR) was begun and external chest compressions were discontinued. A warming gradient of 10 C was maintained between the perfusate and core body temperature until the perfusate temperature was 38 C. The mean perfusion pressure during ECR was 60 mm Hg, and the average blood flow was 2.2 L/sq m/minute. Heparin sodium, mannitol, calcium chloride, and sodium bicarbonate were given while the bypass system was in place. When the core temperature reached 25 C, a single spontaneous gasp and fine ventricular fibrillation occurred. Within a few minutes the child opened her eyes, and her pupils became reactive. When the core temperature reached 37 C, ECR was stopped. The child's neurologic course improved gradually but steadily. At her discharge after 8 weeks of hospitalization, she was noted to have a tremor that interfered with her fine motor skills. One year after the accident, the child was functioning at her age level and her tremor was improving progressively.

The described submersion in cold water for at least 66 minutes is the longest time yet reported. This is the first reported successful use of ECR in a child sustaining accidental hypothermia.

▶ This paper reports what appears to be 2 "world records": First, neurologic recovery after cold water submersion for 66 minutes and, second, a core temperature of 19 C, the lowest reported for a submersion victim who regained intact neurologic survival. More importantly, however, the authors delineate the principles of ECR and emphasize the feasibility of regionalization of care for markedly hypothermic patients similar to triage systems for major trauma. They point out that hypothermic pediatric patients may be stabilized at primary and secondary care centers; however, patients in critical condition should be rapidly referred to pediatric tertiary care centers where ECR and pediatric intensive care are available.—J.S. Torg, M.D.

Muscle Glycogen Utilization During Shivering Thermogenesis in Humans
Martineau L, Jacobs I (Defence and Civil Inst of Environmental Medicine, Downsview, Ont; Univ of Toronto)
J Appl Physiol 65:2046–2050, November 1988   18–23

When humans are exposed to a cold environment, shivering thermogenesis increases oxygen uptake and heat production. In animals there is

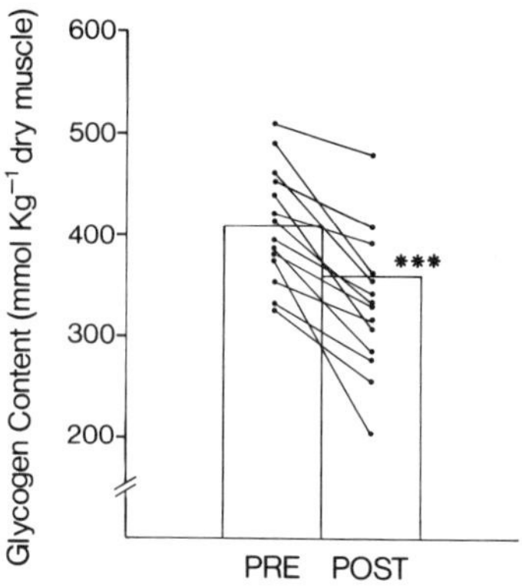

Fig 18–4.—Individual and mean values in 14 persons of glycogen levels before and after cold water immersion at 18 C. ***Significantly different from preimmersion value ($P < .001$). (Courtesy of Martineau L, Jacobs I: *J Appl Physiol* 65:2046–2050, November 1988.)

evidence that shivering thermogenesis is a glycogenolytic process, with intramuscular glycogen depletion accompanying heat production. In an attempt to clarify the importance of skeletal muscle glycogen as a fuel for shivering thermogenesis in humans, 14 healthy persons were immersed to the shoulders in 18 C water for 90 minutes or until rectal temperature decreased to 35.5 C. Venous blood samples and biopsy specimens of the vastus lateralis were obtained before and immediately after immersion.

During immersion the metabolic rate increased to 3.5 times resting values and rectal temperature decreased to 35.8 C. Glycogen concentration in the vastus lateralis decreased from 410 to 332 mmol of glucose per kg of dry muscle (Fig 18–4). A decrease occurred in all 14 individuals. Plasma volume was markedly reduced during immersion. After correcting for the decrease, the blood lactate level increased by 60% and plasma glycerol levels increased by 38%. In contrast, plasma glucose levels decreased by 20% after immersion. The mean expiratory exchange ratio was biphasic, increasing from 0.80 to 0.85 during the first 30 minutes and decreasing toward baseline thereafter.

Intramuscular substrates, as well as circulating substrates, fuel shivering in humans. Skeletal muscle glycogen reserves are used in the transduction of energy to shivering musculature.

▶ Shivering is an important mechanism of heat production during hypothermia, whether caused by immersion in cold water or exposure to cold air under wet conditions. Body metabolism can reach a level of 5 METS with severe shivering, and because the heat is produced by simultaneous isometric contractions of opposing agonists and antagonists, there is a strong tendency to draw upon muscle glycogen reserves. This is important from several perspectives. First, the unfit person with low glycogen reserves may not have sufficient stored fuel to walk down from a cold mountain top and to maintain body heat. Second, as glycogen stores are depleted, the blood glucose level falls and fat metabolism gives rise to a ketosis; this adds to the confusion already induced by the falling core temperature, leading to unwise tactics and an increased risk of accidents.

An increase in muscle glycogen reserves can thus be helpful if exposure to cold conditions is possible; it is also important that expeditions carry sufficient reserves of food to maintain blood glucose levels.—R.J. Shephard, M.D., Ph.D.

Hypothermia and Blood pH: A Review
Swain JA (Natl Insts of Health, Bethesda, Md)
Arch Intern Med 148:1643–1646, July 1988   18–24

Clinicians are well aware of the deleterious effects of hypothermia. The literature was reviewed to summarize the laboratory, theoretical, and clinical evidence that the management of blood pH during hypothermia may change the appearance or magnitude of these deleterious effects.

Resuscitating patients from accidental hypothermia and inducing hypothermia during cardiac surgery requires clinicians to make important choices in the manner in which the blood pH of the patient is managed. Theoretical calculations and experimental laboratory and clinical evidence indicate that constraining pH to 7.4 during hypothermia may be undesirable, whereas maintaining the pH relatively alkalotic to pH 7.4 during hypothermia may be desirable. The relationship between pH and PCO_2 that must occur to maintain a pH in the latter, or alpha-stat scheme, is shown in Figure 18–5. In the future, additional techniques of pH management, such as inducement of a respiratory alkalosis, may prove to be even more efficacious. However, the balance of current clinical and experimental data favors the alpha-stat scheme of pH management during hypothermia.

Clinicians must make important decisions as to the manner in which the blood pH of hypothermic patients is managed. Theoretical calculations, clinical evidence, and laboratory findings currently indicate that the

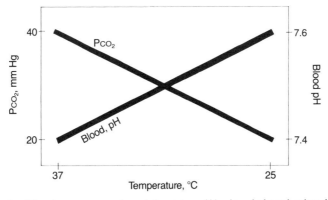

Fig 18–5.—When the temperature of a sealed container of blood in which total carbon dioxide content is constant is decreased, the pH rises and carbon dioxide pressure (PCO_2) falls, as described by Henderson-Hasselbach relationship. (Courtesy of Swain JA: *Arch Intern Med* 148:1643–1646, July 1988.)

most desirable method of managing pH during hypothermia is the alpha-stat scheme.

▶ Although this paper is written from the perspective of hypothermic surgery, some of the principles that are enunciated apply also to recovery from accidental hypothermia occurring during mountain hikes or boating accidents in frigid waters. The problem is indicated in Figure 18–5: If blood is placed in a sealed container and cooled drastically, the carbon dioxide becomes more soluble in the lipid phase, causing a decrease of P_{CO_2} and a rise of pH; if an attempt is made to maintain the pH constant, the CO_2 content of the body must be increased to undesirable levels, with an adverse impact on tissue enzymes such as phosphorylase and phosphofructokinase, particularly during rewarming.

In accidental hypothermia the situation is often complicated by exhaustion of the glycogen reserves from shivering. An excessive reliance on fat metabolism and circulatory failure leads to tissue acidosis despite the low core temperature, and there is a need for substantial infusions of bicarbonate to induce the alpha-stat scheme recommended by Swain.—R.J. Shephard, M.D., Ph.D.

The "Arolla" Index: A Study of 88 Cases of Frostbite During a High Mountain Competition
Reymond M, Rigo M (Hôpital du District, Monthey, Switzerland)
J Chir (Paris) 125:239–244, 1988   18–25

The prestigious Glacier Patrol is a 100-km ski race over high-mountain terrain from Zermatt, Switzerland, to Verbier via Arolla at an altitude ranging from 1,520 to 3,650 m. This competition, which has been open to Swiss and foreign military and civilian groups, was first organized in 1943 and held in 1944 and 1949; it was suspended, however, because of a fatal accident. The race was reinstated in 1984, but in 1986 it was called off halfway through the course because of a sudden change to extreme weather conditions that led to severe frostbite in many competitors. This study was designed to discover why there were so many victims of frostbite and to learn the outcome in those stricken.

A total of 690 men and 6 women started the race in Zermatt. All participants had to qualify for the race and were chosen on the basis of previous experience as mountain guides or participation in alpine skiing clubs or similar groups. Three age classes were defined: 20–32 years, 33–40 years, and older than age 40 years. Eighty-eight (12%) of the 696 participants were affected, including 31 with first-degree frostbite, 38 with superficial second-degree frostbite, 12 with deep second-degree frostbite, and 7 with third-degree frostbite. Frostbite occurred on a single hand in 27 skiers, both hands in 27, a single foot in 8, both feet in 3, and on the face in 65. One skier who had signs of moderate to severe hypothermia was admitted with a rectal temperature of 31.5 C. The presence of a physician and a helicopter on the course saved this patient's life.

Seventy patients were treated at first-aid stations by warming the frostbitten extremities in warm water. Six patients required immediate hospitalization and remained hospitalized for a mean duration of 7.4 days. Sixty-one patients eventually required professional care, but no amputations were necessary. Forty-five patients still had sequelae of frostbite 4 months later.

Most victims attributed their frostbite to the sudden change in weather. However, other factors played an important role, including age, inadequate training, substandard equipment, and, mostly, lack of common sense.

Because the wind-chill index does not denote duration of exposure, the term "Arolla Index" was coined for a formula that links duration of exposure time, defined by both temperature and wind-chill index, with degree of frostbite. The Arolla Index should be useful in future studies of exposure injuries.

▶ Long-distance ski races frequently are occasions when a substantial number of competitors sustain frostbite. If the weather is severe, periodic inspection of competitors over the course of the route is mandatory. The Arolla Index suggested in this report—a combination of the traditional wind-chill index with duration of exposure—should provide a useful aid to future preventive efforts.— R.J. Shephard, M.D., Ph.D.

19 General Medicine and Miscellaneous Topics

Required Physical Activity and Child Development
Shephard RJ (Univ of Toronto)
Aust J Sci Med Sport 20:3–9, June 1988   19–1

There has been increasing concern about the decline in physical activity and low fitness levels in American youth. The impact of regular required daily physical activity programs for elementary school children was studied in rural and urban Canadian school boys and girls who underwent 1 hour of endurance-type physical activity daily in addition to the standard 40-minute weekly physical education program.

In all, 546 children in grades 1 through 6 were enrolled in the longitudinal study. The 5-hour weekly program was supervised by a physical education professional. During the first 2 years the program emphasized mastery of movement skills and socialization, later progressing to cardiovascular and endurance training, and finally to team games. Findings were compared with those in controls.

Over several years, study children made substantial gains in work capacity, aerobic power, muscle force, and performance test scores. The exercise program had no influence on stature or body build, nor was obesity reduced. However, various aspects of psychomotor development were enhanced. Study participants also had significantly higher academic achievement than did control children despite reduced time for classroom instruction.

Further study is warranted to determine long-term implications for health and life-style. However, it is apparent that 5 hours per week of a school day can be allocated to physical education without risk to immediate health or to academic progress.

▶ This is one of the classic longitudinal studies of the impact of daily physical activity on primary school children. Many publications have come from this study, and the present paper summarizes some of the effects on physiology and psychomotor development. It is essential reading for anyone interested in the impact of physical education programs in schools. The work should have significant political impact, especially in areas in which politicians and school boards wish to further emasculate already depleted physical education programs.—J.R. Sutton, M.D.

Exercise Medicine in Medical Education in the United States
Whitley JD, Nyberg KL (California State Univ, Bakersfield)
Phys Sportsmed 16:93–100, October 1988   19–2

Leisure-time physical activity among adults in the United States has increased in the past 20 years. The extent to which United States medical schools offer formal instruction in exercise physiology in their 4-year undergraduate curriculum, the modes of instruction, and whether instruction is elective or required were evaluated.

Medical bulletins were requested from all 125 medical schools in the United States. The return rate was 84%. Each bulletin was analyzed to identify courses, rotations, and research related to exercise physiology and sports medicine. Of the 92 schools studied, 62% did not offer formal instruction in exercise physiology or sports medicine. In the remaining 35 schools, only 13 separate courses are totally devoted to either exercise physiology or sports medicine. Of the 20 exercise topics offered within other courses, 11 dealt with the reactions of the physiologic systems to exercise, 5 were related to physical fitness, and 4 were on specialized topics (e.g., cardiac rehabilitation). Physiology departments alone account for 30% of the total instruction in exercise medicine. Exercise information is part of the required course work in only 4 of the 92 schools sampled.

Most medical students in the United States do not receive formal instruction in the medical aspects of exercise during their 4-year undergraduate training. They should be required to take at least a short course in exercise medicine that emphasizes cardiorespiratory fitness.

▶ This article calls attention to an apparent deficiency in medical education. As the authors point out, endorsement of exercise by its inclusion in the medical curriculum would help to legitimize its inclusion also as a major factor in good health and probably would increase its adoption by the public.—J.S. Torg, M.D.

Sports Medicine Centers: Aspects of Their Operation and Approaches to Sports Medicine Care
Weidner TG (California State Univ, Northridge)
Athletic Training 23:22–26, Spring 1988   19–3

There is at present no uniform system for establishing, operating, or evaluating a sports medicine practice. Because sports medicine is not considered a medical specialty, there are no guidelines for the services or staffing that a sports medicine center (SMC) should provide.

A questionnaire was sent to a random sample of 150 SMCs listed in the 1984 *Sports Medicine Directory*. Sixty-three SMCs (42%) returned properly completed questionnaires. Respondents were asked to indicate

Table 1.—Classification/Description of Sports Medicine Centers

Classification	Description
Physical fitness center	Conduct fitness evaluations, prepare exercise prescriptions, and offer lifestyle counseling
Sports and exercise injury center	Diagnose, treat, and rehabilitate acute injuries
Medical center	Rehabilitate cardiac, pulmonary, diabetic, and asthmatic patients
Primary care sports medicine center	Diagnose and treat medical problems that are related in some way to sport or exercise participation
Special exercise or sport activity sports medicine center	Diagnose, treat, and rehabilitate conditions prevalent in a particular activity—e.g., dancing, running
Sports medicine research center	Generate knowledge concerning the response, adaptations, and clinical aspects of exercise and sport activities

(Courtesy of Weidner TG: *Athletic Training* 23:22–26, Spring 1988.)

which of 6 listed SMC activity categories best described their primary and secondary service efforts (Table 1). Responses were also solicited with regard to initial appointment criteria, profiles of clients seeking care, general operating procedures, staffing, and client reimbursement for services.

The largest number (80.3%) of the surveyed SMCs were Sports and Exercise Injury Centers. Nearly half (45.7%) of the SMC clientele do not come to an SMC because of injury. Clients are most often adult (37.2%) recreation/fitness enthusiasts (28.1%) who consult a SMC for clinical service. Most of the SMCs appear to provide fitness/conditioning programs with little commitment to wellness and health promotion, education, or injury prevention. Most centers reported a fairly even distribution of client care among physicians, physical therapists, and athletic trainers (Table 2), but physical therapists had an overwhelming majority (98.2%) of the total involvement at SMCs. Athletic trainers were more involved than physical therapists only in the area of fitting athletes with protective equipment. Private payment (95.2%) and insurance (87.1%) were the most common reimbursement modes.

These data indicate that SMCs are simply traditional medical care settings that emphasize sports medicine care, as 38.6% of the surveyed

Table 2.—Distribution of Client Injury Diagnosis and
Management Protocols and Sports Medicine Centers

Protocol	Reported at Center	
	Frequency	Percentage
Physician Diagnosis/Supervision of all injuries	27	47.37%
Physical Therapist triage under Physician	25	42.86
Athletic Trainer triage under Physician	21	36.84
Physical Therapist triage — no supervision	14	24.56
Athletic Trainer triage under Physical Therapist	13	21.05
Athletic Trainer triage — no supervision	11	19.30
Physical Therapist triage under Athletic Trainer	6	10.53
Nurse triage under Physician	2	3.51
Nurse triage—no supervision	2	3.51
Other	3	5.26

Note: Most centers reported more than one protocol, so
there were a total 124 protocols reported by 57 centers.

(Courtesy of Weidner TG: *Athletic Training* 23:22–26, Spring 1988.)

SMCs provided less than half of their services to clients with sports medicine concerns.

▶ What is an SMC, and what are the functions of its personnel? Through a questionnaire type survey, the author has attempted to answer these questions and other specifics regarding SMCs. Sports medicine centers offer a wide variety of services. I'm sure that the background and experience of the personnel working in a center determine the type of services offered.—F.J. George, ATC, PT

Athletes' Headaches: Not Necessarily "Little" Problems
McCarthy P (Honolulu)
Physician Sportsmed 16:169–173, October 1988   19–4

Although athletes are often subject to headaches, the incidence and prevalence of sports-related headaches are unknown; however, it is agreed that headaches are often underreported and misdiagnosed. Athletes' headaches can be grouped into 3 categories: trauma-triggered migraines, exertional headaches, and effort headaches.

Exertion can trigger both migraine episodes and muscle-contraction headaches. The exertional headache lasts for only a few minutes, occurs in all parts of the head, and may move around. According to the neurogenic theory, when the monoaminergic system is stimulated, pain centers in various parts of the brain respond with headaches. Stimulation can be through the Valsalva maneuver, which is practiced by weight lifters, or through more subtle dynamic exertion in running or swimming. The long-popular vascular theory holds that constriction and dilation of blood vessels are responsible for headaches.

Systolic pressures in body builders doing leg presses have been measured at more than 400 mm Hg, with diastolic pressures in the high 300s. The increase in blood pressure appears to be related to the size of the muscle mass: the greater the mass, the higher the increase. Single repetitions with maximum weight increase the blood pressure less than more repetitions done to failure with a lower weight. Those who sustain blood vessel injury may have an inherent weakness, possibly an aneurysm. Effort headaches more often occur in individuals prone to migraine. Alcohol consumption can be a contributing factor. A prolonged graded warm-up may help athletes who are prone to headaches.

Some headaches are symptomatic of a more serious condition. Migraine headaches that follow a blow to the head may be indicative of a subdural or epidural hematoma, or a subarachnoid hemorrhage caused by a ruptured aneurysm.

▶ The division here between exertional and effort headaches is artificial. Exertional headaches, first described by Hippocrates, have been discussed previously (1986 YEAR BOOK OF SPORTS MEDICINE, pp 174–176; 1983 YEAR BOOK OF SPORTS MEDICINE, pp 151–152). For athletes with exercise-related headache, the extent of workup is debated; neurologists often recommend a complete neurologic evaluation, including computed tomography scan or magnetic resonance imaging. They argue that, occasionally, exertional headaches can reflect an intracranial lesion such as a glioma or subdural hematoma. They also note that 1 person in 20 has an asymptomatic intracranial aneurysm, and that headache during exercise can signal a subarachnoid hemorrhage from such an aneurysm (1). Cluster headaches, too, can occur in athletes and interfere with their sport (2). Headache can be an early symptom of heat stress or acute mountain sickness. Also, I have seen headache as an early symptom of hyponatremia, presumably occurring from the increased intracranial pressure that can accompany this complication of distance running (3).—E.R. Eichner, M.D.

References

1. Tobin WE, Cantu RC: *Physician Sportsmed* 17:145–148, 1989.
2. Bracker MD, Rothrock JF: *Physician Sportsmed* 17:147–158.
3. Nelson PB, et al: *Physician Sportsmed* 16:78–88.

Epistaxis in the Athlete
Stevens H (Univ Hosp, Vancouver)
Physician Sportsmed 16:31–40, December 1988   19–5

Epistaxis may result from either local or systemic causes. Because they are more likely to sustain facial trauma, athletes may be at greater risk. Epistaxis usually has a local cause. Nasal fracture should be suspected in persistent bleeding, even when deformity is not evident. Hypertension should also be ruled out. Rarely, there may be an underlying bleeding disorder; the cause is more likely to be a platelet disorder or a subtle clotting defect.

About 90% of epistaxis episodes arise from the anterior-inferior septal region. Bleeding secondary to a nasal fracture often occurs in the nasal roof. Posterior epistaxis is generally more severe than anterior epistaxis, and it is always more difficult to manage. Bleeding comes from the larger nasal branches of the internal maxillary artery or from the ethmoidal arteries. In athletes it may be caused by a nasal/facial fracture.

Epistaxis resulting from nasal trauma usually stops spontaneously within a few minutes. Bleeding may begin a few days after swelling from a nasal fracture has begun to subside. Immediate persistent hemorrhage and delayed hemorrhage both require prompt reduction of the nasal fracture for control. After reduction, bleeding usually stops, and packing is rarely necessary.

A well-equipped epistaxis tray should be available in the hospital. For minor anterior epistaxis, nasal blood clots should be suctioned. Kiesselbach's area is usually the source of bleeding. A solution containing an anesthetic and a vasoconstrictor should be applied topically and left in place for 5 minutes. The site can be cauterized with silver nitrate or electrocautery. An antibiotic ointment also should be applied topically. Nasal packing should be avoided. Anterior nasal packing should be used if bleeding is severe or the site is not amenable to cautery. In these patients the nose should be taped with the nostrils pinched together.

▶ This is a masterful review of treatment of nosebleed in the athlete. Epistaxis has been discussed previously (see the 1985 YEAR BOOK OF SPORTS MEDICINE, pp 211–212) in an article that noted the frequency of nosebleeds in skiers, owing to dryness of the nasal mucosa at altitude. In wrestlers, nosebleeds during a match are common and usually can be controlled by inserting a small nasal tampon. After the match direct pressure is effective (1).—E.R. Eichner, M.D.

Reference

1. Harvey J, et al: *Physician Sportsmed* 15:137–143, 1987.

Acne Vulgaris in the Athlete
Conklin RJ (Univ of British Columbia, Vancouver)
Physician Sportsmed 16:57–68, October 1988   19–6

Acne, particularly the pustular and cystic/nodular forms, can be emotionally devastating, affecting athletic performance. Acne treatment is fundamentally the same for athletes and nonathletes. However, certain aspects of sports can affect acne adversely.

In some patients treatment may require caution. The best treatments are topically applied tretinoin for comedonal acne, benzoyl peroxide or topically applied antibiotics and tretinoin for comedonal and mild pustular acne, and combined oral antibiotic therapy and long-term benzoyl peroxide or topically applied antibiotics, with the eventual goal of stopping the oral treatment with antibiotics within 3–5 months, for moderate and severe pustular acne. For patients with severe cystic/nodular acne, high-dose oral antibiotic therapy and intralesional steroid injections or oral isotretinoin therapy should be considered.

▶ Factors tending to exacerbate acne in athletes include heavy sweating; friction associated with the use of shoulder pads, bench presses, or a brace; and (in some high-performance competitors) abuse of androgenic steroids. Dr. Conklin focuses particularly on the female athlete, in whom acne perhaps causes more concern and is thus more liable to interfere with training. However, it is worth noting that acne occurs in both sexes, and that androgen secretion seems a triggering factor. The tendency of endurance training to suppress androgen levels in male athletes could conceivably have a beneficial effect on the skin.

The measures proposed in this article seem rather heroic for what is essentially a cosmetic problem and are a devastating criticism of values in our current society.—R.J. Shephard, M.D., Ph.D.

Grappling With Herpes: Herpes Gladiatorum
Becker TM, Kodsi R, Bailey P, Lee F, Levandowski R, Nahmias AJ (Univ of New Mexico, Albuquerque; Emory Univ; Princeton Univ)
Am J Sports Med 16:665–669, November–December 1988   19–7

Herpes gladiatorum is a skin infection often found in college wrestlers that is caused by herpes simplex virus (HSV). Descriptive data on occurrence, age, and geographic distribution have not been published, and risk factors for acquiring this infection have not been identified.

A study was conducted in which members of 4 college wrestling teams were surveyed and high school and college athletic trainers nationwide were sampled. Serum samples from 1 college wrestling team were studied for HSV antibodies.

Nine of 48 college wrestlers studied reported histories of herpes gladiatorum. Only 1 of these had a history of oral HSV infection, but 7 had at least 1 match with an opponent who had cold sores or vesiculopapular skin rash. Clinical manifestations of herpes gladiatorum included a vesiculopapular rash on the face, upper arm, or trunk. All had tingling or burning sensations before the appearance of the rash. One athlete was hospitalized with fever, malaise, and pain after the first occurrence. The number of recurrences ranged from 1 to 8. All wrestlers were treated symptomatically.

Of 12 members of 1 team, 5 with herpes gladiatorum had serum antibody titers to HSV-1; no HSV-2 antibodies were found. None of the 5 had histories of cold sores or other HSV infections. Of the 94 college wrestling teams surveyed, 64.9% reported at least 1 episode of HSV skin infection during the 1984–1985 season; of 69 high schools, 24.6% reported episodes. Athletic trainers reported that 7.6% of college wrestlers and 2.6% of high school wrestlers had HSV skin infections.

Wrestlers exposed to opponents with cutaneous HSV lesions are at high risk of contracting herpes gladiatorum. Early recognition and diagnosis of HSV skin infection and immediate exclusion of the infected wrestler from competition and practice is the best method of prophylaxis.

► This epidemiologic survey emphasizes how common herpes gladiatorum can be, especially among collegians. It also covers diagnosis and therapy; it presents good color photos of typical lesions, and considers the pros and cons of using oral acyclovir to suppress recurrent herpes gladiatorum. Treatment, including acyclovir, is also covered in a stellar recent review of the medical problems of wrestlers (1). The recent outbreak among 16 wrestlers and a coach in a Wisconsin high school highlights the importance of prompt recognition and treatment of this contagious disease (2).—E.R. Eichner, M.D.

References

1. Harvey J, et al: *Physician Sportsmed* 15:137–143, 1987.
2. Duda M: *Physician Sportsmed* 17:50, 1989.

Pressures in Normal and Acutely Distended Human Knee Joints and Effects on Quadriceps Maximal Voluntary Contractions
Wood L, Ferrell WR, Baxendale RH (The University, Glasgow)
Q J Exp Physiol 73:305–314, 1988   19–8

Previous research has yielded discrepancies in observations on pressure changes in normal, nondistended joints with passive positioning. This discrepancy was investigated and the effects of fluid distention on pressure changes determined in 10 knees of 5 individuals.

Resting intra-articular pressures were subatmospheric, with a mean value of −5 mm Hg. Little variation was noted in intra-articular pressure with changing joint angle in the normal joint. Infusion of a volume as small as 5 ml of sterile saline into the joint cavity caused the intra-articular pressure to increase to supraatmospheric levels. Changing the joint angle then produced clear modulations in intraarticular pressure. The pressure increased as the limb was moved into extension and back to flexion, with a minimum occurring in the midrange. The modulations were more pronounced with active positioning of the joint com-

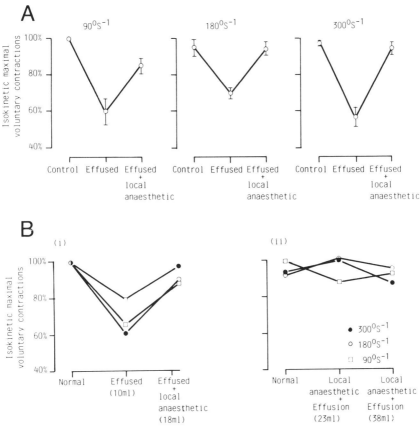

Fig 19–1.—A, mean percentage changes (± SEM) in isokinetic maximal voluntary contraction at different velocities and under different experimental conditions (n = 5). The presence of fluid in the knee resulted in marked reduction in performance at all velocities, which was almost completely restored by further injection of local anesthetic. **B, left,** response fluid infusion followed by local anesthetic. **B, right,** response when local anesthetic preceded fluid infusion. (Courtesy of Wood L, Ferrell WR, Baxendale RH: *Q J Exp Physiol* 73:305–314, 1988.)

pared with passive positioning. Successive increases in intra-articular volume yielded an increase in intraarticular pressure and in the degree of modulation of intra-articular pressure with joint angle. Cyclical flexion-extension movements produced a progressive decrease in the maximum pressure noted in extension. Non-noxious distention of the knee caused substantial reductions in the magnitude of isometric and isokinetic maximal voluntary contractions of quadriceps because of a reflex inhibition from joint mechanoreceptor afferents (Fig 19–1).

The presence of subatmospheric intra-articular pressure in the knee at rest is consistent with previous findings in human beings and animals. The mean value of this subatmospheric pressure is also consistent with the values reported previously. In the normal joint, little variation is observed in intraarticular pressure with changes in joint angle over the ranges of positions examined, either by active or passive positioning.

▶ Patients who have swollen knees as a result of cartilage injury frequently complain that their discomfort is increased by a long flight in an economy-class aircraft cabin. The increase of pressure with sustained flexion of the knee, as demonstrated here, may explain the phenomenon. The impact of the effusion on isokinetic force is very striking, offering interesting proof of the potential negative feedback role of mechanoreceptors about a joint.— R.J. Shephard, M.D., Ph.D.

The Strength of Artificial Ligament Anchorages: A Comparative Experimental Study
Amis AA (Imperial College, London)
J Bone Joint Surg [Br] 70-B:397–403, May 1988   19–9

Much work has been done on artificial ligaments and the clinical use of a range of devices, but little has been published on the design or properties of their anchorages. The holding strength of various commercially available anchorage devices for artificial ligaments was compared. These devices were the Sherman bone screw, Gore/AO screw, Richards staple, bollard, toggle, and grommet. Tensile tests to failure were done on these devices, which were implanted into cadaveric bones. The results of the tests were graphed for comparison (Fig 19–2).

Although some of the fixation devices were designed for use in cancellous bone, the local thickness of the much stronger cortical bone determines the holding strength of these devices. Because the thickness of the cortical shell increases with distance from the joint line, ligament anchorages should be placed as far from it as possible, subject to constraints such as those imposed by incision and length of implant.

The forces imposed on ligaments during athletics and by trauma are unknown, thus using anchorages that are at least of similar strength to the implants seems prudent. The only device tested that can achieve this was the transcortical grommet. When used around an AO screw, this grommet had significantly greater holding strength than the other devices tested.

The Use of Fibrin Adhesive in the Repair of Chondral and Osteochondral Injuries
Kaplonyi G, Zimmerman I, Frenyo AD, Farkas T, Nemes G (Natl Inst of Traumatology, Budapest)
Injury 19:267–272, July 1988   19–10

Repair of osteochondral and chondral injuries has been accomplished with screws, wires, and staples, but these can further damage the cartilage. In the case of small or thin fragments, tissue adhesives are success-

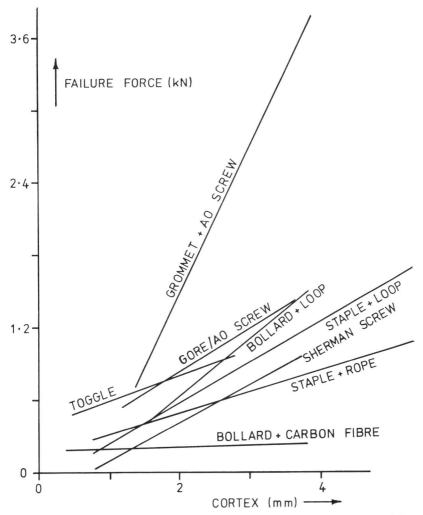

Fig 19–2.—Comparison of results of strength test for all fixation methods examined shows the benefit of placement in thicker cortical bone. The grommet had significantly greater fixation strength than the other methods when used away from the joint line. The toggle is a convenient device if fixation close to the joint line is necessary. (Courtesy of Amis AA: *J Bone Joint Surg [Br]* 70-B:397–403, May 1988.)

ful. The most useful bonding agent consists of concentrations of human fibrin. A series of 29 patients had 39 fragments replanted.

The patients were injured at various joints: knees, ankles, elbows, and hands. Arthroscopic examination allowed direct view of the joint surfaces and assessment of cartilage damage. A thin layer of fibrin adhesive provided initial stability and allowed rapid revascularization of the osteochondral fragment. A plaster cast was required for 3 weeks to increase stability. Patients were advised to avoid bearing weight on the knees and ankles for 6–12 weeks.

At radiologic examination, healing was seen in 15 patients. In 5 patients the fracture was not visible. Nine of 12 who were examined arthroscopically showed signs of healing at 6 months. In 1 case loosening of the cast caused fragment displacement. Three patients had limited movement and 2 experienced pain.

There is a potential for bloodborne diseases from fibrin adhesive, but careful screening of donors has avoided this complication. On the whole, fibrin adhesive is successful, relatively easy to use, and has little risk of complication.

▶ This interesting paper describes the exciting potential for the use of fibrin adhesive in the repair of chondral and osteochondral fractures. Apparently, fibrin adhesive has had widespread use by cardiologists, otorhinolaryngologists, and plastic surgeons for a variety of procedures. It is interesting to note that the authors state: "Out of 1 million cases where fibrin adhesive was used, there have been no reported cases of hepatitis-B, HIV infection or any other form of blood-borne disease." Also, although somewhat premature, the authors conclude that, "In view of our results fibrin adhesive can be recommended for the operative management of cartilage injuries."—J.S. Torg, M.D.

The Poor Quality of Early Evaluations of Magnetic Resonance Imaging
Cooper LS, Chalmers TC, McCally M, Berrier J, Sacks HS (Harvard School of Public Health; Mt Sinai School of Medicine of City Univ of New York; VA Med Ctr, Bronx)
JAMA 259:3277–3280, June 10, 1988   19–11

Fifty-four articles on magnetic resonance (MR) imaging, published in English-language journals from 1980 to 1984, were reviewed using commonly accepted criteria of research methodology. Nearly two thirds of the articles reviewed appeared in *Radiology* and the *American Journal of Radiology*.

Only 1 study gave evidence of previous planning by describing a protocol. Histopathologic findings were presented in only 22% of the articles. No article contained evidence of randomization of the sequence of the imaging procedures or blinding of the readers to other sources of information. There was some quantitation of the findings in 44% of the articles. None of the articles included more than 5 of 10 procedures that were considered optimal, and there was no indication of improvement over time.

Health care professionals who pay for expensive diagnostic technology should require better research on its diagnostic efficacy. The need for proper quantitative methods is clear. Research in MR imaging has largely been limited to descriptive studies. None of the present studies can be considered high-quality assessments by current criteria of research methodology.

▶ Certainly, scientific writing in the radiologic journals, as in other specialty journals, requires improvement. However, the papers included in this review were those published between 1980 and 1984, which represents the extreme infancy of MR researching and a period during which the main goal was to share experience and knowledge. Also, although this review is based on 54 articles, when the overlap of authors is considered it represents only approximately 18 different investigating groups. It is therefore not surprising that the format of the research is similar throughout. It would be interesting to subject this review paper to the commonly accepted criterion of research methodology.—J.S. Torg, M.D.

Detection of Muscle Injury in Humans With 31-P Magnetic Resonance Spectroscopy
McCully KK, Argov Z, Boden BP, Brown RL, Bank WJ, Chance B (Univ of Pennsylvania; Univ of Oregon)
Muscle Nerve II:212–216, March 1988   19–12

Exercise-induced muscle injury affects athletes at all levels. To determine whether a completely noninvasive procedure, ^{31}P-labeled magnetic resonance spectroscopy (MRS), can detect evidence of muscle injury in humans, 5 healthy persons performed lengthening contractions of the wrist flexor muscles and 3 jogged backward down a flight of stairs to produce calf-muscle lengthening contractions. They underwent MRS be-

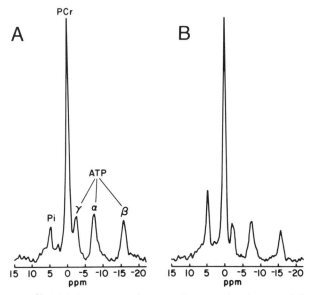

Fig 19–3.—The ^{31}P-labeled MRS spectra from wrist flexor muscles of 1 person before (**A**) and 24 hours after (**B**) 60 lengthening contractions. Each spectrum consists of 60 scans collected over 5 minutes. The 5 major peaks are (from left to right): inorganic phosphate *(Pi)*, phosphocreatine *(PCr)*, and the 3 peaks from adenosine triphosphate *(ATP)* (gamma, alpha, and beta). For comparative purposes, the height of each spectrum was normalized to the same value of PCr. Compared with PCr, Pi is elevated, and ATP is reduced after the lengthening contractions. (Courtesy of McCully KK, Argov Z, Boden BP, et al: *Muscle Nerve* II:212–216, March 1988.)

fore and 1 hour after exercise and once daily on days 7 through 10. Selected patients with destructive neuromuscular disorders were tested for comparison without undergoing the exercise protocol.

One hour after the arm exercise there was a significant increase in the inorganic phosphate to phosphocreatine ratio (Pi/PCr) (Fig 19–3). The maximum increase occurred 1 day after exercise and remained elevated for 3–10 days. Results were similar after the leg exercises. The adenosine triphosphate (ATP)/(Pi+PCr) increased in all arm exercisers but decreased in 2 of 3 leg exercisers. Exercise protocols that did not involve lengthening contractions did not result in changes in either Pi/PCr or ATP/(Pi+PCr). Patients with various neuromuscular diseases also had increased Pi/PCr at rest.

Elevated Pi/PCr at rest can reflect nonspecific muscle damage in both normal and diseased persons. Because ^{31}P-labeled MRS is a reliable noninvasive method of measuring Pi/PCr in skeletal muscle, it can be used to determine the status of muscle injury in active persons and in patients with neuromuscular disease.

▶ The authors describe a sophisticated, noninvasive technique for determining response to "exercise-induced muscle injury" on an intracellular level. It would appear, at this point in time, that the technique is limited to investigational purposes and has as yet untapped potential for adding to our understanding of problems in this area.—J.S. Torg, M.D.

Stress Fractures: MR Imaging
Lee JK, Yao L (Albany Med College; Albany Med Ctr Hosp, NY)
Radiology 169:217–220, October 1988   19–13

Radionuclide bone scanning is the definitive imaging modality for the diagnosis of stress fracture. Five patients with stress fracture were studied with high-field-strength MRI. The examinations were performed 1½ to 4 weeks after onset of symptoms. Results of initial radiographs were negative for stress fractures.

In all cases, MRI consistently showed thick intramedullary bands of very low signal intensity that were continuous with the cortex (Fig 19–4). These bands corresponded in location to areas of new bone formation or fracture noted on radiographs. The T1-weighted images also consistently showed surrounding areas of decreased signal intensity in the marrow space. In 3 patients prominent intramedullary areas of high signal intensity were also noted on T2-weighted images when MRI was performed within 3 weeks of onset of symptoms, but were much less prominent when imaging was performed 3½ to 4 weeks after onset of symptoms. In 2 patients T2-weighted images demonstrated juxtacortical or subperiosteal areas of high-signal intensity when imaging was performed within 2 weeks after onset of symptoms.

These data show that MRI may prove as sensitive as bone scintigraphy in the early phase of evolving stress fracture while providing more spe-

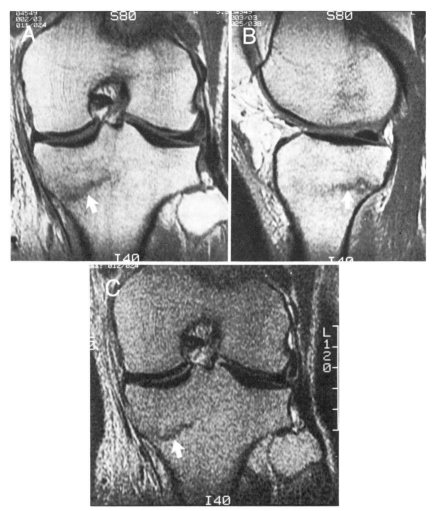

Fig 19–4.—Images of a 44-year-old male surgeon who had knee pain for 3½ weeks after starting a jogging routine. Appearances on initial plain radiographs were normal. **A,** coronal proton density (1,500/20) image shows a 3-cm linear band of very low density *(arrow)* in the medial proximal tibial metaphysis. **B,** sagittal proton density (2,300/20) image shows the same band of low intensity *(arrow)* seen on **A,** which is continuous with the tibial cortex. **C,** coronal T2-weighted (1,500/80) image shows minimally increased signal intensity in the marrow space adjacent to the low-intensity band *(arrow)* but no high-density juxtacortical findings. (Courtesy of Lee JK, Yao L: *Radiology* 169:217–220, October 1988.)

cific information. The characteristic MR findings of stress fracture distinguish it from occult intraosseous fracture.

▶ The purpose of the authors is to distinguish MR findings of stress fractures from occult intraosseous fractures, a diagnosis described by the same authors in a previous publication. The validity of these being 2 separate entities has not yet been substantiated.

Of the 5 stress fractures reported, 3 occurred in conjunction with athletic pursuits; these patients' ages were 50, 44, and 11 years. Of the 2 nontraumatic fractures, 1 occurred in a lactating woman and the other in a patient aged 87 years. As would be expected in this population, all of the stress fractures were in cancellous bone, as opposed to the more typical cortical stress fractures occurring in the shafts of the long bones. Cancellous stress fractures are typically difficult to see radiographically and, although MR is a useful method to document the injury, bone scan is less expensive and equally, if not more, sensitive. The specificity of the MR findings is not yet established and radiographic confirmation is still essential in the follow-up of these patients to exclude necrosis, tumor, or infection.—J.S. Torg, M.D.

Stress Fracture of the Metacarpal in an Adolescent Tennis Player
Murakami Y (Miki Orthopedic Hosp, Imabari, Japan)
Am J Sports Med 16:419–420, July–August 1988   19–14

In athletes stress fractures of the weight-bearing lower extremities occur much more frequently than stress fractures of the upper extremities. Stress fracture of a metacarpal occurred in an adolescent tennis player.

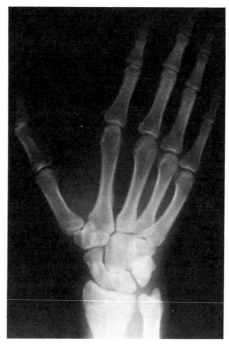

Fig 19–5.—Roentgenogram 2 weeks after initial roentgenogram of hand of adolescent tennis player. (Courtesy of Murakami Y: *Am J Sports Med* 16:419–420, July–August 1988.)

Boy, 16 years, had practiced tennis 2–3 hours a day for the previous year. He recalled no injury to the hand, but he experienced a gradual onset of pain that became so severe he could no longer practice. He had point tenderness over the base of the second metacarpal without swelling. The wrist and fingers moved through full range of motion. Initial roentgenograms showed a faint periosteal elevation of the ulnar aspect of the base of the second metacarpal, was consistent with a stress fracture. A 4-week rest period with a gradual return to tennis was recommended.

Roentgenograms obtained 2 weeks later showed periosteal new bone and a hairline crack in the cortex (Fig 19–5). At 6 weeks the patient was symptom free. He began playing tennis again, but he used a different grip. At 9-month follow-up roentgenograms showed solid union with remodeling at the area of the stress fracture.

Apparently the repeated strike of the handle of a tennis racket against the palm can be traumatic enough to fracture a carpal bone. Hand injuries may be related to improper grip or to poor stroke technique, and players with such problems should seek instructional help.

▶ This interesting and unusual injury was previously reported more than a decade ago (1). Poor technique is suggested to be the mechanism!—J.R. Sutton, M.D.

Reference

1. Stark HH, et al: *J Bone Joint Surg [Am]* 59A:575–582, 1979.

Delayed Unions and Nonunions of Stress Fractures in Athletes
Orava S, Hulkko A (Deaconess Inst and Univ of Oulu, Finland; Keski-Pohjanmaa Central Hosp, Kokkola, Finland)
Am J Sports Med 16:378–382, July–August 1988   19–15

Stress fractures may not unite promptly in athletes who remain too active. In a series of 369 athletes who sustained stress fractures in a 14-year period, 37 (10%) had delayed union or nonunion. All were competitive athletes or joggers. In some patients symptoms and signs occurred only after a hard training session. The primary radiologic findings frequently were minimal or nonexistent. The mean diagnostic delay was 3½ months.

Twenty-two patients were treated surgically. Nonoperative management was based on avoiding provocative training and, when indicated, casting or the use of special footwear. One patient required reoperation because of refracture. The time from surgery to full athletic activity ranged from 3 months to 6 months. Twenty of 22 patients had excellent or good results from surgery, as did 12 of 15 medically managed patients.

More intense training programs may result in more delayed unions and nonunions of stress fractures in athletes. Stress fractures at risk sites should be observed closely to insure adequate primary healing. Established nonunions call for surgical treatment, as do some delayed unions in top-level athletes.

▶ In addition to defining a stress fracture with delayed union or nonunion as being one that has not healed clinically or roentgenographically during a 3-month period, delayed union can be distinguished from nonunion by roentgenographic findings. Unfortunately, the authors do not proceed to define the distinguishing radiographic features. Of the group of 369 fractures reviewed, those identified as being predisposed to delayed nonunion involved the sesmoid, midtibia, base of the fifth metatarsal, tarsal navicular, and olecranon.—J.S. Torg, M.D.

Perineal Nodular Indurations ("Accessory Testicles") in Cyclists: Fine Needle Aspiration Cytologic and Pathologic Findings in Two Cases
Vuong PN, Camuzard P, Schoonaert M-F (St Michel Hosp, Paris)
Acta Cytol 32:86–90, January–February 1988   19–16

A pathologic condition that is widely recognized by professional cyclists but has not been thoroughly studied is the nodular induration of the perineum, also referred to as accessory testicles, third testis, or ischial hygroma. Cytologic and histologic examinations were carried out on fine-needle aspiration material obtained from lesions in 2 cyclists.

Man, 28, a professional cyclist for more than 1 year, complained of 2 nodules that developed in a 10-month period. Clinical examination showed 2 cystic formations, each measuring 2 cm in diameter, situated just posterior to the scrotum and on each side of the midline. The cysts were covered with normal skin and were painless when palpated. Fine-needle aspiration of the nodules was performed. Perioperatively, the lesions were 2 poorly delineated cystic formations located in the inner aspect of ischial tuberosities. They were not clearly separated from the connective tissue of the perineal superficial fascia. Incision revealed a fibrinous material. The aspirates contained few cellular elements, consisting of a few vacuolated histiocytes within a background of fibrinous material. There were some microcalcifications but no synovial cells.

Accessory testicles seen in cyclists consist of localized aseptic areas of necrosis with pseudocyst formation involving connective tissue in the superficial fascia of the perineum. The lesions develop as a result of repeated microtrauma to the perineum, caused by the vibrations of the bicycle seat. These indurations are a genuine handicap for professional cyclists. Their presence is a contraindication to cycling in men who cycle for recreation.

▶ This is an interesting pathologic entity of which I was unaware and thought you might likewise not know.—J.R. Sutton, M.D.

Subject Index

A

Abdomen
  fitness testing, evaluation criteria, 221
Abrasions
  hydrocolloid dressings for, 78
Abuse
  drug, in athletes, 303
Accidents
  cycling, urban, study of, 92
  diving, causing gastric rupture, 354
  ski chairlift, 108
  skiing, study of, 102
Acetabular
  labrum tear, arthroscopy of, 148
Acetazolamide
  in mountain sickness, 351, 352
Acid
  -base states, altered, and acute altitude
    exposure, 228
Acne
  vulgaris in athlete, 372
Acromioclavicular
  separation, complete, shoulder analysis
    after, 135
Adhesive
  fibrin, in chondral and osteochondral
    injury repair, 376
Adolescence
  adolescent gymnast (see Gymnasts,
    adolescent)
  female
    athletes, eating attitudes and body
      weight in, 316
    dancers, iron deficiency in, 286
    readiness to participate in sports, 24
    tennis during, stress fracture of
      metacarpal in, 382
    weight loss and regain in, repeated, in
      wrestlers, 328
α Adrenoceptors
  in coronary flow during exercise (in
    dog), 245
Aerobic
  capacity during pregnancy and exercise,
    32
  dancing, heart rate and caloric cost in,
    27
  power
    of senior citizen, xvi-xvii
    training and, high-velocity resistance
      circuit, 85
    training, and submaximal exercise
      effects on sleep, 337
Age
  -related changes in arm movements, 4

Aged
  (See also Senior citizen)
  walking, muscle strength in triceps
    surae during, 4
Airway
  response, dichotomous, to exercise in
    asthma, 234
Alcohol
  coronary artery disease and exercise,
    258
Alcoholism
  chronic, withdrawal, exercise response
    after, 260
Allograft
  tendon for reconstruction of anterior
    cruciate ligament, 178
  tendon transplant into knee, 177
Alpha adrenoceptors
  in coronary flow during exercise (in
    dog), 245
Altitude(s)
  acute altitude exposure and altered
    acid-base states, 228
  high (see High altitude)
  intermediate, mountain sickness at,
    incidence, 350
  oxygen transport during exercise at,
    345
Alveolar
  bronchoalveolar lavage in mountain
    sickness and pulmonary edema,
    348
Amenorrhea
  athletic, cyproterone acetate and
    osteoporosis, 334
Amenorrheic runners
  body composition of, 324
Anabolic steroids
  self-reported use by power lifters, 306
  use by athletes, 303
  use by male high school seniors, 308
Anaerobic
  power
    of senior citizens, xv-xvi
    tests, factor analysis, 211
Analog
  recording system and Cybex II
    isokinetic dynamometer, 222
Androgenic steroids
  self-reported use, by power lifters, 306
Angina
  exertional, cardiac output in, and
    nifedipine, 254
  stable, diltiazem vs. nifedipine in, 247
Ankle
  arthroscopy, long-term follow-up, 209

Author Index